Assembly of the Executive Mind

Assembly of the Executive Mind

Evolutionary Insights and
a Paradigm for Brain Health

Michael Hoffmann
University of Central Florida

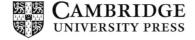
CAMBRIDGE
UNIVERSITY PRESS

CAMBRIDGE
UNIVERSITY PRESS

University Printing House, Cambridge CB2 8BS, United Kingdom

One Liberty Plaza, 20th Floor, New York, NY 10006, USA

477 Williamstown Road, Port Melbourne, VIC 3207, Australia

314–321, 3rd Floor, Plot 3, Splendor Forum, Jasola District Centre, New Delhi – 110025, India

79 Anson Road, #06-04/06, Singapore 079906

Cambridge University Press is part of the University of Cambridge.

It furthers the University's mission by disseminating knowledge in the pursuit of education, learning, and research at the highest international levels of excellence.

www.cambridge.org
Information on this title: www.cambridge.org/9781108456005
DOI: 10.1017/9781108589246

First published 2019

Printed in the United Kingdom by TJ International Ltd. Padstow Cornwall

A catalogue record for this publication is available from the British Library.

ISBN 978-1-108-45600-5 Paperback

For Bronwyn, Jenna Leigh, and Michael.

Contents

Acknowledgments

The singling out of individuals for thanks no doubt will leave out many others that were instrumental in my training and conceptualization of brain health and fitness, and for this I apologize in advance. The evolution of my thinking and ultimately this book is a tribute to many friends and colleagues that helped me in my formative years. I was very fortunate to have Professor Phillip Tobias as my anatomy professor and Dean of the medical school at the University of Witwatersrand. He taught us human anatomy from not one, but three large books called *Man's Anatomy,* Parts 1, 2, and 3, but more importantly enkindled in his students a fascination for human origins that he was so famous for. Professors Pierre Bill and John Cosnett of the University of Kwa-Zulu Natal, Durban for their patient and expert teaching in clinical neurology, guiding my early career development. Professor John Robbs, head of surgery and vascular surgery, University of Kwa-Zulu Natal, Durban for his enthusiastic support and promotion of my early forays into cerebrovascular medicine and helping form the Durban Cerebrovascular Group. Professor Bill Pryse-Phillips helped land my first neurology job at Memorial University, Canada while he researched and wrote his book, *Neurology Dictionary*. Professors J.P. Mohr and Ralph Sacco enthusiastically guided me through my stroke fellowship and instilled the fervor for computerized registry analyses at Columbia University, New York. I am very fortunate to have continued guidance and mentorship in cognitive neurology and cognitive neuroscience from Professor Frederick Schmitt of the Sanders Brown Aging Institute at the University of Kentucky and Professor Ken Heilman of University of Florida. I am grateful to Dr. Fiona Crawford and Dr. Michael Mullen for providing me with a platform for launching neuro-archeological seminars at the Roskamp Institute in Sarasota and promoting clinical cognitive neurology to flourish side by side with their high-level neuroscience research. The Cambridge University Press team, Noah Tate, Gary Smith, Anna Whiting, and Emily Jones, that so enthusiastically guided this book to fruition, were exceptional in their efficiency and professionalism. At the center of my life are my family, Bronwyn, Jenna Leigh, and Michael, whose support is inestimable.

Registry data used

Clinical examples and radiological images were sampled from the following IRB-approved registries of which the author was the principal investigator. These registries pertained to the collection of clinical investigative, radiological, and management data of consecutive stroke and cognitive impairment patients, aged 18–90 years, accrued through prospectively coded dedicated stroke and cognitive disorders registries in tertiary referral centers. These were approved by the relevant University Institutional Review Boards and the latter two registries were also in compliance with HIPAA (Health Insurance Portability and Accountability Act) regulations when this was enacted.

1. The NIH-NINDS Stroke Data Bank (New York)

Under the following contracts: N01-NS-2-2302, N01-NS-2-2384, N01-NS-2-2398, N01-NS-2-2399, N01-NS-6-2305.
Status: Stroke Research Fellow (1990–1991)

2. The Durban Stroke Data Bank

IRB approval: University of Natal, Durban, South Africa (approved by the Ethics Board of the University of Kwa-Zulu Natal).
Status: Principal Investigator (1992–1998)

3. The USF-TGH Stroke Registry

IRB #102354 (University of South Florida).
Status: Principal Investigator (2002–2006)

4. The USF-Cognitive Stroke Registry

IRB #106113 (University of South Florida)
Status: Principal Investigator (2007–2010)

Consent

All patients signed informed consent for the evaluation and the collection of the their neurological, medical, and neurocognitive data.

Cover Image

Cover image designed and drawn by Michael S. Hoffmann, MS ISOM, Washington DC, USA, adapted from artwork © Can Stock Photo Inc. / woodoo.

Introduction

Deciphering the natural environment, including human form and function, is best achieved by interdisciplinary study. The differing sciences inform each other and there is often two-way or bidirectional information exchange between disciplines. For example, evolution informs neuroscience and neuroscience has the power to inform evolution. This was well described by David Lewis-Williams in his interpretation of cave rock paintings in which certain artistic depictions reflected different stages of hallucination in the human mind. In his elegant overview of how ancient art helps understand the neuroscience of our minds, presented in his book *The Mind in the Cave*, he describes how the intensified trajectory of altered consciousness level of visual hallucinations (fully fledged hallucinations) in ancestral humans was recognized as being identical to migrainous fortification spectra (jagged lines), familiar to contemporary neurology [1].

The Nobel prize-winning physiologist Eric Kandel eloquently portrayed how neuroscience and art inform each other, detailed in his two exceptional books, *The Age of Insight* [2] and *Nature's Reductionism: Bridging the Two Cultures* [3]. The parent field of medicine, biology, is often instrumental in the understanding of human brain mechanisms, such as theories of how we developed superb color vision. Isbell's snake-detection theory helped inform current-day neurology and psychiatry about snakes having acted as a primary selective pressure operating on primates and expanding their visual systems. In brief, evolutionary exposure to venomous snakes, which are usually patterned and colored, induced trichromacy in the African primates, as opposed to the mere dichromacy of the South American primates, the latter having had minimal venomous snake exposure. The third component of the theory, the Madagascar lemur, which has the worst color vision of the primates, had no exposure to venous snakes at all [4]. Many arts and sciences are therefore valuable in helping to understand the evolution of the human executive mind. From my perspective, the discipline of clinical neurology, which is concerned with brain lesions and their consequences, or fractured brain circuits, can inform the discipline of archeology that deals with the analysis of fractured skulls. Hence, fractured minds and brain circuits can similarly be regarded as a two-way process in the study of neuro-archeology. As can be seen from Figure 0.1, many disciplines helped inform the assembly of our frontal lobes and our minds. There are, of course, numerous disciplines in the arts and sciences. Perhaps increased interaction among them will lead to ever-greater insights. Clinical medicine just happens to be a discipline that is among the least interdisciplinary at the present time, as we shall see in Chapter 12. The great visionary and biologist Edward Wilson coined the term *consilience* in his book of the same name, emphasizing the unity of all knowledge and disciplines, and conceived of all the arts

1

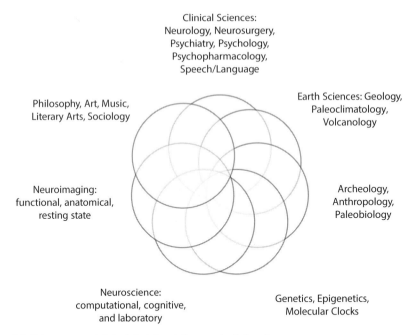

Clinical Sciences:
Neurology, Neurosurgery,
Psychiatry, Psychology,
Psychopharmacology,
Speech/Language

Philosophy, Art, Music,
Literary Arts, Sociology

Earth Sciences: Geology,
Paleoclimatology,
Volcanology

Neuroimaging:
functional, anatomical,
resting state

Archeology,
Anthropology,
Paleobiology

Neuroscience:
computational, cognitive,
and laboratory

Genetics, Epigenetics,
Molecular Clocks

Figure 0.1 Science, art and clinical disciplines inform our brain functions.

Piecing together the components from
fractured skulls

Piecing together the components from
fractured minds

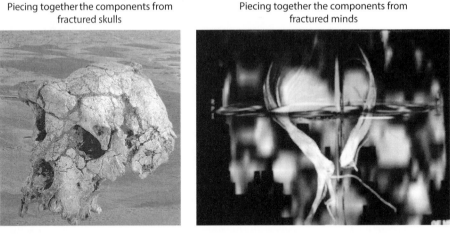

Figure 0.2 The unravelling of the human mind: a method of studying human cognitive evolution.
Reprinted by permission from Springer Nature from Wood B. Hominid revelations from Chad. *Nature* 2002;418:133–135.

and sciences as being innately bound by a small number of natural laws in physics and chemistry [5].

One can either gather fractured skulls and bones or study fractured brain circuits in deciphering brain function and how it evolved (Figure 0.2). Similar to the approach of Vilayanur Ramachandran and Oliver Sacks, individual case reports and sometime case series can be very illuminating, as have the recent spate of *n*-of-1 trials that are gaining momentum as part of the precision medicine movement. This book is woven around key case reports, case series, case control studies, and cohort studies, most of them published by the author, emanating from four different stroke and cognitive neurology registries cited in the acknowledgments. These are used throughout the book to highlight how the multitude of frontal lobe presentations and related cognitive and behavioral syndromes, after various brain lesions, illuminate the unraveling of the mind, together with an evolutionary perspective. From a terminological perspective, frontal lobes refer to the anatomical entity Brodmann areas (BA) 4, 6, 8, 9, 10, 11, 12, 13, 32, 14, 44, 45, 46, and 47. The executive mind, strictly speaking, refers the lateral prefrontal cortex or areas BA 9 and 46 and the behaviorally relevant frontal regions BA 11, 12, 13, and 14. *Frontal network systems* (FNS) refers to the frontal-type syndromes that may be due to frontal lobe lesions, but are actually more often due to lesions of the expansive networks throughout the brain that the frontal lobes are part of. For the purposes of this book, *the executive mind* is used to refer to the frontal lobes, both executive and behavioral, and their expansive networks in their entirety.

Hence, neuro-archeology has been used as an overarching term to refer to the relationship of mind functioning as it pertains to archeological finds [6]. Archeologists delve in material remains and infer past human behavior. The discipline has spawned a number of fields of study, including cognitive archeologists who endeavor to infer mental capabilities and modes of thought processes from reconstructed behaviors. Cognitive neuroscientists are concerned with the neurobiological circuitry of behaviors associated with psychological processes. Neuroscientists pursue molecular chemistry, genetics, and cellular structures largely by studying extant neural organisms. Clinical neurology capitalizes on a vast array of neurological diseases and conditions that lead to relatively stereotyped syndromes that in their own way disentangle the mind and illuminate some of its workings. In the vast majority of these clinical cases and series there lies hope. Not only does precise diagnosis elucidate the – sometimes bewildering – presentations, but through the diagnosis lies the potential for management and treatment. At times it is nature that heals and sometimes with treatment and intervention there is marginal benefit and sometimes there are dramatically positive results. Frontal lobe lesions and their brain behavior relationships is a relatively new science; it was launched by the seminal Boston Crowbar case in 1864 in the USA and the Broca's aphasia report from France, but only blossomed in the mid-1980s [7,8].

In the 1950s, the neurosurgeon Penfield performed intraoperative stimulation experiments and made the important observation that frontal lobe stimulation revealed no response at all, other than a movement response when stimulating the motor cortex [9]. Luria's important frontal lobe function observations, mostly from traumatic brain injury (TBI) patients, still profoundly influence neuropsychology today. He was the first to make the crucial distinction between behavior from frontal lobe damage and cognitive function impairment from frontal lesions. For example, he reported the case of a man seen in his office who caught the next train out of Moscow's central station without any consideration for its destination [10]. The behavioral syndromes of frontal lobe pathology later expanded and were elegantly demonstrated by Lhermitte's innovative style of frontal testing and description of various field-dependent behaviors, in differing environments. These methods were key to understanding the syndromes and how very simple techniques may be illuminating in discerning frontal lobe behavior. He described how field-dependent behavior syndromes frequently emerge following disruptions of the mirror neuron network in the brain [11,12].

People with frontal lesions or pathology seldom seek evaluation; if they do, initial cognitive screening tests commonly employed, such as the Mini-Mental State Examination (MMSE), are insensitive to frontal cognitive syndromes, while the Montreal Cognitive Assessment (MOCA) is impervious to frontal behavioral syndromes [13,14]. Yet, the presentations may include those with profane, puerile, irascible, or facetious behaviors that are difficult to quantify and have no devised metric tests.

Mesulam belabored the common and astonishing paucity of formal neuropsychological test scores, often normal, associated with frontal lobe lesions [15]. Specific behaviorally oriented tests – such as Frontal Systems Behavioral Evaluation, Frontal Behavioral Inventory, Bar-On Emotional Intelligence Test, and the Behavioral Rating Inventory of Executive Function – are more likely to elicit the salient abnormalities [16–18]. Another major contribution by Mesulam was the introduction of the concept of an FNS, rather than frontal lobe syndrome. As subcortical infarcts, multiple sclerosis, TBI, toxic metabolic encephalopathies, and other multifocal processes are more common causes of frontal syndromes as opposed to lesions of the anatomical frontal lobe themselves, this becomes a preferable designation [19–21].

Things have changed for the better. Isolated case reports or case series are unable to provide insights with regard to frequencies of cognitive syndromes and FNS, the solution being computerized registry-based analyses. In addition, the protracted period associated with autopsy-verified lesion locality has been supplanted by increasingly sophisticated neuroimaging methods. Magnetic resonance imaging (MRI) nowadays has at least a dozen different imaging sequencing modalities that can detail acute strokes, arteries, veins, fiber tracts, neurovascular activity, and spectroscopy, all with superior resolution. Most importantly, intrinsic connectivity analyses by fMRI have yielded insights into brain network function. A registry-based approach for analyses of specific higher cortical function deficit (HCFD) subtypes, in particular FNS, determined that the latter were important and pervasive cognitive syndromes, the most common and ubiquitous in neurological and psychiatric disease. However, testing of HCFD by the three major clinical brain disciplines – neurology, psychiatry, and neuropsychology – differs markedly, that is with respect to discipline culture, historically, and philosophically. At the same time, each has unique contributions and so all complement each other. Certain brain disease processes such as stroke, epilepsy, meningitis, and encephalitis, however, require emergent evaluation.

Clinical cerebrovascular decision-making is constrained by a 4.5-hour thrombolytic therapy window or, even more demanding, the so-called *golden first hour* of intervening with clot-busting agents [22]. Multiple concurrent procedures, including neuroimaging and laboratory and cardiac investigations leave only a few minutes for clinical assessments, and no place for neuropsychological testing. Despite the challenge of performing cognitive evaluations in the emergency situation, at least a cursory appraisal of FNS is pertinent as these are the most common clinical neurological impairments. Clinical monitoring of FNS is crucial for appreciating any improvement or deterioration of the patient. A typical stroke damages approximately two million neurons and 14 billion synapses each minute [23]. The degree of attention and cooperation by the person is also severely limited in such a scenario. Yet the relevance of FNS testing is that the expansive supervisory cognitive network (metacognition) may be the most sensitive indicator of cognitive status once emergent evaluation has been accomplished. Based on one of the stroke registries, a system was devised that incorporated (1) behavioral neurological assessment of the myriad known syndromes quantified in ordinal and nominal data terms; (2) a neuropsychiatric syndrome evaluation according to pre-specified criteria (DSM-IV), configured to nominal data; and (3) a neuropsychological battery approach recorded in predominant numerical, normed evaluations. The semi-quantitative bedside test was devised, incorporating cognitive, neuropsychiatric, and behavioral syndromes, and enabling assessment within approximately 20 minutes. By incorporating the extensive testing of syndromes germane to behavioral neurology and neuropsychiatry, in addition to brief neuropsychological batteries, a reasonable appraisal of FNS was accomplished by the development of the COCONUTS evaluation (**co**mprehensive, **co**gnitive test **neu**rological **t**est in **s**troke) [24].

Other registry-based research revealed that HCFD, including FNS, were not only very common in acute and subacute stroke, but that FNS were evident regardless of lesion localization. Hence, frontal, subcortical, posterior parietal, or occipital, and even subtentorial and brainstem strokes often had associated FNS. The frequency was surprising, with approximately half of people with subtentorial stroke manifesting with FNS [25–27]. In retrospect, as the frontal lobes and their networks connect to all areas of the brain, this now seems less surprising. Further research into the neurobiological mechanisms of these processes in isolated brainstem or cerebellar stroke by SPECT brain scanning has suggested a neurotransmitter perturbation to be a likely candidate [28]. These findings were corroborated by a subsequent clinical analysis of stroke patients with minimal or no long tract signs (one-sided weakness, numbness, or vision disturbance) with FNS caused by isolated subtentorial (brainstem or cerebellum) stroke [29].

Sometimes we find simple tests that may discern and diagnose complex processes. The mirror neuron system (MNS), for example, evolved in stages during our primate history from about 60 million years ago and can be affected by cerebral lesions. We can test for the MNS by documenting syndromes such as echopraxia, utilization behavior, and environmental-dependency syndromes. These are not commonly employed tests, yet they offer an important opportunity to improve neurological evaluation and monitoring of complex FNS [30]. Such an example proved to be a most decisive one in my formative years in neurology registrar (resident) training in the large modern subtropical city of Durban, South Africa, largely serving the Zulu population. During this time and even today, tuberculosis (TB) and human immunodeficiency virus (HIV) related neurological illness was rampant, to the extent that many neurological syndromes we encountered were often considered TB-related until proven otherwise. TB neurology can be immensely protean and can be a great masquerader, much like luetic disease was in earlier European history. This was probably an important reason why the young, well-educated Zulu man, a teacher, I encountered presenting initially with a seizure captivated our attention one morning on clinical rounds. Whatever we did, he did. For example, on completing the tendon reflex examination with the traditional Queen's Square reflex hammer, he picked it up and proceeded to elicit all his own reflexes. He also imitated actions, words, and gestures faithfully, without instruction to do so and even when asked not to do so, with his mystified physicians looking on. For example, he spontaneously started teaching the resident physicians when asked to accompany them into a room that was reminiscent of a classroom in which he took on the role of a teacher – the environmental-dependency syndrome. He displayed many different field-dependent behavioral syndromes, since described more precisely by Professor Lhermitte of Paris in 1986, which he termed imitation behavior, utilization behavior being the environmental-dependency syndromes [11,12]. The cause was an unusual bifrontal stroke, attributed to TB-related

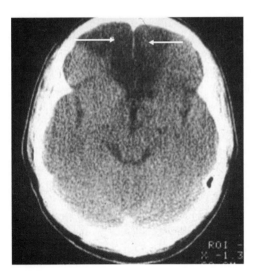

Figure 0.3 Bilateral frontal infarcts (strokes) decoupling brain circuits that hint at our evolutionary past (arrows).

vasculitis (inflammation) of his frontal brain arteries (Figure 0.3). The brain circuitry that had been lesioned, with the various field-dependent behaviors as the predominant clinical syndrome and without other neurological sequelae, had "uncoupled" his mirror neuron circuitry [31]. The MNS and its relevance to human cognition (language, praxis, theory of mind, learning) has only relatively recently been appreciated [32]. From an evolutionary perspective, the MNS is viewed as a fast-track learning mechanism, forgoing learning by trial and error, and is viewed as the neurobiological substrate of our cultural revolution, prompting Ramachandran to expound that "The MNS will do for psychology what DNA has done for biology" [33].

Studies of people with MNS uncoupling yields unique insights into brain functions. In a large clinical study some 25 years after the event of the Durban Zulu man with pervasive field-dependent behaviors, a series of 73 MNS-uncoupled patients derived from a registry of 1436 people with stroke were evaluated, and a much wider range of presentations was uncovered. The loss of personal autonomy that occurs may take many forms and is described in more detail in Chapter 11 [34]. Fortunately, the majority of people beset with sudden field-dependent behavior syndromes recover within days to weeks. During primate and subsequent human evolution, progressively increasing frontoparietal integration became the foundation of exaption (using a device or feature for another purpose) for a more elaborate MNS, one of the functions enabled being the conversion of visual data into knowledge within the general cognitive domains of attention and memory, as well as more specialized domains such as language and tool use [35].

Convergent evidence accumulating from research in archeology, evolutionary neuropsychology, genetics, and linguistics has advanced a hypothesis that working memory may be the "cognitive missing link" that enabled intra-connectivity of the various intelligence domains (social, natural history, technical), with cognitive fluidity and cross-modal connectivity culminating in increased creativity. Working memory may be viewed as a kind of "operating system of our brain" and the "engine of cognitive connectivity" and

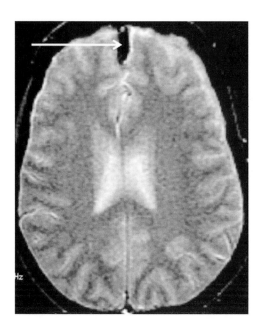

Figure 0.4 Isolated frontopolar lesion (midline dark area, indicated by arrow) due to a discreet brain hemorrhage.

executive function [36]. The working memory circuit and the mirror neuron circuitry are both extensive frontoparietal cerebral circuits and are key circuits that make us human and constitute core frontal systems today. These can both be assessed clinically relatively rapidly by simple bedside tests.

Emotional intelligence (EI) is an important subcomponent of frontal function and has rarely been addressed in neurological patients, including those suffering from TBI, stroke, dementia, and multiple sclerosis. Emerging evidence has indicated that EI is a critical "intelligence" for success, whether intrapersonal, interpersonal, or with career achievements. In analysis of stroke data, EI was found to be negatively affected by diverse brain lesions. However, areas most impactful were frontal, temporal, and subcortical, as well as subtentorial regions [29,37].

At times the heralding of a stroke is nonspecific, such as a seizure or severe headache without discernible neurological deficit. The rapid access to high-volume comprehensive stroke centers in many parts of the world today, with imaging mandatory within 30 minutes, often depicts a stroke that is unexpected or has no obvious clinical accompaniment. Such was the case with a middle-aged, well-educated woman with a very unusual stroke lesion location with a rather unusual cause. The most anterior aspect of her brain, called the frontopolar cortex (FPC), BA 10, was damaged by a ruptured dural arteriovenous malformation (abnormal blood vessel) with discrete hemorrhage measuring 2.3 cm^3. BA 10 is one of the few brain areas that is dramatically enlarged in humans in comparison to the closest extant primate, the chimpanzee. FPC functions arbitrate our most apical human cognitive qualities, such as the simultaneous consideration of diverse options and task switching, elaborated on in more detail in Chapter 11 [38,39]. This study remains, to date, the sole, isolated FPC lesion analysis reported (Figure 0.4). Cognitive testing was normal with the exclusive impairment in EI subtest scores. This medial FPC lesion was

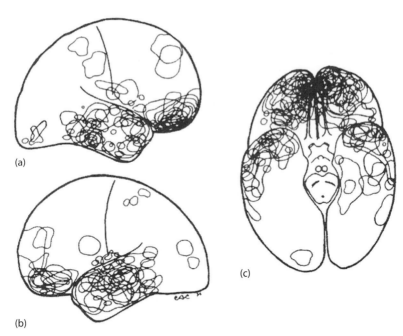

(a)

(b)

(c)

Figure 0.5 Silent neurological lesions, silent neuropsychological lesions, and often silent neuroimaging (unless using DTI, PET, IFC): TBI and the frontotemporal predilection. (a) sagittal right brain; (b) sagittal left brain; (c) horizontal from below. Distribution of contusions in 40 consecutive autopsy cases.
Sources: Courville CB. *Pathology of the Nervous System: Part 4.* Pacific, Mountain View, CA, 1937; Courville CB. *Trauma of the Central Nervous System.* Williams and Wilkins, Baltimore, MD, 1945.

consistent with being a necessary component involved in the emotional processing of internal states of a person [40].

Frontal lobe presentations can be enigmatic, bewildering, covert, and silent. Standard clinical neuroscience texts typically list two dozen or more differing presentations. The first frontotemporal dementia, Pick's disease, was described in 1892 [41]. Although it could have served as a very revealing pathology of differing frontal functions, it was largely ignored, with a possible explanation that it could be the existence of several different types of pathology, in addition to Pick bodies, that cause the so-called frontotemporal lobe dementia (FTD). Pick's disease happened to be associated with very infrequent pathology, while the generic FTD was a common dementia. This pathology–clinical mismatch deprecated FTD and related frontotemporal lobe syndrome (FTS) over the next century, and consequently they were trivialized as clinical syndromes.

TBI syndromes today are reminiscent of the Pick's/FTD debacle. TBI has a predilection for the frontotemporal lobes and associated circuitry (Figure 0.5), and was first described pathologically in 1937 [42] and has been corroborated by neurosurgical studies since. Predictably, they are relatively "blind" to standard neuropsychological testing (NPT) that samples differing brain circuits, and often to neuropsychiatric assessments, including depression. Many seminal neurological cases published in the last 100 years have repeatedly alerted clinicians to the dramatic cognitive–behavioral dissociation after frontal lobe lesions. Frontal lobe patient reports have persistently emphasized the profound behavioral impairments in the context of otherwise normal (NPT) patients in the last few decades. Arnold Pick, in his landmark description of Pick's disease, also noted presentations principally with inhibition and abulias (poverty of thought, action, and speech), not cognitive impairment as a rule. The commonly used screening tests such, as the MMSE, MOCA, and even those specific to frontal lobe function, such as the Frontal Assessment Battery (FAB), are often within normal range and hence they may miss the entry criteria of NPT [43]. In-depth NPT testing itself is often normal or only mildly impaired. Various degrees of abulia, however, are a common and pervasive accompaniment of frontal and subcortical lesions and may hinder adequate behavioral and NPT testing.

The marked clinical cognitive–behavioral dissonance accounts for some enigmatic justifications offered by patients, such as "driving through a red light is wrong but I may do so." This clinical cognitive–behavioral sundering may also further delay diagnosis because their language skills and cognitive skills are often remarkably convincing. At the cost of possible oversimplification of intricate frontal lobe function, the wide array of frontal behavioral presentations can be understood in terms of two broad categories: abulia (A) and disinhibition (D). For example, the FTD-behavioral variant (bv) syndrome may be divided into FTD(bv)-A and FTD(bv)-D. Abulia, as an overarching deportment, includes episodic dysmemory due to inattention, impaired registration and impaired retrieval, self-neglect, emotional flatness, lack of empathy, stereotyped behavior and ritualistic behavior – humming, hand rubbing, foot tapping, grunting, lip-smacking, clock watching, counting, punding, and feasting on the same foods. Disinhibition, on the other hand, accounts for the syndromes of socially inappropriate behavior, abnormal eating behaviors (eating off other people's plates), and impulsivity. Most, if not all, may originate in the network defraying caused by mirror neuron network disruption and uncoupling.

For too long neuroimaging has been unhelpful. The pervasively vague, polysymptomatic presentations, and borderline NPT results are characteristic of mild TBI patients. Buttressed by the frequently so-called "normal" anatomical brain scans, this generally cements the notion that there is "nothing significantly wrong with the brain." Newer neuroimaging techniques are changing this quagmire. Diffusion tensor imaging (DTI), in particular, has been instrumental in being able to zero-in on the fiber tracts that bear the brunt of the damage, which amount to about 100 000 miles in the human brain. Functional imaging with metabolic positron emission tomography (PET) brain scans often reveal hypometabolic (decreased activity) areas in both frontal and anterior temporal lobes. More promising are the newer MRI-based network scans. Resting-state networks (default mode network, salience network) or intrinsic connectivity network (ICN) imaging have shown a more extensive brain connectomal disruption after TBI. This gels fittingly with the concept of hub vulnerability hypothesis discussed in Chapter 12. In brief, the human connectome (the brain's entire fiber network) has "hotspots" that are susceptible to traumatic, vascular, and metabolic injury. These critically important hubs subserve higher cognitive processes and are the most energy-consuming regions of the brain [44].

Evaluation with the FTS criteria of Rascovsky et al. [45] or the Daphne criteria [46] are important for deficit estimation and to guide further treatment responses. Thereafter, assessment for FTS with behavioral neurological testing – such as the Frontal Behavioral Inventory (FBI), Frontal Systems Behavioral Examination (FRSBE), or Behavior Rating Inventory of Executive Function (BRIEF) – may provide more insightful appreciation of the range, extent, and gravity of the manifold syndromes [16,18,47]. Behavioral neurological tests that interrogate the inferior frontal, anterior temporal lobes and uncinate fasciculus and frontotemporal circuitry are required for a more representative evaluation of TBI. Pertinent syndromes may include partial or complete forms of the Geschwind-Gastaut and Klüver–Bücy syndromes, not captured by NPT (see Chapter 11). TBI is now seen as a progressive inflammatory, apoptotic, and vascular disease that may progress for months to years [48].

Perhaps the preponderance of the diagnostic challenges may be ascribed to the inherent difficulty pertaining to the assessment of the most intricate aspect of human behavior. Historically, the memory-centric focus associated with Alzheimer's disease likely overshadowed frontotemporal behavioral presentations, where memory is mostly spared. New insights from a pathophysiological point of view inform us that mild and moderate TBI is a chronic inflammatory response with the activation of several inflammatory and apoptotic pathways [49,50]. Recent findings point to a process that may progress and worsen over several years. This is in direct contradistinction to the classic teaching of rapid recovery over weeks to months after "concussion" [51]. Furthermore, it is also a "microvascular disease" process with vasospasm (narrowing of brain arteries) described in the initial phases with neurovascular uncoupling. An alarming 4.43 hazard ratio for developing FTD after TBI has since been reported, and data from a rat model indicate that behavioral impairments are likely due to TDP-43 short fragment accumulation [51].

Why the diagnostic and syndromic concern? With more precise diagnosis, treatment prospects become more discerning and effective. The nature and extent of TBI diagnosis is important in view of emerging treatments that may help our patients. These include computerized exercises such as BrainHQ and Cogmed, which facilitate working memory and attention, pharmacotherapy (amantadine, methylphenidate), and specific attention to an omega 3/6 ratio diet. Lindelov et al. presented important data that hypnosis in TBI improves working memory, fundamental to all other brain functions [52]. Kitagishi et al. showed that supplementation with natural compounds such as dietary fish oil (rich in polyunsaturated fatty acid) induces PTEN expression (activation of peroxisome proliferator-activated receptor). This has a key role in neuroprotection, stimulates cell proliferation, and enhances cell survival [53]. Neuroplasticity-centered treatments are a particularly exciting prospect, with the first positive trial reported during November 2017 by the Helius group on cranial nerve noninvasive neuromodulation with mild-to-moderate TBI in 122 randomized subjects [54,55].

At times subtle or covert frontal syndrome presentations are key to avoiding fulminant irreversible brain disorders. During my first months as a newly graduated neurologist, a call from the emergency room was for evaluation of a middle-aged man whose wife was concerned that on arriving at their long-established home that day, after a routine outing, he stated that their bedroom was unfamiliar to him. Examination revealed a mild pyrexia without other accompanying general medical or neurological examination abnormalities. Magnetic resonance brain scan imaging revealed classic medial temporal and inferior frontal lobe abnormalities, consistent with herpes simplex encephalitis 1 (HSV-1), cerebrospinal fluid (CSF) indicative of viral infection, and subsequent confirmation by brain biopsy. The heralding neurological presentation was a relatively sudden onset of "jamais vu" or feeling of unfamiliarity in relation to his own bedroom. This could also be regarded as a delusional misidentification syndrome for place, as will be discussed in more detail in Chapter 10. HSV-1 presentation is more often fulminant, associated with headache, fever, seizures, and altered mental status. When the presentation is covert,

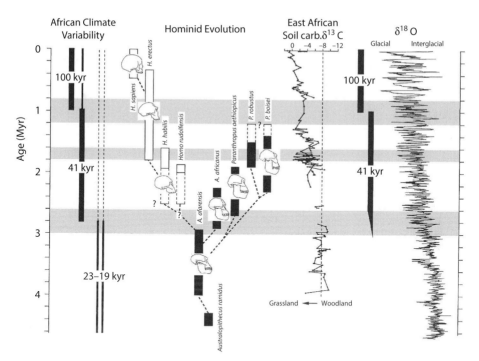

Figure 0.6 More recent hominin proliferation and brain enlargement, paleoclimate changes, and ice ages (horizontal gray bands) over the last three million years.

From deMenocal PB, Bloemendal J. Plio–Pleistocene climatic variability in subtropical Africa and the paleoenvironment of hominid evolution: a combined data-model approach. In: Vrba ES, Denton GH, Partridge TC, Burckle LH (eds.), *Paleoclimate and Evolution with Emphasis on Human Origins*. Yale University Press, New Haven, CT, 1995. Reprinted with permission from AAAS.

as with this man, a delay in correct diagnosis may easily occur and may have tragic consequences. With improved MRI functions, polymerase chain reaction CSF evaluation, and antiviral treatment available today, the majority of people afflicted survive with good recovery, as did the our man [56,57].

Another key clinical realization is that diffuse brain lesions are more common causes of frontal lobe syndromes than frontal lobe lesions themselves. In addition to TBI, there are other diffuse types of brain lesions that preferentially affect the frontal systems via the extensive frontal subcortical connections. This is certainly the case and includes many disorders, most notably multiple sclerosis, small-vessel cerebrovascular disease, and neurotoxicological disorders such as Gulf War Illness.

A frequent headline-grabbing topic, climate change, is featured almost monthly in leading science journals such as *Nature* and *Science*. This prevailing feature reminds us of how fragile our existence is in the universe and how dramatically climate can impact humanity, something we are oblivious to until it's too late. What may be less known is that severe climate alterations had a direct role in forging the human brain and its complex circuitry in the first place (Figure 0.6). A 2016 report in *Science* concerns the Atlantic Meridional Overturning Circulation (AMOC) flow slowing from 20 Sverdrups in 2004 to 15 Sverdrups in 2014. One Sverdrup is one million cubic meters of water per second, or the same as all the Earth's rivers combined [58]. Why would this be important? The

AMOC is the pulse of the planet's climate system, in a sense. Any slowing and we can get whiplash climate changes, also called Dansgaard–Oeschger (D–O), Heinrich, and Bond events that are associated with sudden cooling events within decades or sometimes just a few years. These lead to sudden ice ages even at a time of global warming, for example, which has happened many times over the last few million years [59,60].

References

1. Lewis-Williams D. *The Mind in the Cave.* Thames and Hudson, London, 2002.

2. Kandel ER. *The Age of Insight.* Random House, New York, 2012.

3. Kandel ER. *Reductionism in Art and Brain Science: Bridging the Two Cultures.* Columbia University Press, New York, 2016.

4. Lynne A. Isbell. *The Fruit, the Tree and the Serpent.* Harvard University Press, Cambridge, MA, 2009.

5. Wilson EO. *Consilience: The Unity of Knowledge.* Vantage Books, New York, 1999.

6. Renfrew C, Frith, C, Malafouris L. *The Sapient Mind: Archeology Meets Neuroscience.* Oxford University Press, Oxford, 2009.

7. Harlow JM. Recovery from the passage of an iron bar through the head. *Publications of the Massachusetts Medical Society* 1868;2:327–347.

8. Broca P. Nouvelle observation d'aphémie produite par une lésion de la moitié postérieure des deuxième et troisième circonvolution frontales gauches. *Bulletin de la Société Anatomique* 1861;36:398–407.

9. Penfield W. Mechanisms of voluntary movement. *Brain* 1954;77:18.

10. Luria AR. *Higher Cortical Functions in Man.* Basic Books, New York, 1972.

11. Lhermitte F, Pillon B, Seradura M. Human autonomy and the frontal lobes. Part 1: imitation and utilization behavior – a neuropsychological study of 75 patients. *Ann Neurol* 1986;19:326–334.

12. Lhermitte F. Human autonomy and the frontal lobes. Part II: patient behavior in complex and social situations: the "environmental dependency syndrome." *Ann Neurol* 1986;19:335–343.

13. Folstein MF, Robins LN, Helzer JE. The Mini-Mental State Examination. *Arch Ger Psychiatry* 1983;40:812.

14. Nasreddine ZS, Phillips MA, Bedirian V, et al. The Montreal Cognitive Assessment MoCA: a brief screening tool for mild cognitive impairment. *J Am Geriatr Soc* 2005;53:695–699.

15. Mesulam M-M. Large scale neurocognitive networks and distributed processing for attention, language and memory. *Ann Neurol* 1990;28:597–613.

16. Grace J, Malloy PF. *Frontal Systems Behavior Scale.* PAR, Lutz, FL, 2002.

17. Bar-On R. *The Bar-On Emotional Quotient Inventory (EQ-i): Technical Manual.* Multi-Health Systems, Toronto, 1997.

18. Roth RM, Isquith PK, Gioia GA. *BRIEF-A: Behavior Rating Inventory of Executive Function – Adult Version.* PAR, Lutz, FL, 2005.

19. Kramer JH, Reed BR, Mungas D, Weiner MW, Chui HC. Executive dysfunction in subcortical ischemic vascular disease. *J Neurol Neurosurg Psychiatry* 2002;72:217–220.

20. Tullberg M, Fletcher E, DeCarli C, et al. White matter lesions impair frontal lobe function regardless of their location. *Neurology* 2004;63(2):246–253.

21. Wolfe N, Linn R, Babikian VL, Knoefel JE, Albert ML. Frontal systems impairment following multiple lacunar infarcts. *Arch Neurol* 1990;47:129–132.

22. Del Zoppo GJ, Saver JL, Jauch EC, Adams HP. Expansion of the time window for treatment of acute ischemic stroke with intravenous tissue plasminogen activator: a science advisory from the American Heart Association/American Stroke Association. *Stroke* 2009;40:2945–2948.

23. Saver JL. Comments, opinions and reviews: time is brain – quantified. *Stroke.* 2006;37:263–266.

24. Hoffmann M, Schmitt F, Bromley E. Comprehensive cognitive neurological assessment in stroke. *Acta Neurol Scand* 2009;119(3):162–171.

25. Hoffmann M, Sacco RS, Mohr JP, Tatemichi TK. Higher cortical function deficits among acute stroke patients: the Stroke Data Bank experience. *J Stroke Cerebrovasc Dis* 1997;6:114–120.

26. Hoffmann M. Higher cortical function deficits after stroke: an analysis of 1000 patients from a dedicated cognitive stroke registry. *Neurorehabil Neural Repair* 2001;15:113–127.

27. Hoffmann M, Schmitt F. Metacognition in stroke: bedside assessment and relation to location, size and stroke severity. *Cogn Behav Neurol* 2006;19(2):85–94.

28. Hoffmann M, Watts A. Cognitive dysfunction in isolated brainstem stroke: a neuropsychological and SPECT study. *J Stroke Cerebrovasc Dis* 1998;7:24–31.

29. Hoffmann M, Benes Cases L. Etiology of frontal network syndromes in isolated subtentorial stroke. *Behav Neurol* 2008;20:101–105.

30. Rizzolatti G, Fabbri-Destro M, Cattaneo L. Mirror neurons and their clinical relevance. *Nat Clin Pract Neurol* 2009;5:24–34.

31. Hoffmann M, Bill PLA. The environmental dependency syndrome, imitation behaviour and utilisation behaviour as presenting symptoms of bilateral frontal lobe infarction due to Moyamoya disease. *S Afr Med J* 1992;81:271–273.

32. Rizzolatti G, Fadiga L, Fogassi L, Gallese V. Resonance behaviors and mirror neurons. *Arch Ital Biol* 1999;137:85–100.

33. Ramachandran VS. *The Tell-Tale Brain.* W.W. Norton, New York, 2011.

34. Hoffmann M. The panoply of field dependent behavior in 1436 stroke patients: the Mirror Neuron System uncoupled and the consequences of loss of personal autonomy. *Neurocase* 2014;20(5):556–568.

35. Subiaul F. Mosaic cognitive evolution: the case of imitation learning. In Broadfield D, Yuan M, Schick K, Toth N. (eds.), *The Human Brain Evolving.* Stone Age Institute Press, Gosport, IN, 2010.

36. Wynn T, Coolidge FL. The implications of the working memory model for the evolution of modern cognition. *Int J Evol Biol* 2011. doi:10.4061/2011/741357.

37. Hoffmann B, Chen R. The impact of stroke on emotional intelligence. *BMC Neurology* 2010;10:103.

38. Koechlin E, Hyafil A. Anterior prefrontal function and the limits of human decision making. *Science* 2007;318:594–598.

39. Burgess PW, Durmontheil I, Gilbert SJ. The gateway hypothesis of rostral prefrontal cortex (area 10) function. *Trends Cogn Sci* 2007;11(7):290–298.

40. Hoffmann M, Bar-On R. Isolated frontopolar cortex lesion: a case study. *Cogn Behav Neurol* 2012;25:50–56.

41. Josephs KA, Hodges JR, Snowden JS, et al. Neuropathological background of phenotypical variability in frontotemporal dementia. *Acta Neuropathol* 2011;122:137–153.

42. Courville CB. *Pathology of the Nervous System: Part 4.* Pacific, Mountain View, CA, 1937.

43. Dubois B, Slachevsky A, Litvan I, Pillon B. The FAB: a frontal assessment battery at the beside. *Neurology* 2000;55:1621–1626.

44. Crossley NA, Mechelli A, Scott J, et al. The hubs of the human connectome are generally implicated in the anatomy of brain disorders. *Brain* 2014;137:2382–2395.

45. Rascovsky K, Hodges JR, Knopman D, Miller BL, et al. Sensitivity of revised diagnostic criteria for the behavioral variant of frontotemporal dementia. *Brain* 2011;134:2456–2477.

46. Boutoleau-Bretonniere C, Evrard C, Benoit-Hardouin J, et al. DAPHNE: a new tool for the assessment of the behavioral

variant of frontotemporal dementia. *Dement Geriatr Cogn Dis* 2015;5:503–516.

47. Milan G, Lamenza F, Iavarone A, et al. Frontal behavioral inventory in the differential diagnosis of dementia. *Acta Neurol Scand* 2008;117:260–265.

48. Giza CC, Hovda DA. The neuro-metabolic cascade of concussion. *J Athl Train* 2001;36:228–235.

49. Byrnes KR, Wilson CM, Brabazon F, et al. FDG-PET imaging in mild traumatic brain injury: a critical review. *Front Neuroenerg* 2014. doi: 10.3389/fnene.2013.00013.

50. Fagerholm ED, Hellyear PJ, Scott G, Leech R, Sharp DJ. Disconnection of network hubs and cognitive impairment after traumatic brain injury. *Brain* 2015;138:1696–1709.

51. Wang H-K, Lee Y-C, Huang C-Y, et al. Traumatic brain injury causes frontotemporal dementia and TDP-43 proteolysis. *Neuroscience* 2015;300:94–103.

52. Lindelov JK, Overgaard R, Overgaard M. Improving working memory performance in brain-injured patients using hypnotic suggestion. *Brain* 2017;140:1100–1106.

53. Kitagishi Y, Matsuda S. Diets involved in PPAR and PI3K/AKT/PTEN pathway may contribute to neuroprotection in atraumatic brain injury. *Alzheimers Res Ther* 2013;5:42.

54. A double-blind, randomized, sham-controlled study of the safety and effectiveness of the PoNS™ device for cranial nerve noninvasive neuromodulation ("CN-NINM") training in subjects with a chronic balance deficit due to mTBI. ClinicalTrials.gov ID: NCT02429167.

55. Leonard G, Lapierre Y, Chen J-K, Wardini JC, Ptito A. Noninvasive tongue stimulation combined with intensive cognitive and physical rehabilitation induces neuroplastic changes in patients with multiple sclerosis: a multimodal neuroimaging study. *Mult Scler J Exp Transl Clin* 2017. doi: 10.1177/2055217317690561.

56. Sili U, Kaya A, Mert A; HSV Encephalitis Study Group. Herpes simplex virus encephalitis: clinical manifestations, diagnosis and outcome in 106 adult patients. *J Clin Virol* 2014;60(2):112–118.

57. Grydeland H, Walhovd KB, Westlye LT, et al. Amnesia following herpes simplex encephalitis: diffusion-tensor imaging uncovers reduced integrity of normal-appearing white matter. *Radiology* 2010;257(3):774–781.

58. Hand E. New scrutiny for a slowing Atlantic conveyor. *Science* 2016;352: 751–752.

59. Dansgaard, W, Johnson SJ, Clausen HB, et al. Evidence for general instability of past climate from a 250-kyr ice-core record. *Nature* 1993;364(6434):218–220.

60. Heinrich H. Origin and consequences of cyclic ice rafting in the Northeast Atlantic Ocean during the past 130,000 years. *Quat Res* 1988;29:142–152.

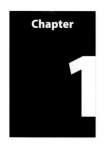

The Evolution of Larger Brains since the Vertebrate–Invertebrate Divide

Chapter 1

Plants don't move. Movement requires brains. Tracking brain size from fish, to amphibians, reptiles, mammals, and eventually primates reveals which areas enlarged and the reasons why. The implications why the evolution of progressive brain size and complexity is important for us today is analyzed and lessons for our treatments today.

The building blocks of all cells, communication between them, and neural circuitry at micro-, meso-, and macroscales are central to the study of cognition. With neurochemistry as a subset of chemistry pertaining specifically to the neural systems, the evolutionary origin of neurochemistry goes back about 3.5 billion years. Primordially, cosmochemistry supplied the first stellar elements of hydrogen and helium, from which formed the building blocks of currently known, increasingly heavier elements of the periodic table. Thereafter planetary and Earth-based evolution (origin 4.6 bya), in terms of petrochemistry (rock chemistry) evolved through phases of the black Hadean Earth (meteorite, volcanism, lava flows), Blue Earth (oceans arise), and Gray Earth, with granite forming and the rise of continents. Petrochemistry, or the formation of rocks, yielded six principal elements comprising ~98 percent of the Earth: silicon, oxygen, magnesium, calcium, aluminum, and iron. Further chemical evolution proceeded in terms of geochemistry. With the living Earth (3.8 bya) came organic chemistry, DNA and RNA, and finally neurochemistry. With Red Earth and the catalysis of the great oxygen event came multicellular life forms and further mineral evolution. Three separate episodes of Snowball Earth or White Earth occurred from 650 to 580 mya, eventually leading to Green Earth with the Cambrian explosion of animal and plant life [1].

From Cellular Complexity to Neural Network Complexity

The remodeling from small to larger brains can be traced back to the first life forms that evolved from unicellular (3.5 bya) organisms, at which time our most ancient cells (prokaryotes) contained circular, free-floating DNA with 64 possible codons, enabling the production of 20 amino acids for protein building. Mostly unicellular prokaryotes at times aggregate into an amorphous (shapeless) form, seen in blue green algae and slime molds, and are capable of cell-to-cell signaling [2].

Complex Cells (Eukaryotes) and Multicellular Life Forms (Metazoans)

The three earliest life forms were the archaea, bacteria and eukaryotes. A presumed eukaryote symbiosis with prokaryotes allowed the acquisition of the cellular powerhouse – mitochondria – in eukaryote cells at about 1.7 bya, with the universal energy current – ATP generation.

Cellular Agility

A key evolutionary attribute of eukaryotic cells was their ability to change shape in response to the environment, seen in nature's simplest organisms, the amoebae. These use the key signaling molecule that our brains and bodies use today, cyclic AMP, in response to stressors which cause dispersed amoebae to aggregate. These organisms show how an extant life form can be representative of the transition from unicellular to multicellular. They were also equipped with the cellular machinery of receptors – neurotransmitters and ion channels – that we target and attempt to manipulate for therapeutic gains today [3].

The Oxygen Catalyst

Before the great oxygen event (GOE) at 2.4–2.1 bya, the atmosphere contained about 0.001 percent of the oxygen levels present today (21 percent in air). About 600 mya, multi-cellular life forms (metazoans) arose, delayed by the approximately three billion year wait for an adequately oxygenated atmosphere. With photosynthesis producing atmospheric oxygen, the next steps in evolution proceeded, with the building of bigger bodies, neural tissue, and brains, thanks to the formation of collagen, which is a more energy-expensive tissue that only became possible with higher oxygenation levels [4]. Oxygen allowed chemical desaturation reactions that promoted polyunsaturated fatty acids (PUFAs) from shorter to longer chains and synthesis and emergence of the six double bonds found in docosahexaenoic acid (DHA). Such lipids are the building blocks of complex cellular structures, mitochondrial electron transport systems, nuclear envelopes, reticular endothelium and plasma membranes that incorporate antioxidant enzymes, receptors, transporters, and signaling systems.

The DNA dictionary operates with four-letter words that are translated into proteins, using about 20 words (amino acids) that are ultimately assembled into three-dimensional active proteins. Thus, proteins within a cell can be viewed as existing in five dimensions: covalent bonds, hydrogen bonding, metal coordination (three dimensions), phi–phi interactions (fourth dimension), and electrochemical (lipophilic and hydrophilic) and van der Waals type forces (fifth dimension). In comparison to DNA's four words (nucleotides) and proteins (20 amino acids), lipids are immensely more complex, with 364 common "lipid words" with greater potential for expression and subtlety of signal or promulgation. The creation of 32 phyla during the Cambrian explosion is ascribed to the enhanced cellular energy production powered by oxygen, with metabolic processes accelerated and DNA able to mutate more rapidly. Aerobic metabolism also increased the complexity of lipids, leading to the organization of membrane lipids that could then respond to varying environmental conditions (e.g., temperature, pressure, chemistry). Importantly, lipids facilitated change at the chemical and molecular levels in the context of an otherwise stable genome. This has direct relevance to epigenetic mechanisms and is discussed in Chapter 4.

The Evolution of Multicellular Systems

After being held in a frigid state by Snowball Earth ~600 mya when glaciation reached close to the equator, the early metazoans, represented by the 1 cm long worm-like ancestral urbilaterian, heralded the attainment of cephalization (head formation), the centralization of the nervous system from the hydra-type neural net arrangement, and bodily bilateral symmetry. Neuronal complexity and increasing response options soon followed, with the addition of an intervening interneuron to the basic two-layer nervous system, having been composed of a sensory and motor neuron [5]. The 600 million year marine environment legacy at this stage yielded a basic nervous system that was the beginning of our current neurotransmitters and intracellular signaling. Bilaterians soon evolved from the urbilaterians, in turn branching into the protostomes that gave rise to arthropods (insects), flatworms, and annelids, and the deuterostomes that included the chordates from which the 520 million year old extant lancelet (amphioxus) evolved, from which the first vertebrates and ultimately mammals arose [6].

Eyes first evolved ~543 mya, during the Cambrian explosion when all major phyla appeared over a five million year period. The "Light Switch Theory" proposed by Parker relates to the Cambrian explosion whereby he proposed that the abrupt evolution of vision and eyes occurred in response to life lived in the light [7]. Atmospheric changes allowed increased amounts of light to reach the Earth, and consequently the benefits of seeing were so compelling that eyes evolved independently in several lineages. This in turn led to more active predation in that animals can not only identify by vision but can actively pursue and kill. The concomitant evolution of harder body parts such as teeth and jaws, and shells to protect smaller animals from being eaten, evolved rapidly in response. The overall result was an explosive diversification of life forms [8]. Vision has a close association with predator–prey interactions and is something that primates, in particular, developed expansively during their evolution.

The archetypal vertebrate, amphioxus, sporting a notochord and dorsal nerve cord, with the swelling at one end, is a living representative of the first brain. From this arrangement arose the vertebrates, with the addition of a backbone to the notochord. By the time of the Early Cambrian period (541–485 mya), the vertebrate structure of the brain and neurotransmitter systems that jawless fishes and we have in common with jawed vertebrates was represented by the now extinct galeaspid (435–370 mya). The distinguishing feature was the identification of twin nostrils instead of one on their cranium, which implied vertebrate cranial development before jaw development [9].

Networking the Early Nervous System

There was a close association between the development of jaws and complex head structures that coincided with the evolution of predation. The evolutionary advantage of possessing a head and eyes with myelin-assisted brisk nerve conduction for improved bodily control constituted features leading to vertebrate success. The size of the organism was important; for the relatively smaller invertebrates with unmyelinated nerves, conduction velocities of 1 m/s sufficed. Body size increases demanded nerve conduction speed increases for both effective evasion and predation, with up to a 100-fold conduction velocity increase to 50–100 m/s along the nerve fibers. Myelinization also facilitated advantageous placement of key sensory organs, in particular the eyes, allowing extended optic nerves. Both metabolic efficiency and compaction of the nervous system were possible, with more proficient nerve impulse propagation that constituted 50 percent of metabolic energy demands. Not surprisingly, myelin evolution was concomitant with jaw development and the neural crest [10]. This period was represented by the first jawed fish, the placoderms, and the fearsome 11 m, four ton superpredator *Dunkleosteus* (380–360 mya) during the Devonian period [11]. Hence, the physical space constraint imposed by the development of a skull and vertebral column was solved by the exponential conduction velocity increase afforded by myelination, with a consequent surge in body size [12].

Migration and Adaptation from Water to Land

Perhaps fish arms races or the catastrophic Hangenberg event, near the end of the Devonian period (358 mya), associated with a rapid sea-level fall and anoxic period, attributed to Southern Hemisphere glaciation, prompted the move to land by the first vertebrates [13]. The subsequent void in the tetrapod fossil record (360–345 mya), referred to as Romer's gap, was a consequence of these massive extinctions, including both primitive and armored fishes, the placoderms and *Dunkleosteus*. The vertebrates with recognizable limbs, represented by *Panderichthys* (397 mya), *Tiktaalik* (375 mya), and *Acanthostega* (365 mya), were intermediate between the lobe-finned fishes and first terrestrial tetrapods, with their anatomical transitional limbs, termed "fishapods" by Neil Shubin, the discoverer of *Tiktaalik* [14–16].

Although measured in geological timescales of tens of millions of years, soon after this gap, ray-finned fish, including sharks, dominated and further amphibian terrestrial invasion followed. The most devastating extinction of all followed, the Permian–Triassic extinction event of 252 mya that obliterated ~96 percent of marine and ~70 percent of terrestrial vertebrates. The most proximate cause was the volcanic eruption of the massive Siberian Traps, a continent-sized, 7 000 000 km^2 area of land covered in basaltic lava from which earthly life needed about 30 million years to recover [17]. More recently a similar geological process involving the Deccan Traps on the Indian subcontinent was involved in the terrestrial dinosaur extinction and the rise of mammals.

The next wave of animals soon followed, with archosaurs and reptilian evolution that in turn ultimately gave rise to dinosaurs, pterosaurs, birds, and crocodiles [18]. Together with the archosaurs, the synapsids, the early mammal-like reptiles, were the dominant terrestrial vertebrates during the Permian period (299–251 mya), but most disappeared during the Permian–Triassic extinction save for *Lystrosaurus*, which survived on several continents. Both early mammals and dinosaurs evolved at similar times at 250–199 mya during the Triassic period, from the synapsids and archosaurs respectively [19]. Superior water conservation by the archosaurs, by virtue of excreting uric acid as a paste rather than a fluid, allowed them to tolerate the aridity of the ancient continent of Pangea, whereas synapsids excreted urea and so required water for excretion [20]. Another proposal includes the comparatively more rapid erect limb development with respect to the synapsids, leading to improved stamina and circumventing "carrier's constraint" [21]. These metabolic and skeletal advantages helped the archosaurs become dominant during this time period [22].

The Reign of the Dinosaur

The protracted period of dinosaur dominance was significant and, had astrological forces not intervened, mammal proliferation would not have taken place, nor ours. With mammals still small, relatively insignificant, and confined to a nocturnal existence for protection in the Jurassic period (201–145 mya), Earth differed markedly also from a geographic perspective. The continents were clustered together in assemblages termed Gondwanaland in the Southern and Laurasia in the Northern Hemisphere, separated by the vast, ancient

Tethys sea, with palm trees and tropical trees in Antarctica. The rearrangement to form our nowadays familiar continents first began with the fissuring of the ancient supercontinent of Pangea, which in turn arose from even earlier tectal arrangements of the continents Rodinia and Panotia. The Jurassic period was associated with a near-global tropical climate in part due to the then equatorial ocean circulation as opposed to the current north–south configuration. The most common terrestrial vertebrate at the time was the lizard *Lystrosaurus*, whose fossils have been found in the majority of continents, including Antarctica, and whose unique physiology allowed it to endure the Permian–Triassic period which saw the most severe extinction event on Earth, with markedly elevated CO_2 levels [23]. The remarkable success of the 200 million year dinosaur reign was terminated by a particularly catastrophic event, thought to be an asteroid impact 66 million years ago, itself in turn perhaps coupled to the 35 million year comet cycle and compounded by the secondary geothermal events it set in motion, namely the Deccan Traps with associated volcanism [24]. The Deccan Traps, comprising continental flood basalts in India of 300 000 km^3 of erupted lava, lasting 750 000 years, occurred around the time of mass extinction at 65 mya at the end of the Cretaceous period, coincident with the disappearance of the non-avian dinosaurs [25].

The long-term mammalian coexistence with the dinosaurs is worthy of scrutiny. Dinosaur success may have been partly due to their unique ability of mesothermia, a transitory ability between mammalian endothermy (self-regulation of body temperature) and reptilian ectothermy (environmentally regulated body temperature). It has been postulated that this type of intermediate thermoregulation allowed the dinosaurs to grow to their uniquely enormous size and mass due to lower energy costs in the tropical environment they occupied. This may also have been advantageous in competition with both endothermic and ectothermic animals at the time [26,27].

Early Mammals

Mammals were initially small and nocturnal, and relied on smell and hearing more than vision. They had larger brains than the antecedent reptiles and amphibians, and a six-layer cortex (Figure 1.1). The synapsids, which initially diverged from the reptilian tetrapods about 300 mya, during the Carboniferous period, featured relatively low-resolution olfaction (smell) and hearing, limited vision, coarse tactile reactivity, and crude motor coordination [28]. Their cerebral circuitry for sensorimotor integration in their brains was relatively impoverished in comparison to the sensorimotor integration circuitry of later mammals, primates, and subsequently humans.

The extensive brain frontoparietal integration and circuitry would eventually support key cognitive facilities such as working memory and mirror neuron systems and other higher cortical functions characteristic of humans. Mammalia arose about 200 mya in the Early Jurassic period, represented by *Morganucodon*, that by this time featured greater olfactory resolution and tactile sensitivity, the latter attributed to body hair. Relative to earlier synapsids, *Morganucodon* featured improved sensorimotor coordination, lengthy cochlea (hearing organ), and reduced middle ear ossicle size, which nevertheless remained attached to the lower jaw. *Morganucodon*, as the basal member of the Mammaliaformes, is representative of the first pulse in encephalization, with an estimated encephalization quotient (EQ) of ~0.32, approximately 50 percent larger than the basal cynodonts. EQ is a more precise evaluation, allowing for allometric effects of relative brain size or the ratio,

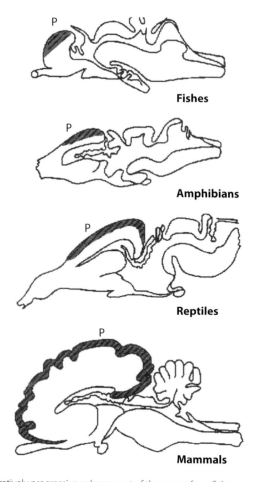

P

Fishes

P

Amphibians

P

Reptiles

P

Mammals

Figure 1.1 The comparatively progressive enlargement of the cortex from fish to amphibian to reptile to mammalian cortex. P = pallium, refers to both paleocortex and neocortex.

Source: Fuster JM. *The Prefrontal Cortex.* 5th ed. Elsevier, Amsterdam, 2008. Reproduced with permission from Academic Press; *See also:* von Bonin G. *Essays on the Cerebral Cortex of Man.* Charles C. Thomas, Springfield, IL, 1948.

between actual brain mass and the predicted brain mass in an animal of a certain size. The formula is represented as:

$$EQ = \text{brain weight}/0.12 \times \text{body weight}^{2/3}$$

and the mean EQ for mammals is 1. The EQs of carnivores, cetaceans, and primates are all above 1, with elephants at 1.1, chimpanzees at 2.2, bottlenose dolphins at 4.1, and humans at 7.4.

During this time, the mammalian third eye or parietal eye – that would eventually become the current pineal gland in humans – formed. The evolutionary living fossil of the parietal eye is still seen in the lizard-like tuatara found in New Zealand as a miniature dot at the vertex of the head that is reactive to light. The tuatara is a representative tetrapod from over 200 mya, when tetrapods were evolving into lizards, turtles, crocodiles, and dinosaurs. In mammals and humans it became the light-responsive pineal gland, which secretes melatonin for sleep maintenance and thermoregulation. Progressive brain enlargement among these animals was principally due to enhanced olfaction, better represented by *Hadrocodium* (~150 mya), whose middle ear ossicles were separate from the lower jaw. Further progressive sensorimotor integration is suggested by spinal cord and cerebellum enlargement.

The Crown Mammalia represented a third pulse of mammalian evolution, with further increase in olfactory neural circuitry and ossified ethmoid turbinals, enabling a tenfold increase of olfactory epithelium in the nasal cavity. Further progression was also present in auditory apparatus and sensorimotor integration, both drivers of increased encephalization (brain enlargement). Several other mammalian attributes were now in place, including more nutritious feeding habits of insectivory, miniaturization, viviparity, parental care, elevated metabolism, and milk associated with the origin of the neocortex. Endothermia was suggested by early mammalian fur, which in turn had exapted from hair, originally for tactile function. It would later be a critical factor in maintaining endothermia in future planetary cooling and glacial cycles. A requisite for the enlarging brain was a higher-quality diet and elevated metabolism, which in turn benefited from endothermia [28].

Bolides and the Catastrophic Cretaceous–Tertiary Event

An asteroid impact is the most likely proximate cause of the Cretaceous–Tertiary extinction (KT event) ~66 mya, with supportive evidence being the underwater Chicxulub crater discovered in the Gulf of Mexico. This provided new opportunities for mammals to become diurnal and proliferate following non-avian dinosaur extinction. Additional geological evidence bolstered this premise through bands of iridium, a signature of asteroids that is rarely of earthly origin. Bands of iridium, dated to this time, have been found in many parts of the world, both marine and terrestrial rock strata [29]. The Alvarez bolide impact theory states that catastrophic global climactic perturbations were precipitated by various aerosols including ash, sulfuric acid, and dust permeating the atmosphere, reducing solar radiation for decades and causing an "impact winter" [30]. Because of evidence for a more gradual dinosaur extinction process over several millions of years, current theories support a combination of the bolide (meteor) impact, which may have triggered massive volcanic eruptions of the Deccan Traps in India, with the developments of super-plumes [31,32]. Overall, the combined events led to the extinction of the non-avian dinosaurs, as well as ~75 percent of animal and plant life. One group that was spared was the branch of dinosaurs that had invested in miniaturization, similar to some mammals, over the last 200 mya. At least four orders of mammals had diversified before this impact, but much more rapid mammalian diversification ensued in the millions of years thereafter, with the earliest ancestral primate, *Archicebus achilles* dating to about 55 mya [33]. Arboreal habitation selects for smaller size and provided improved safety and feeding opportunities. The only surviving dinosaurs occupied this niche, developed feathers for insulation, as well as nocturnal living, which led to further evolution of flight and birds. Notably, ancestral primates also occupied the arboreal environment [34,35].

Mammalian Evolution

We retain many of the characteristics that developed nearly 300 million years ago. Mammalian evolution equipped us with a six-layer cortex during our residence in Laurasia and Gondwanaland. Interestingly, bipedalism was also evident in some animals, notably *Tyrannosaurus rex*. Brain growth was fueled by the higher-quality insectivorous diet and later by nectar and fruit consumption. A notable discovery is that of seven west Malaysian rain forest mammalian species that consume up to 3.8 percent (vol/vol) alcohol concentration (mean 0.6 percent) as part of their natural diet, on a daily basis. The pentailed tree shrew in particular (*Ptilocercus lowii*) regularly consumes nectar containing alcohol doses from clusters of flowers (inflorescences) from the bertram palm in amounts that humans would find intoxicating, yet the small squirrel-sized mammal shows no signs of inebriation, even though the estimates of 36 percent probability would lead to a drunken state every third night in these small creatures. Perhaps the mammals that feed on bertram palm nectar eliminate a significantly larger proportion of ingested alcohol via the glucuronic acid conjugation pathway rather than alcohol dehydrogenase, as in humans. The pentailed tree shrew is representative of a living model of now extinct mammals from which all extinct and extant tree shrews and primates evolved. In these a moderate to high alcohol intake was part of their diet and denotes a penchant for alcohol in mammals prior to primate evolution. In addition, plant saps high in sugar (phloem sap) and nectar are prone to fermentation and alcohol production, and remain part of the dietary intake of current-day primates and in traditional human cultures today [36].

This evolutionary metabolic trait may be important for our understanding of current-day human alcohol-related maladaptive conduct, which evolved in the context of protracted selection for low-level alcohol availability in conjunction with frugivory (fruit eating) among mammal, primate, and then human ancestral species. Ripening fruit and its associated variable alcohol concentrations is a valuable nutrient for mammals, as well as some insects and birds. This came under genetic selection and intake hampered by natural availability. Current-day alcoholism can be regarded as yet another example of an evolutionary mismatch condition or evolutionary hangover, in that gene protection against potential harmful effects was not present initially. Modern alcohol availability allows an intake that is too rapid for appropriate evolutionary responses [37,38].

Placental mammals evolved during the Cretaceous period, estimated at about 80 mya, and developed the mammalian fear module, specifically for detection and avoidance of their three principal predator groups: carnivores, snakes, and raptors that may threaten survival. Later in evolution, primates elaborated this fear module and upgraded its efficiency with the addition of with trichromatic vision [28]. Clinical neurological and psychiatric syndromes such as post-traumatic stress disorder (PTSD) and anxiety are among the more common and challenging neural disorders recognized today that pertain to this ancient neural circuitry. Visual neural systems that allow rapid and accurate, visually guided actions were under the control of the brain's superior colliculus (SC) and pulvinar system, primarily for predator detection and avoidance. Substantia nigra connections in the midbrain of the brainstem, at the same time, allowed these mammals to instantly abort their current activity, in preference for the identified threat. The brain therefore has a two-tier system, with the initial system a more fundamental, unconscious circuit critical for survival, being able to process large amounts of basic sensory information, which is a feature of vertebrates. The SC enables freezing in relation to rapidly advancing objects. Both dogs and bears, for example, have difficulty identifying motionless objects. The later addition of the conscious component, a mammalian feature, with the lateral geniculate nucleus (LGN) of the thalamus now part of the circuitry, improved overall perception, but was slower. However, this system featured extensive cortical connections that lead to superior identification of predators with downstream decision options such as the option of attack, flee, or warn others. Importantly, primates evolved their visual apparatus further with the incorporation of the amygdala and the extensive fear module as part of the vision circuitry [39]. Nowadays we recognize this part of the evolutionary process as relevant to PTSD-related flashbacks and vivid dreams. The LGN-P pathway expanded in primates in particular, where it featured in snake detection by providing focused selection to the lower visual field. Both the LGN visual system and SC pulvinar visual system were influenced by predator pressures and had complementary functions for predator detection. The LGN system and SC system both evolved in primates; the former is more involved with details and the latter more with unconscious, automatic responses such as avoiding predators and hand–eye coordination. Hence, our visual brain circuitry has been wired for rapid, preconscious detection of snakes by the fear module comprising the amygdala, SC, locus coeruleus, and pulvinar [40].

Impairments of this circuitry are seen nowadays in people with SC damage, which is rare but more commonly in people with Parkinson's disease, who have slower reaction times to peripherally placed stimuli. Isbell's conception of this circuitry is particularly well depicted. The koniocellular or K pathway links the retina to the SC nucleus for automatic grasping and visually guided reaching. A second route links the retina to the pulvinar, mostly involved with the fear module. A third pathway links the retina to the LGN, with links thereafter to the middle temporal (MT) region in the posterior superior temporal area, involved with motion. The SC pathway, amygdala, and pulvinar link the visual and motor deficits in people with Parkinson's disease, who sometimes freeze for no reason [41,42]. Loss of dopamine from the substantia nigra could be causing freezing in the automatic visual SC system to peripheral distractors where the K pathway appears most responsive. Further insights of the evolutionary process for Parkinson's disease include the freezing responses frequently seen. Freezing is a natural response in mammals to objects that suddenly appear in the periphery. Patients with Parkinson's disease may be assisted by following visual lines or patterns on the floor, whereby cortical vision centers override the SC pathway. In addition, the fear module is impaired in Parkinson's disease whereby patients no longer respond to fearful facial expressions.

Evolutionary Explanations of Blindsight

People with primary visual (V1) lesions frequently retain some visual capacity but are relatively devoid of perceptual awareness or the ability to acknowledge the percept. Navigating a route with avoidance of strategically placed obstacles can be successfully performed, as can the recognition of emotional facial expressions [43–45]. In some people with left visuospatial neglect due to a lesion of the right parietal region, often by stroke, blindsight in the hemifield may occur. Marshall and Halligan's experiment of an intact house and a house on fire was profound in that the majority with such lesions showed a preference for the house not on fire, suggesting unconscious processing of the images [46].

Summary

The fundamentals of a brain and body plan that early and later mammals bequeathed us include the following.

Brain anatomy
Six-layer cortex
Fear module
Three-tier visual processing

Brain circuitry
Frontoparietal, progressive integration of sensorimotor systems
Grasping enhanced by fine-branch habitat
Transition from primarily olfactory sense to vision as the primary sense
Blindsight
PTSD flashbacks
Parkinson's disease freezing, gait disorders, altered emotional processing

Skeletal
Cranial size increase to an EQ of ~0.5
Inner ear ossicles separating from the lower jaw
Ossified ethmoid turbinals

Diet and metabolism
High-quality diet (insectivory)
Frugivory
Penchant for alcohol in mammals prior to primate evolution?

References

1. Hazen RM. *The Story of the Earth: The First 4.5 Billion Years, from Stardust to Living Planet.* Penguin, New York, 2013.

2. Fuqua C, White D. Prokaryotic intercellular signaling: mechanistic diversity and unified themes. In Fairweather I (ed.), *Cell Signalling in Prokaryotes and Lower Metazoa.* Kluwer Academic Publishers, Dordrecht, 2004.

3. Caveney S, Cladman W, Verellen LA, Donly C. Ancestry of neuronal monoamine transporters in the Metazoa. *J Exp Biol* 2006;209:4858–4868.

4. Lyons TW, Reinhard CT, Planavasky NJ. The rise of oxygen in Earth's early ocean and atmosphere. *Nature* 2014;506:307–315.

5. Squire LR, Berg D, Bloom FE, et al. *Fundamental Neuroscience*, 4th edn. Academic Press, Amsterdam, 2013.

6. Denes AS, Jekely G, Arendt D, et al. Conserved mediolateral molecular architecture of the annelid trunk neuroectoderm reveals common ancestry of bilateral nervous system centralization. *Cell* 2007;129(2):277–288.

7. Parker A. *In the Blink of an Eye.* Perseus, Cambridge, MA, 2003.

8. Briggs DE. The Cambrian explosion. *Curr Biol* 2015;25(19):R864–R868.

9. Gai Z, Donoghue PC, Zhu M, Janvier P, Stampanoni M. Fossil jawless fish from China foreshadows early jawed vertebrate anatomy. *Nature* 2011;476:324–327.

10. Zalc B, Goujet D, Colman D. The origin of the myelination program in vertebrates. *Curr Biol* 2008;18:R511–R512.

11. Anderson PSL, Westneat MW. Feeding mechanisms and bite force modeling of the skull of Dunkleosteus terelli, an ancient apex predator. *Biol Lett* 2007;3:77–80.

12. Zalc B. Origins of vertebrate success. *Science* 2000;288:5464.

13. Sandberg CA, Morrow JR, Ziegler W. Late Devonian sea level changes, catastrophic events and mass extinctions. In: Koeberl C, MacLeod KG (eds.), *Catastrophic*

Events and Mass Extinctions: Impacts and Beyond. Geological Society of America, Boulder, CO, 2002.

14. Daeschler EB, Shubin NH, Jenkins FA Jr. A Devonian tetrapod-like fish and the evolution of the tetrapod body plan. *Nature*. 2006;440:757–763.

15. Boisvert, CA. The pelvic fin and girdle of Panderichthys and the origin of tetrapod locomotion. *Nature* 2005;438:1145–1147.

16. Niedzwiedzki G, Szrek P, Narkiewicz K, Narkiewicz M, Ahlberg P. Tetrapod trackways from the Early Middle Devonian period of Poland. *Nature* 2010;463:43–48.

17. Campbell IH, Czamanske GK, Fedorenko VA, Hill RI, Stepanov V. Synchronism of the Siberian traps and the Permian Triassic boundary. *Science* 1992;258(5089):1760–1763.

18. Nesbitt SJ. The early evolution of archosaurs: relationships and the origin of major clades. *Bull Am Mus Nat Hist* 2011:352;1–292.

19. Kemp TS. The origin and early radiation of the therapsid mammal-like reptiles: a palaeobiological hypothesis. *J Evol Biol* 2006;19:1231–1247.

20. Benton, MJ. *Vertebrate Paleontology*, 3rd edn. Blackwell Science, London, 2005.

21. Carrier DR. The evolution of locomotor stamina in tetrapods: circumventing a mechanical constraint. *Paleobiology* 1987;13:326–341.

22. de Bakker MA, Fowler DA, den Oude K, et al. Digit loss in archosaur evolution and the interplay between selection and constraints. *Nature* 2013;463:445–448.

23. Sahney S, Benton MJ. Recovery from the most profound mass extinction of all time. *Proc Biol Sci* 2008;275:759–765.

24. Fan J, Katz A, Randall L, Reece M. Dark-disk universe. *Phys Rev Lett* 2013;110(21):211302.

25. Schoene B, Samperton KM, Eddy MP, et al. U-Pb geochronology of the Deccan Traps and relation to the end-Cretaceous mass extinction. *Science* 2015;347:182–184.

26. Grady JM, Enquist BJ, Dettweiler-Robinson E, Wright NA, Smith FA. Evidence for mesothermy in dinosaurs. *Science* 2014;344:1268–1272.

27. Balter M. Dinosaur metabolism neither hot nor cold, but just right. *Science* 2014;344:1216–1217.

28. Rowe TB, Macrini TE, Luo ZX. Fossil evidence on origin of the mammalian brain. *Science* 2011;332:955–957.

29. Alvarez LW, Alvarez W, Asaro F, Michel HV. Extraterrestrial cause for the Cretaceous–Tertiary extinction. *Science* 1980;208:1095–1108.

30. Vellekoop J, Sluijs A, Smit J, et al. Rapid short term cooling following the Chicxulub impact at the Cretaceous–Paleogene boundary. *PNAS* 2014;111:7537–7541.

31. Brusatte SL, Butler RJ, Barrett PM, et al. The extinction of the dinosaurs. *Biol Rev Camb Philos Soc* 2014. doi: 10.1111/brv.12128.

32. Lin SC, van Keken PE. Multiple volcanic episodes of flood basalts caused by thermochemical mantle plumes. *Nature*. 2005;436:250–252.

33. Springer MS, Murphy WJ, Eizirik E, O'Brien SJ. Placental mammal diversification and the Cretaceous–Tertiary boundary. *PNAS* 2003;100:1056–1061.

34. Benton MJ. How birds became birds: sustained size reduction was essential for the origin of birds and avian flight. *Science* 2014;345:508–509.

35. Lee MSY, Cau A, Naish D, Dyke GJ. Sustained miniaturization and anatomical innovation in the dinosaurian ancestors of birds. *Science* 2014;345:562–566.

36. Wiens F, Zitzmann A, Lachance M-A, et al. Chronic intake of fermented floral nectar by wild treeshrews. *PNAS* 2008;105:10426–10431.

37. Dudley R. Evolutionary origins of human alcoholism in primate frugivory. *Q Rev Biol* 2000;75:3–15.

38. Dudley R. Fermenting fruit and the historical ecology of ethanol ingestion: is alcoholism in modern humans an

evolutionary hangover? *Addiction* 2002;97:381–388.

39. Kaas JH. The evolution of brains from early mammals to humans. *Wiley Interdiscip Rev Cogn Sci* 2013;4(1):33–45.

40. Kalin NH, Shelton SE, Davidson RJ. The role of the central nucleus of the amygdala in mediating fear and anxiety in the primate. *J Neurosci* 2004;24:5506–5515.

41. Bender DB, Butter CM. Comparison of the effects of superior colliculus and pulvinar lesions on visual search and tachistoscopic pattern discrimination in monkeys. *Exp Brain Res* 1987;69: 140–154.

42. McDowell S, Harris J. Irrelevant peripheral visual stimuli impair manual reaction times in Parkinson's disease. *Vis Res* 1997;37:3549–3558.

43. Weiskrantz L. *Blindsight: A Case Study and Implications*, Oxford University Press, Oxford, 1986.

44. Weiskrantz L. Blindsight revisited. *Curr Opin Neurobiol* 1996;6:215–220.

45. Heywood CA, Kentridge RW. Affective blindsight? *Trends Cogn Sci* 2000;4(4): 125–112.

46. Marshall JC, Halligan PW. Blindsight and insight into visuospatial neglect. *Nature* 1988;336:766–767.

The Profound Increase in Primate Gray Matter Growth

Dancing across the tectonic plates, the vertebrate lineage ultimately led to early mammals and primates in Gondwanaland. Thereafter the "planet of the apes" took place mostly in present-day Europe, from which our ancestors were derived. Every important step or phase shift, such as frugivory (fruit eating) and bipedalism, during these epochs encompasses rules and lessons we need to abide by today.

Primate Evolution on the Early Continents in Geological Time

A review of the complicated history of primate evolution may be likened to a hop, skip, and jump across the tectonic plates over the last 65 million years. During this time the Earth was tropical, with palm trees in Antarctica, the angiosperm evolution had begun about 125 mya, and the Paleo-Eocene Thermal Maximum (PETM). Following the asteroid impact in Chixulub 66 mya, combined with subsequent volcanism from the Deccan Traps eruptions, mammal proliferation began, with over 20 new orders recognized [1]. The angiosperm evolution was in full swing, having begun about 125 mya, and the Paleo-Eocene Thermal Maximum (PETM) was about to start, at about 55 mya, with global temperatures rising 6°C, an event that lasted about 200 000 years. A global tropical and subtropical climate ensued and was the backdrop against which primate evolution transpired. Initially, the early primates inhabited the fine-branch arboreal canopies and were predominantly nocturnal and diminutive. A variety of ecological niches were filled, dictated by the primate's adaptability and suitability to the amount of sunlight and darkness. Some thrived as cathemeral species (neither nocturnal nor diurnal, with irregular activity at any time of night or day) as some prosimians are today. Others became crepuscular (active primarily during twilight, after dawn or before dusk). Yet others became matutinal or only active before dawn and some pursued the vespertine niche, being only active after sunset [2].

Early primates were equipped with large frontally directed eyes, enabling stereoscopic vision, and corticospinal tract development that allowed grasping, head, neck, and mouth orientation for manipulation of objects, with a visual frame of reference paramount among the senses. Further elaboration of the premotor area, Brodmann area (BA) 6, and the posterior parietal region developed in concert as one of the many examples of progressively expanding frontoparietal circuitry.

The Six-Layer Mammalian Cortex in Primates

The initial development of granular cortices (characterized by the presence of layer four) of the caudal prefrontal cortex (PFC) or BA 8, as well as the granular components of the orbital PFC (parts of BA 11, 13, and 14) appeared thanks to the challenging arboreal environment of tropical forests in which most primates lived. *Granular cortex* refers to layer four of the six-layer mammalian cortex. The cortex is 2–4 mm thick and 80 percent of neurons in general are excitatory and 20 percent inhibitory. The outermost layer is layer one, the molecular layer; layer two is the external granular; layer three the external pyramidal layer; layer four the internal granular layer; layer five the internal pyramidal layer; and layer six the multiform layer. Primate cortical pyramidal cells comprise more than 70 percent of cortical neurons and up to a 30-fold difference has been documented with respect to the number of dendritic spines on primate pyramidal cells in the PFC compared to the other lobes [3]. Computational abilities are therefore presumed to be enhanced considerably among the circuits they subserve [4]. The granular cortex is not present in non-primate mammals and most researchers in this field agree that the thickness of layer four determines whether or not a granular layer exists at all. An increase in cell density of this layer also increases with caudal to rostral (from back to front) progression within the frontal lobes. The measurements are not absolute, however, with dysgranular and agranular existing on a continuum. Mackay and Petrides consider that cortical areas with layer four densities below a certain threshold are agranular [5].

Lesions seen in clinical neurology in reference to these areas include conditions presenting with clumsiness of the hands and arms, which were critical for grasping and in negotiating the challenging fine-branch habitat of primates. These include limb ataxia (missing the target due to erratic pointing), apraxias (clumsiness of fine finger and hand movements), and simple imitation behavior syndromes related to a disturbance of the frontoparietal circuitry underlying the mirror neuron system. Hand–eye coordination, vital to life in the high forest canopies, when disturbed or impaired is represented by the forced eye deviation in epileptic seizures and visuospatial abnormalities seen as components of Balint's syndrome. This dramatic syndrome may be seen among pregnant women with eclampsia or various stroke syndromes, for example, and comprises the triad of simultanagnosia (piecemeal vision not able to see all the parts of an object in the field of view), optic ataxia (missing the target when reaching with the hand), and optic apraxia (being unable to voluntarily move the eyes in a particular direction). Other "lesions" seen today include the top five causes of mortality today: cardiovascular disease, cerebrovascular disease, dementia, cancer, and metabolic syndromes and obesity, which can all be significantly reduced by a regular fruit intake. Ever more high-level scientific studies support fruit intake for reducing our most pervasive and costly diseases [6,7].

The majority of primates live in tropical forests, deemed the most complex ecosystems on our planet, containing thousands of different plant species, several hundred types of vertebrates, and many more invertebrates (Figure 2.1). Primary rain forests are up to 80 m (260 feet) high and secondary forests with abundant leaves and fruit are often concentrated around rivers, called gallery forests. These complex ecosystems feature high-quality diets with frugivory (fruit), folivory (leaves), insectivory (insects, arthropods), gummivory (gums), gramnivory (seeds), and nectivory (nectar) on the menu. This complex environment also allowed for experimentation with various forms of locomotion

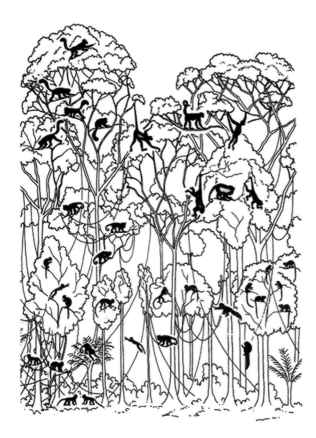

Figure 2.1 The vast three dimensional environment of the equatorial forests and primate evolution.

Source: adapted from Feagle J. *Primate Adaptation and Evolution*, 3rd edition. Academic Press, New York, 2013. Reproduced with permission from Academic Press.

in which primates engaged. All of the following may be found among extant primates: arboreal quadrupedalism, terrestrial quadrupedalism, knuckle walking, leaping, suspensory climbing, and bipedalism – the latter uniquely maintained by the eventual human lineage [2].

During the PETM warm period, the first split occurred among primates, the strepsirrhines (wet-nosed primates, lemurs, lorises) and haplorhines (dry-nosed primates, tarsiers, monkeys, apes) at about 55 mya. Adaptive radiation occurred during this time, a process by which one species evolves into two or more species with a relatively rapid expansion and diversification of an evolving group adapting to their new ecological niche. These new primate species resembled modern prosimians (lemurs, lorises, and tarsiers) and comprised two main families, the Adapidae (similar to lemurs and lorises) and the Omomyidae (tarsiers and galagos). This occurred during the Eocene epoch, and they were widely distributed in Asia, America, Europe, and Africa, with much greater prosimian diversity than today. Notably the Adapidae fossil from the Messel pit in Germany, named *Darwinius*, from 47 mya was near-perfectly preserved due to a unique combination of events that allows us to study these early primates. They also reached the nascent island of Madagascar, born of two major rifting events during the break-up of Gondwanaland: the initial separation from Africa ~160 mya and subsequently from the combined Seychelles and India land mass 66–90 mya. The fissuring of Gondwanaland

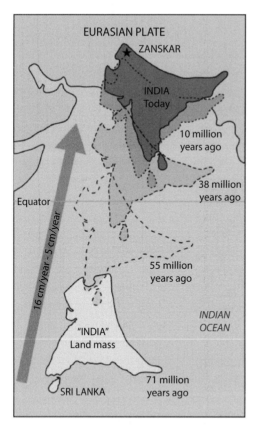

Figure 2.2 Indo-Madagascar, Himalayan Mountains, and Tibetan Plateau formation. Collision of the Indian continent with Eurasia occurred at about 55 mya, with most of the uplift occurring ~8 mya. Atmospheric circulation over Africa changed with drier summer air and loss of two moisture-bearing winds.
Source: U.S. Geological Survey.

along the Davie Fracture Zone commenced ~182 mya, with East Gondwana – including Madagascar, the Antarctic, and Indian plates – separating from the African plate. East Gondwana in turn subsequently broke apart 115–120 mya, with the unusually expeditious transition of India northward and collision with the Asian plate forming the Himalayas and Tibetan plateau, the highest mountains on Earth (Figure 2.2). India and the Seychelles then separated from Madagascar 84–95 mya. This India–Asia collision and the active orogenic zone continues today, with about 5–50 mm estimated increase in the height of Mount Everest each year. In addition, the instability of this zone is associated with more frequent earthquakes than in more stable mountain regions such as the Alps. In a current review of plate tectonic speed and its earthquake associations, or "plate rate controls quake theory," the recent Zagros Mountain quake with tragic loss of life was such a reminder of the relatively rapid 1–5 cm collision rate of the Himalayan systems [8].

Primate Origins and Indo-Madagascar Eden Hypothesis

Fossil primates (plesiadapiforms) were widespread in Europe and North America, Asia, and South America, but not in Madagascar. The plesiadapiforms or stem primate attributes help explain our burgeoning frontoparietal circuitry that was subsequently adapted for working memory, our brain's fundamental operating system. How did they do this? By leaping from branch to branch in the high canopies of tropical forests at heights of around 30 m (~100 feet), a premium was placed on catching that next branch. These were the fine-branch specialists. They also were capable graspers, and had three-dimensional, but not yet trichromatic, color vision. Prosimians were common in Europe and North America until 55 mya and diversified during the Eocene at 55–34 mya, with 60 different genera known to date. Prosimians then appear to fade from the fossil record in what is today Europe and North America during the subsequent Eocene and Oligocene epochs of 34–23 mya [9].

The split between anthropoid primates and tarsiers appeared about 45 mya and subsequently the Old World and New World primates, the catarrhines and platyrrhines, at about 34 mya. By this time global cooling had accelerated with the formation of the Antarctic ice sheet. Apes and Old World primates split at about 23 mya and humans split from the ape lineage at about 7 mya. While platyrrhine monkeys diversified in South and Central America, catarrhines, with their two premolars, appear in the fossil record in the Fayum depression, nowadays Egypt, at about 34–32 mya [10]. These subsequently spread to Europe and Asia, but not to North America or South America.

With the separation of Africa and South America ~100 mya, the venue of origin of primates has been postulated to be the "Indo-Madagascar Garden of Eden" by Isbell. To help explain this part of primate evolution, two land bridges between Antarctica and Indo-Madagascar are implied. Relatively undisputed is the Kerguelen plateau, mostly underwater currently, but which was above water 90 mya. A second land bridge that may have been relevant to primate migrations was the Gunnerus ridge, connecting Madagascar to Antarctica up to 82 mya, which supports similar fossil dinosaurs and extant and extinct animals that have their closest relatives found in South American, India, and Madagascar. The land bridge connecting South America to India and Madagascar via Antarctica and subsequent Indo-Madagascar Eden hypothesis with temporary docking with Africa on the way to the eventual collision with the Asian land mass, helps explain prosimian and early primate evolution from a biogeographic point of view [11]. Strepsirrhines and haplorrhines had diverged early in primate evolution, between 60 mya (fossil data) and 90 mya (genetic data). All that remains of this key geological event in primate evolution is the remote Kerguelen Islands, among the most isolated places on Earth, also known as Desolation Islands, in the vast southern Indian Ocean over 2000 miles (3000 km) from Africa. Rarely visited today except by the occasional round-the-world ocean yacht racing vessels such as the Jules Verne maxi-catamaran races, they are beyond the reach of helicopter range should mishaps occur.

The strepsirrhines featured both a rhinarium and a toothcomb, the latter of which provides fossil evidence of grooming that had emerged among primates 40 mya and that continued to have increased importance into the human lineage [12]. Tactile grooming eventually transformed into vocal grooming or language in the human lineage [13].

Global Cooling and the Origin of the Premotor and Ventral Premotor Motor Cortices

The primate brain had already doubled in size relative to mammalian brains by the end of the Paleogene period (60–25 mya), attributed to high-quality diets, frugivory in particular, and challenging polyadic relationships. The latter were a consequence of increased sociality that in turn helped counter predation risk.

After the intensely tropical PETM phase of 55 mya, increasing global cooling and associated aridity at ~34 mya was precipitated in large part by Antarctic glaciation. After the ancient Tethys ocean and its warm equatorial ocean circulation were expunged due to tectonic plate movements, a global change of the ocean circulations from an equatorial to an interpolar, meridional configuration took place (Figure 2.3). A consequence was that the cold dense water formed by sea ice peregrinated northwards from Antarctica, via sea troughs and basins, with global cooling first precipitated ~50 mya but with acceleration at 34 mya and even more so by ~6 mya. The latter event coincided with northern glaciation and the formation of the Arctic Pond [14,15]. These caused profound challenges in climate unpredictability, with fickle food sources. Primates benefited from frontal lobe specializations, with a reduction in the number of errors incurred, when faced with challenging environmental choices. However, not all anthropoid encephalization can be attributed to austere climate change [16]. Other drivers of increased brain size included predation, sociality, and a higher-quality diet. Much later in the human lineages, chemical food processing (fire) and protolanguage became additional drivers [17]. All were, however, adaptations and flexible responses to environmental unpredictability. Climate remains a major factor today, including intermittent global cooling, increased glaciation, and aridity episodes in relation to the four different Milankovitch cycles – orbital forcing events – measured for example in marine isotope stages. In addition, unpredictable and erratic fluctuations in cooling occur periodically, termed Heinrich and Dansgaard–Oeschgar events. These are precipitated by freshwater influx into the Atlantic Meridional Overturning Circulation (AMOC), where down-welling in the northern Atlantic may be associated with whiplash-type climate changes from warm to cold spells [18]. In addition to glaciation and orbital Milankovitch forcing events, the closure of the Panama isthmus, Indonesian seaway closure, the opening of the Drake passage, African Rift valley formation (formation of complex topography), Himalayan formation, and Tibetan Uplift all influenced the biogeography of primate evolution at various stages [19].

Early primates (anthropoids) developed both visual and frontal cortices. The fine-branch habitation of the early primates took advantage of the angiosperm evolution, with initially nocturnal feeding on insects, fruits, nectar, flowers, and seeds. Reaching, grasping, capturing, and feeding on fine branches exerted particular demands in terms of vision and balance. This period of evolution developed the premotor cortex (BA 6), the frontal eye fields (BA 8), and the ventral premotor (VPM) cortex (BA 44 and 45). In conjunction with the elaboration of these frontal regions was the origin of the corticospinal tracts that enabled fine reaching and manipulation [16]. The VPM cortex is involved in the coordinated movements of the arm, head, and mouth together with the corticospinal and brainstem projections onto motor neurons that provide muscular control to the jaw, lip, head, and upper extremity. This facilitated hand to mouth feeding while at the same time successfully balancing in potentially precarious, arboreal, unstable fine-branch habitats. Lesions of the corticospinal tracts are today seen as praxis deficits, particularly melokinetic or limb kinetic apraxias. Lesions of the ventral premotor cortex and their posterior parietal connections are seen as syndromes of ideomotor apraxias (object and tool use deficits).

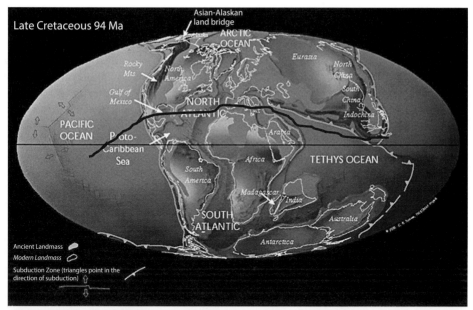

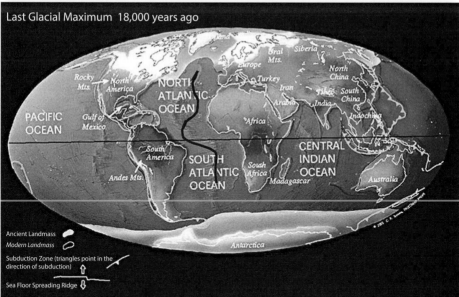

Figure 2.3 The change from an equatorial to a polar circulation. The ancient Tethys ocean was associated with a warm equatorial ocean circulation that changed with tectonic plate movement that slowly obliterated it with a change to interpolar meridional-type circulation (curvilinear lines).

Source: adapted from Prof. Christopher R. Scotese, PALEOMAP Project, 134 Dodge, Evanston, Illinois 60202 with permission.

Further Anthropoid Prefrontal Cortex Development: The SMA, Pre-SMA, Motor Programs, and Imitation

With a move to diurnality for most primates came a frontal orientation of the eyes from a more lateral position for three-dimensional vision, fovea development for improved visual acuity, and sociality. A number of physical, morphological, brain, and metabolic changes also ensued. Anthropoids became arboreal quadrupeds, became larger, and became very dependent on angiosperm products such as fruits rather than those of the fine-branch niche such as nectar, flowers, and insects. With this change came challenges such as increased predation risk and volatile food availability. Because of the predation risk, group living was adopted but with the inherent consequences of managing group interactions and conflicts. Soon thereafter the divergence into haplorrhines and platyrrhines occurred at ~34 mya, coincident with maximal Antarctic glaciation with precipitous global cooling, aridity, and environmental challenges in terms of food and tree scarcity in certain regions. Faced with inconstant resources, made more unpredictable by the global cooling and climate changes, learning rapidly even from a single experience was advantageous. This curtailed pursuing choices for securing nourishment that were improvident or potentially perilous, including predation risk. The development of the new prefrontal granular cortical areas improved foraging during times of meager food availability. More specifically, the ventral PFC guided choices by auditory as well as visual information (foveal vision, trichomacy) that allowed food signs and signals to be acquired by distant and more proximal regions. The dorsal PFC augmented foraging preferences based on visually experienced events and the ability to sequence actions. The dorsomedial PFC enabled choosing and evaluating actions based on the previous experience that in turn was derived from both external and internal sensory inputs. The polar PFC or frontopolar cortex improved foraging choice by analogical reasoning, that is the basis for making inferences and adaptation to novelty. Overall these new granular cortices, together, allowed anthropoids to adapt to new situations by learning quickly, including abstract rules, sometimes after a single event, and gave anthropoids advantages over their ancestors [16].

The capacity of differentiating not only the self from others, but also other features and characteristics from others, appeared during this new era of sociality. Neurons in the dorsomedial PFC and adjacent pre-supplementary motor areas (pre-SMA) have been shown to be important in distinguishing oneself from others in a group. The complexity of social interactions allows behavioral observation of others providing fictive actions, outcomes, and rewards, and the opportunity for the individual to learn directly from such events without being directly involved. The dorsomedial PFC encodes for such events, and a key node of the neurobiological substrate of social learning was in place [20]. In addition, gaze-specific cells, located in the superior temporal gyrus, and facial recognition enlarged in these anthropoids. Overall, these new granular areas in the prefrontal cortex and superior temporal cortex improved foraging efficiency during an epoch of increasingly unstable food availability (Figure 2.4).

Pyramidal cells in primate species with larger granular PFC were also more spinous compared to species with smaller granular PFC. As a comparison, human granular PFC pyramidal cells have been shown to be 70 percent more spinous than the macaque monkey, and threefold more spinous than the baboon and vervet monkey. The relatively recent and profound expansion of the granular PFC among primates had therefore developed both by additional neurons and also by more complex neurons that were more spinous. This allowed a dramatic escalation in branching complexity, particularly in the human

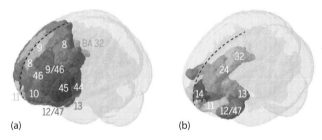

(a)   (b)

Figure 2.4 The frontal cortex evolved in a number of steps: pre-frontal cortex components. (a) Lateral view; (b) medial and ventral views.
From Carlen M. What constitutes the prefrontal cortex? *Science* 2017;358:478–482. Reprinted with permission from AAAS.

granular PFC, enabling more excitatory inputs compared to other primate species. These features enabled a sampling of increasing numbers of inputs and so more connectivity complexity. The inordinately branched, spinous neurons of the human granular PFC might be one of the factors contributing to human intelligence [21].

Development of the Retinal and Tactile Fovea in Primates

Tarsiers and anthropoid primates have a 0.7 mm fovea with about 250 000 cone-shaped photoreceptors per square millimeter, but no rod-shaped photoreceptors. In strepsirhines there is no fovea, but tiny rods are found in the central retina. Foveas did, however, evolve independently in vertebrates, fish, birds, and reptiles; cats developed a visual streak that resembles a fovea [22]. The haplorrhine fovea is unique among mammals and allowed for improved manipulation of objects and reaching under visual guidance [23]. This was later to be supplemented by routine trichromacy as opposed to the polymorphic trichromacy of platyrrhines with two and not three cone receptors. The majority of mammals, as well as strepsirhines, possess two cone receptors subserving short-wavelength light and one for long-wavelength light reception. The catarrhine gene long-wavelength cone receptor gene was duplicated, resulting in the three different kinds of cones. The haplorrhines ultimately developed trichromatic vision, with platyrrhines remaining with relatively poorer color vision and the least color vision among strepsirhines. Isbell hypothesized that trichromacy allowed for improved venomous snake detection [11].

The caudal (posteriorly placed) area of the PFC that includes the frontal eye field and BA 8 represented a new area in the frontal region among anthropoids. This region receives cutaneous inputs from a somatosensory receptor, the sensitive Meissner corpuscle, which is found in the epidermis of the fingertips. These respond to skin deformation and relay minor pressure differences in the finger tips that would have enabled assessment of ripeness of fruit by gauging the softness or hardness of the fruits. Highly sensitive receptors respond to skin deformation with a rapidly adapting response. This allows precision in the manipulation of objects and for discerning shape, weight and texture [24]. This has been termed *tactile fovea development*. Clinical neurological deficits seen in these capabilities include the cortical sensory syndromes such as agraphesthesia, astereognosis, abaragnosis, and two-point discrimination ability.

Diurnality and development of the fovea had occurred already in the haplorrhines (55 mya) after their split from the strepsirrhines. In addition, the orbital ridge behind the frontally oriented eyes had evolved, but with a decrease in the overall size of the orbit (nocturnality requires bigger eyes for maximum light perception). The visual cortex had reached maximal proportions as represented by *Aegyptopithecus* 33 mya, but the frontal lobes had not yet enlarged in the earlier anthropoids. Brain enlargement occurred with the split between platyrrhines (nostrils facing sideways, "flat nose" or the New World monkeys) and catarrhines (nostrils facing downward, "down nose" or the Old World monkeys) about 34 mya. Anthropoids also developed larger bodies (*Parapithecus* and *Aegyptopithecus* estimated weight of 6.4–8.5 lb or 3–4 kg), foraged over a much wider range, became more frugivorous than the previous omnivory of the earlier primates, and adopted arboreal quadruped locomotion on the larger branches within the arboreal environment. The high-energy fruit available to them, thanks to the angiosperm evolution, came with some caveats, with dispersion both in place and time. The act of foraging and coping with wider ranges also placed them under increased predation risk. Passingham and Wise portend that resource volatility in terms of widely fluctuating seasonality of fruits and young leaves was one of the major driving forces in the expansion of the anthropoid PFC with new granular cortices [16].

Primate evolution can only be understood in the context of climate and plate tectonics [25]. Progressive polar climate evolution and associated further global cooling steps took place during the Eocene (56–33.9 mya), Oligocene (33.9–23.0 mya), Miocene (23–5.3 mya), and Pliocene epochs (5.3–2.58 mya). The most proximate cause was the formation of the three principal expansions of the Antarctic ice sheet. Termed polar cryospheric expansion, these developed as follows:

- Middle Miocene: development of the East Antarctic ice sheet;
- Late Miocene: development of the West Antarctic ice sheet;
- Late Pliocene and Quaternary: development of the Northern Hemispheric ice sheets.

These, in turn, were due to plate tectonic movements with the circumpolar ocean circulation in the Southern Ocean that effectively isolated Antarctica from warmer equatorial waters, and the obliteration of the Tethys Ocean, with its equatorial circulation being replaced by the formation of a north-to-south interpolar ocean circulation [26].

While rafting to India, habituating on the Indo-Madagascar Garden of Eden, about 55 mya, the haplorrhines evolved their trichromatic vision and increased several PFC granular areas. The biogeography of subsequent primate and ape evolution is complex and spread over the three continents of Africa, Asia, and Europe. The often-confusing terminology is also worth revising:

- Primates: differentiated from mammals due to larger brains, opposable thumbs, and vision being the dominant sense; vision is stereoscopic and trichromatic among some primates;
- Anthropoids: New World and Old World monkeys;
- Hominoids or hominoidea: small apes (gibbons or hylobatids);
- Hominids or Hominidea: great apes, Asian (orangutans) and African (chimpanzees, gorillas);
- Hominins or hominini: modern humans and their extinct ancestors from *Sahelanthropus tchadensis*, australopithecines, *Homo ergaster*, *Homo heidelbergensis*, and *Homo neanderthalensis*;
- *Hominina*: *Homo sapiens*.

The catarrhine primates originated in Africa and Arabia and the subsequent ape-monkey divergence took place in Africa during the Oligocene at 34–25 mya. The earliest members of the stem hominoids, the proconsulids are abundant in the African Miocene fossil record. However, there is only fossil evidence of the crown hominids from the Late Miocene, Pliocene, and Pleistocene in Africa, without any evidence of hylobatids, pongines, or chimpanzee or gorilla ancestors from the African Miocene fossil record. Therefore, it has been presumed that it was in Eurasia that one or more of the stem hominoids diverged into hylobatids and pongines, and thereafter an early African ape dispersed back to Africa to give rise to chimpanzees, gorillas, and hominoids. This premise is supported by the large amounts of fossil hominids that stem from the Eurasian Middle and Late Miocene periods that are not only different to African Miocene apes but also appear to be part of the crown group [2].

David Begun's expertise in primates helps us understand that the earliest mammalian group that has been attributed to the order Primates are the Plesiadapiformes. There is a single lower molar tooth that has been attributed to *Purgatorius ceratops* that was found in a Late Cretaceous deposit. Apes evolved in Africa from *Aegyptopithecus*, dating to 33 mya, with many specimens found in the Fayum depression in modern-day Egypt. By about 20 mya, primitive apes, resembling monkeys more than apes, were prolific in Africa. Among these some had attributes that allowed them to explore Eurasian territories that were more seasonal. This important migration allowed ecological conditions in Eurasia to select for new ape attributes such as diet, behavior, and locomotion, with a subsequent split into the Asian pongines and European hominines. No fossils have been found for this period in Africa, while in Eurasia further developments occurred with increases in brain size and suspensory, locomotory adaptations of the hylobatids, for example. These larger-brained suspensory apes flourished until the progressive global cooling caught up with them and drove them back to equatorial regions in Africa and Southeast Asia, the latter evolving into orangutans and gibbons. The ancestors of the former included the African apes, with gorillas separating at 10 mya from the common chimp, human ancestor, and eventually humans [25].

The extensive faunal exchange between Europe and Africa could only occur after the Tethys Ocean retracted sufficiently during the Miocene by about 19–20 mya. The Tethys seaway closure occurred due to continental plate movement of Africa rotating counter-clockwise to the European plates, causing intermittent land route prospects between the two continents. Catarrhines were present on ancient Paratethys Sea shorelines in Asia by 18 mya and in Europe by 17 mya. With the plate collisions, orogeny (mountain building) ensued with new mountain ranges, including the Pyrenees, Alps, Dinaric, Taurus, and Zagros mountains all forming at a similar time. By about 13 mya there was restricted exchange between Eurasia and Africa, and by 15 mya, after their appearance in Europe, Gripopithecines appeared in Africa as far south as present-day Namibia (*Otavipithecus*). Extensive faunal migrations occurred between Eurasia and Africa during this time. However, by 13 mya the African fossil record became barren. Interestingly, at the same time there was a burgeoning of the fossil record in Eurasia that persisted until approximately 7 mya. The implication is that the crown hominid lineage developed in Eurasia. Further support comes from the Afrotheria, which refers to a clade of mammals of common ancestry, including elephants, tenrecs, hyraxes, aardvarks, and sea cows (Sirenians), with several extinct species that either originated in Africa or are currently living in Africa. This has been related to Africa's long isolation from other continents. Between 14–7 mya there are fossil sites in Africa that yielded abundant remains of forest-dwelling animals – yet not one contains great ape fossils [27]. Molecular evidence supports this cluster of endemic African mammals, the Afrotheria, emerging, but importantly this does not include primates, which therefore had to have evolved elsewhere [28].

The dryopithecines inhabited subtropical Europe 12–13 mya, discovered in 1856 by Edouard Lartet who recommended that *Dryopithecus* (oak forest ape) was a precursor to both African apes and humans. Another important European ape discovery was *Oreopithecus bambolii*, dating to 8 mya, whose fossils were found in coal deposits off the islands of Tuscany and Sardinia, which were swampy forests at the time. *Oreopithicus* had a short and broad pelvis, similar to the australopithecines that appeared very much later, and were bipedal but with a relatively small brain case. Another ape was *Nyanzapithecus alesi*, with several features in common with the enigmatic *Oreopithecus* from 8 mya in Italy. Oreopithecus is considered a close relative of modern apes and part of the human ancestral tree whose ability to walk upright evolved in parallel with that of the human ancestral lineage [29]. During the Late Miocene, Eurasia cooled with accompanying food shortages and Eurasian apes diminished and became extinct by 9 mya, and *Rudapithecus*, *Quranopithecus*, and *Dryopithecus* dispersed south to tropical Africa as the ancestors of the African apes and humans. *Sivapithecus* migrated to Asia, giving rise to the gibbons and orangutans. There is no evidence for any presence of hominines in Africa for the time hominines appeared and proliferated in Europe 12.5–9 mya. About two million years after they disappear from the European fossil record the hominins appear in Africa, now in hominin form, the human ancestors. This two million year gap remains a mystery. However, a possible explanation lies in the Danakil Island bipedality hypothesis advanced by La Lumiere and the aquatic ape hypothesis. The two million year hiatus prompted David Begun to comment that "One thing the record of Miocene apes does not reveal clearly is the reason for the origin of bipedalism, one of the first things to occur in human evolution" [25].

Archeological Insights: The Missing Link and the Late Miocene Fossil Silence

Although "missing link" may be an overused term, perhaps it should really refer to the link between hominoids and bipedal hominids in the time from 14 mya to 6 mya. There are currently no fossils from the time spanning this hominoid to hominid transition. There are also no fossils of African apes from that time period, although molecular dating places gorilla origins at ~8 mya and Asian apes (orangutans and gibbons) splitting from the African hominoids by 14 mya. As humans are closer to African apes compared to any other animal in the hominoid group, they most likely migrated from Eurasia, where hominoids were common at the time of the Late Miocene, yet still absent in Africa.

Obliteration of the Tethys Ocean and the Origins of Bipedalism

Bipedalism is a discerning trait of humans and pre-dated brain enlargement by millions of years. Its importance was perhaps best encapsulated by Montgomery: "Man's habitual and irrevocable bipedalism is unique in the mammal kingdom. Its uniqueness is possibly more strange and noteworthy than our extraordinary intelligence. Our intelligence is a matter of degree, bipedalism is absolute" [30]. Obligate bipedalism is rare among animals, pursued only by the extinct *Tyrannosaurus rex*, kangaroos, penguins, ostriches, gorillas, and hopping mice. There is mounting fossil, nutritional, and biogeographic evidence that bipedalism among hominoids occurred in the littoral setting. Wading engages bipedal walking among extant primates such as bonobo chimpanzees, gorillas in the Congo, and Okavango Swamp baboons [31]. Limited bipedality is also evident among gibbons, atelids, and sifakas. Conventional belief for many years was that East African drying and desiccation of the forest environment forced arboreal hominoids to become terrestrial – the so-called Savannah hypothesis, succinctly presented as the East Side Story [32]. This hypothesis has since been jettisoned, most notably by long-time supporter Phillip Tobias, revered researcher of australopithecines, who declared ruefully at a prominent lecture to the Royal College in London in 1995 that the Savannah hypothesis was dead [33,34].

Littoral zone evolution now seems much more likely, as detailed by Verhaegen, an avid proponent of the aquatic ape hypothesis, first presented by Hardy [35] and subsequently elaborated further by Morgan and Verhaegen [36,37]. Verhaegen developed his view and version, summarized as an aqua–arboreal, littoral, and wading phase of our evolution. In brief, the theory proposed is that our Miocene and Pliocene ape ancestors may have pursued an aqua–arboreal existence within swampy mangrove-type forests and wetlands, feeding on plants, hard-shelled foods, crustaceans, fish, and shellfish in littoral zones. Indian Ocean coastal regions would have been the most likely littoral zone for Pleistocene *Homo* ancestors. A subsequent wading phase is proposed in the later Pleistocene epoch with migration inland from the coast, presumably along the river valleys imbued with convenient gallery forest, associated with less diving, but with predominant wading activities assisted by an orthograde posture and longer legs. After the initial ocean habitat, then riverine occupation, subsequent lacustrine habitation in the East African Rift Valley is postulated, still pursuing shallow-water fish and riverine or lacustrine aquatic foods [38].

Without the need for mutations, Verhaegen's view presumes a sequence of events termed mosaic evolution, characterizing the transition from the ape to the human form. Primates are postulated to have evolved from a so-called above-branch pronograde (walking with the body parallel to the ground) arborealism during the Miocene/Pliocene epochs to an orthograde (upright, vertical) below-branch aqua-arborealism, and subsequently to archaic *Homo* species that partook in shallow diving within a littoral environment. Wading in shallow waters presumably favored bipedality developing in early *Homo* species. Walking and running was subsequently favored in the predominant land dwellers [39]. This is counter to the bipedal origin views of Bramble and Lieberman's Savannah hypothesis with human running on the plains occupying an endurance running niche and "born to run" concept [40]. Verhaegen contends that the aqua–arboreal hypothesis is a more parsimonious explanation, with savannah mammals far exceeding our relatively limited sprint speed of ~20 km/h. In his view, *Homo* locomotion most likely sequentially evolved from tree climbing to swimming to diving and wading and eventually walking and running.

Evidence of Miocene 21–16 mya fossil primates with orthograde posture with both arboreal and terrestrial abilities appeared in apes such as *Nacholapithecus* (orthograde climbing ability) and *Kenyapithecus*, with scansorial activities (adapted or specialized for climbing). The shift from quadrupedalism to bipedality may best be perceived as an initial quadruped ape that was part-arboreal, part-terrestrial quadruped, that engaged in bipedal wading after descending from gallery forests adjoining riverine, lacustrine, or marine environments. Bipedalism is likely to have evolved soon after our ancestral separation from the gorilla and chimpanzee clades [41]. Further support for bipedal evolution comes from the study of extant Atelids, who use their tails for suspension but have the features of lumbar lordosis and full extension of their hind limbs with upright stance. Their anatomy reveals the telltale reduction of iliac height and broad sacral alae, viewed as an early component of hominid bipedality. Both the tailless Proconsul and *Ekembo nyanzae* had broad alae. This supports some primitive Miocene hominoids as being in-between suspensory activity with extension ability as well as early bipedal capabilities [42].

Several researchers support the view that habitual terrestrial bipedality, together with arboreal hand-assisted bipedality seems kinetically more parsimonious [43]. Likewise, the aqua–arboreal (semi-arboreal, semi-aquatic) theory of Miocene hominoids descending from large branches into mangrove-like swamp forests appears similar to what Congo lowland gorillas and bonobo chimpanzees practice nowadays [44]. The vertical aqua-arborealism phase gains support from findings of broad thoraces, dorsal scapulae, tail loss, and more vertical spines of Miocene hominoids such as *Morotopithecus* and *Griphopithecus* 18 mya, which have lumbar vertebrae more similar to human lumbar vertebrae to support orthogrady [45]. Review of human lower limb features such as a wide pelvis (platypelloidy), flattened femurs (platymeria), and vertebral changes (platyspondyly) and generally heavy skeletons are not optimal features for running and are best explained by wading activity. Many other archaic hominoid fossil features such as platycephaly, platymeria, brain expansion, ear exostoses, pachyosteosclerotic bones (more suited to ballast control), protruding nose (mid-facial prognathism), wide bodies, and enlarged paranasal sinuses (perhaps for buoyancy) support shallow littoral diving and wading rather than a cursorial lifestyle. There is also a craniocaudal subcutaneous fatty tissue arrangement in humans for thermoregulatory exchange in the upper part of the body and insulation of the abdomen and lower limbs that may have evolved for thermoregulation while wading [46]. Bipedalism antedated australopithecines fossils discovered from ~3.5 mya onwards, all found in water-based environments but with dental and cranial support of a predominantly vegetarian diet. Evolutionary stasis of Australopithecines, with their relatively small brain size of 400–500 cc, has been attributed to their land-based diet. Meat eating is presumed to have evolved 1–2 million years later, but the partially arboreal australopithecines were not suited to compete with larger carnivores (felines, canid, hyaenid) on the savannah. They also were not suited physiologically, without sun-reflective fur, with a subcutaneous fat layer about tenfold thicker than extant chimpanzees, and their sweat gland method of cooling being more wasteful of water and sodium, as well with low urine concentration competence, none of which are traits suited to the challenging hot savannah habitat [39]. Marine aquatic animals, as well as human infants, feature reniculated kidneys, characterized by multipyramidal medullas and adaptation for avoiding saline water dehydration by facilitating first the concentration and then the excretion of urinary salts, which recedes in childhood [47].

The most likely site of this phase of evolution was within the early Mediterranean and/or the Indian Ocean continental shelves and coastal littoral associated with prolific shellfish and fish (Figure 2.5). Further support comes from the findings of numerous archaic *Homo* species discovered in the adjoining Turkana Basin (East Africa) and marine stingray evidence deposits, also in the last two million years, implying that the Turkana Basin was connected to the Indian Ocean [48]. Pachyosteosclerosis (POS) bones help with buoyancy control and are seen in semi-aquatic animals, and are also a feature in early *Homo* species, such as *Homo erectus*, suggesting this species dined on sessile foods in the littoral zone [49].

Paleo-Climatological Support for Bipedality

During the Late Miocene period of 7–11 mya, termed the Tortonian stage, aridification of North Africa and formation of the Sahara Desert occurred, with shrinking of the Tethys Sea and a weakened African summer monsoon, through orbital forcing (Milankovitch cycles). These predications were formulated through climate model simulations by Zhang

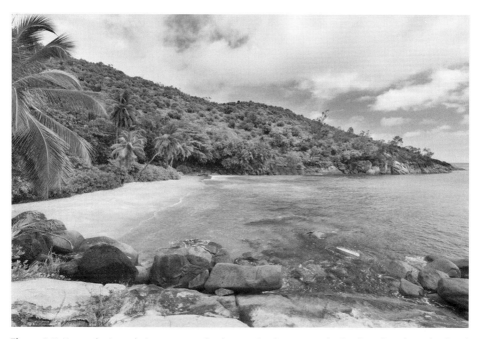

Figure 2.5 Human brain evolution: a new wetlands scenario – humans evolved in the rich ecological niche of the land–water interface. Image: IndustryAndTravel/Shutterstock

et al. and these climatic events caused major African and Asian plant and animal fluxes that included the early hominins in North and East Africa [50].

Geophysical Support for Bipedality

Tectonic plate movement was also relevant, with the most plausible scenario for the evolution of human bipedalism to me, suggested by La Lumiere. He postulated a scenario whereby the complex tectonic plate movements in the tri-plate Afar region, comprising three converging crustal blocks, resulted in a geographic island around 14–9 mya – the Danakil Horst/Alps in the southern Red Sea during the later Miocene period. From ~7 mya, a marine basin was established until 70 kya, with sea flooding into Afar that has never left, instead having evaporated, with the northern part remaining as the Dead Sea in Israel and the eastern end, the Danakil Alps, previously the Danakil Island. Rather than being viewed as a geographic island, it was more appropriately seen as a biological island with regard to the animals caught up in the tectonic plate turmoil. This remains speculation, and the "biological island" may not have been Danakil Island specifically, but any other near shore island within the north-eastern part triplate area, during the Late Miocene period. Perhaps a group of ancestral hominoids stranded on such an island, encircled by ample littoral zones for about two million years, was the appropriate scenario for bipedalism and later surging brain growth (Figure 2.6) [51–53].

Geographic speciation due to geographic separation of this kind provides ideal conditions for rapid evolutionary change, with more rapid change corresponding to more absolute isolation. Support for such mercurial change comes from studies of fish speciation

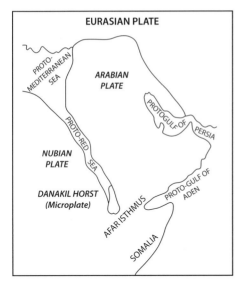
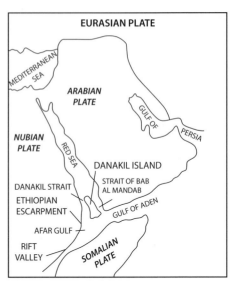

Figure 2.6 Danakil Island and Danakil Alps during the Late Miocene (left) and Early Pliocene (right). The Afar isthmus land bridge that allowed animals to traverse between Africa and Arabia and the Danakil horst (540 km × 75 km wide) are both important aspects of the theory.

Source: La Lumiere LP. Evolution of human bipedalism: a hypothesis about where it happened. *Phil Trans R Soc Lond B* 1981;292:103–107. Reproduced with permission of the Royal Society (Great Britain); permission conveyed through Copyright Clearance Center, Inc.

in isolated small bodies of water that have been recorded to occur ~1000 times faster than in the open ocean [54]. This theory gains support for a very similar scenario for *Oreopithecus bambolii* on the islands of Tuscany and Sardinia, adjacent to modern-day Italy. Notably, *Australopithecus afarenesis* or Lucy, dated to 3.2 mya, was subsequently found in the Afar region of north-east Africa by Donald Johanson in 1976 [55]. No other previously proposed theories of bipedalism explicate this unique human attribute. The many theories of bipedality proposed over the years remain unsubstantiated. Examples include the following hypotheses:

- watching out hypothesis;
- freeing of hands hypothesis;
- throwing hypothesis;
- infant crying hypothesis;
- reaching for food hypothesis;
- carrying of food or provisioning hypothesis;
- display hypothesis;
- orthograde scrambling hypothesis;
- scavenger hypothesis;
- thermoregulation hypothesis.

In summary, a number of features have been proposed in support of the aqua–arboreal bipedalism hypothesis by the proponents, with variable degrees of substantiation (Table 2.1).

Table 2.1

Musculoskeletal and craniofacial	• Upright posture attributed to shallow-water foraging; longs legs and straightened body facilitated diving. • Endurance running is regarded as a more recent adaptation, with foot arch development and short toes. • Eccrine sweat glands have the highest concentration in the upper body so generally presumed not submerged. • Paranasal sinuses facilitated buoyancy for floating the head. • Downwardly directed nostrils helped avoid inhalation of splattering water. • Philtrum of the upper lip enabled sealing off nostrils during submersion or diving.
Physiological	• Diving reflex with bradycardia and peripheral vasoconstriction. • Multipyramidal kidneys excrete salt from sea water. • Sweat and tears excrete salt from sea water.
Skin, hair, and fat	• Hair loss due to it being superfluous in water, with most aquatic mammals being hairless due to drag effects. • Extensive subcutaneous fat layer ~10 times that of chimpanzees for buoyancy, conserving heat, and streamlining.
Metabolic	• Sweat removes excess salt. • High output of salt and water in sweat and tears. • Immersion diuresis removes salt. • Enhanced diving reflexes including bradycardia during dives, peripheral vasoconstriction. • Voluntary breath holding, descended larynx that subsequently became adapted for speech.
Infant data	• Infants display natural swimming ability prior to crawling or walking capability. • Infant floating reflex (at 4–12 months) displayed by rolling onto their back for breathing and flotation. • The infant diving reflex with breath holding, eyes open, rhythmic arm/leg movements for propulsion.

Source: [47,56–62].

Supportive Data

Molecular Virology and Ancient Metabolic Attributes

Molecular Clock Data

The infectious type C retrovirus that previously havocked primates remains endogenous in baboons, as well as all African monkeys and apes, but is no longer deleterious to them. However, it is not present in humans, gibbons, and orangutans, nor anywhere else. Hence an Asian origin of humans was postulated by Todaro. Old World monkeys, apes, and humans possess particular gene sequences, termed virogenes, as part of their normal cellular DNA. Some of these virogenes are related to the RNA of a virus that was isolated from baboons. Viral gene comparison sequences can distinguish Old World monkeys and apes of African origin from those evolved in Asia. Only gorillas and chimpanzees are African by these criteria. Gibbons, orangutans, and man are identified as Asian. This supports the premise that a large part of early human evolution occurred outside Africa [63].

Biochemical Insights

Elevated uric acid levels often present with gout, which is increasing in frequency together with the rising epidemic of hypertension, diabetes, cardiovascular disease, obesity, metabolic disease, and chronic kidney disease. Uric acid has antioxidant, neurostimulatory, immune activation effects as well as pro-inflammatory actions. Evolutionary insights help us understand these functions in relation to its role in instigating foraging in response to starvation and its intricate association with fructose and vitamin C in this regard. Both fructose and uric acid promote the foraging response, while vitamin C counteracts this activity response. Uric acid is degraded by uricase, an enzyme that was gradually decreased and eventually silenced by mutations 15–9 mya, during the Miocene period, when the prolific ape species was profoundly diminished by climate- or bolide (asteroid)-related events. The uricase mutation may have promoted survival through its effect of sodium preservation, blood pressure maintenance, and foraging stimulation [64] during this Miocene crisis period with food scarcity [65].

Uric acid, rather than being a consequence or secondary feature, may have a causal role in the development of the metabolic syndrome, non-alcoholic fatty liver disease, hyperinsulinemia, diabetes, and obesity as elevated uric acid levels usually precede these syndromes [66–69]. Fructose ingestion (corn syrup, refined sugars) has a close relationship to the metabolic syndrome obesity epidemic [70,71], and leads to elevated blood pressure, fatty liver, and triglycerides elevation in humans [72,73], as well as raising serum uric acid. Phosphorylated by fructokinase, fructose is not regulated by ATP depletion as occurs with glucose. A consequence is that local ATP depletion ensues with resultant cell ischemia and the generation of uric acid levels that rise promptly within minutes. Through evolutionary mechanisms, uric acid level increases in the context of fasting, which promotes fat storage, weight gain and the metabolic syndrome. Humans lack a key enzyme in vitamin C synthesis following genetic mutations of the gene L-gulono-lactone oxidase, estimated to have occurred 20–40 mya. This may be the reason why the uricase mutation, with increased uric acid, emerged as the antioxidant replacement to counter the decrease in vitamin C availability during the Miocene crisis [74]. The foraging stimulation provided by elevated uric acid levels may have promoted survival as well as a move from quadrupedalism to bipedalism in the process of wider foraging ranges due to the climactic aridity, dwindling forests, and habitat opening up 15 and 5.2 mya [75]. Both the uricase and ascorbate mutations thus played significant roles in human evolution and perhaps bipedality [76].

Nutritional and Dietary Factors

Darwin made an important prediction in this regard, stating that together with natural selection, conditions of existence are the two forces of evolution. He termed conditions of existence as "pangenes" and regarded them as the more significant of the two factors [77]. Since his deliberations, more have been discovered in the form of reverse transcriptases and the science of epigenetics. Crawford and Marsh since proposed that although variability occurs in both genetics and chemistry, the chemical variation is the more impactful factor. Nutrition is able to induce change in both form and genetics. Differing nutritional principles are implicated, with body component growth on the one hand and brain growth on the other. Once a dietary or food choice and associated behavior become established, DNA is also altered and evolution escalates. Oxidative metabolism eventually appeared about 600 mya, and since then animal neural and visual systems evolved in a docosahexaenoic acid (DHA) abundant environment enabled by oxidative metabolism. DHA has a 600 million year history, which in itself is cogent evidence for its criticality. DHA is an integral component of cell membranes, cell signaling, synapses, neural receptor domains and gene expression, the latter of which also confer protection from oxidative stress within the brain. Of all the fatty acids, DHA is the most biosynthetically restricted of the brain-selective fatty acids as it must be acquired in a preformed state for optimal nutritional value. This is especially important during reproduction, pregnancy, lactation, and infant brain development. Despite its profound importance, DHA acquisition is suboptimal in the terrestrial food chain, with the richest sources being the marine food chain. The fact that DHA has been part of our neural building blocks and circuitry for the last 600 million years, without any change, which is an extraordinary conservation, prompted Michael Crawford to reflect that "DHA was actually dictating to DNA rather than the more conventional view of evolution occurring the other way around" [78].

Specific seafood nutrients are among the most powerful ingredients capable of expanding the mammalian neural systems. Apes under duress of climate and geological changes happened to exploit seashore food chains, and could have become engaged in a multiplicative positive feedback phase. Adding to the support for DHA, arachidonic acid (AA) and eicosapentanoic acid (EPA) are also fundamental and critical PUFAs required for boosting brain growth. None of these can be acquired in sufficient numbers on the savannah. Brain-selective nutrients other than DHA, EPA, and AA include iodine, iron, copper, selenium, and zinc. These are also found in abundance in marine and freshwater shellfish, crustaceans, and fish, more so than in any other habitat. Higher-quality diets that supply copious amounts of protein and energy but not more brain-selective nutrients would not have sufficed to support human brain expansion and evolution [79].

Mammalian marine evolution that occurred from ~50 mya yielded unlimited DHA, with the consequence of a markedly higher brain to body weight ratio compared to large terrestrial mammals. The dolphin (*Tursiops truncates*), for example, has a 1800 g brain in comparison to the land-based zebra (*Equus quagga*) brain weighing a mere 350 g, despite similar overall body weights. The terrestrial mammals that evolved larger bodies on the basis of high protein intakes nevertheless outstripped the ability to secure adequate DHA for adequate brain growth. As both DHA and AA are required for optimal brain function, the marine food web does have some constraints on brain development. A solution is provided by the littoral ecosystem, with abundant access to both DHA and AA [80].

The overpowering nutritional and dietary implications for the aqua–arboreal, littoral evolutionary locality, particularly from DHA and the five key brain-essential nutrients, led Phillip Tobias to declare in 1995 that the Savannah hypothesis was dead, as noted earlier. It has been established now that the genome is exquisitely responsive to the environment, much more than previously thought. Not all transmissible variation is dictated by genetic differences; rather, evolution is multidimensional. The four-dimensional model of genetic, epigenetic, behavioral, and symbol-based evolution proposed by Jablonka and Lamb can each contribute variations by which natural selection may act. It is now appreciated that non-DNA-based transmitted variations play major roles [81]. Additional dimensions may be relevant and include solar radiation, magnetic inversions, and astrophysical and geological factors.

The Wetland Durophage League

The otter, a semi-aquatic mammal, provides some clues to human evolution. Extant carnivores that include mammals such as otters, marsh mongoose, and crab-eating raccoons are representative of the so-called durophagy ecotone (durophagy = hard-shelled food object consumption; ecotone = transition area between two biomes, water and land) as well as species similar to the Australopithecine called *Paranthropus robustus* (2.0–1.2 mya). Robust australopithecines, too, were opportunistic patrons of hard-shelled foods in littoral zones. Fossil *Aonyx* and *Atilax* otters have also been discovered at the same sites where robust australopithecines have been excavated in the South African Swartkrans sites and East African Olduvai sites. Both featured "robust" skulls that characterize animals feeding on hard objects – durophagy at the land–water interface. Consuming such high-value foods as mollusks, crabs, and eggs is permitted in these biomes [82].

The Pinniped Brain and Human Brain Evolution

A review of the current literature gives the distinct impression of a chimpanzee-centric view of evolution, with the last common ancestor similar to an extant chimpanzee. However, a significant point of departure is the perhaps more enduring aquatic phase of our evolution. Current-day bonobo chimpanzees still practice some degree of wading and collection of aquatic foods. Pinnipeds are semi-aquatic animals, numbering about 30 species including gray and harbor seals (Phocidae), walruses (Odobenidae), and Otariidae (Cape fur seals, California sea lions) that have several brain capabilities that far exceed those of chimpanzees. These include much more vocal flexibility, rhythmic ability, and vocal production learning. Harbor seals have been recorded imitating both human words as well as phrases [83]. Their vocal production learning capabilities stem from their relatively unique habitat and social organization, rendering them candidates for musicality and elementary speech production. The core brain processes that allow such abilities include a number of anatomical and brain circuitry features. These include, for example, imitation behavior, the pinniped vocal anatomy in terms of larynx and upper vocal tract air flow being similar to that in humans, and their ability to process both speech and music, the latter entrained in subcortical structures that are involved in rhythm perception and production. Perhaps most importantly, pinniped working memory, covering both visual and auditory working memory, is particularly advanced. Auditory working memory is critical for speech and language, and pinniped auditory working memory exceeds that of non-human primates [84]. These findings imply that the pinniped brain would be a more appropriate comparative, extant model to study some of the unique human features such as speech, vocal learning, and rhythm production (allowing flexibility in vocalization), than primates [85].

The fundamentals of a brain and body bauplan that our primate lineage endowed us with include the following:

Brain anatomy
- multicomponent granular prefrontal cortex (Figure 2.7);
- expanded visual cortex and trichromatic vision.

Brain circuitry
- frontoparietal, further integration of sensorimotor systems;
- mirror neuron system.

Skeletal
- cranial size increase to ~450 cc;
- bipedalism.

Diet and metabolism
- frugivorous diet;
- fall-back foods – tubers;
- marine, riparian, lacustrine, riverine aquatic diet.

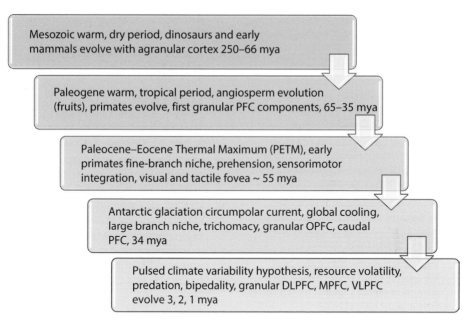

Figure 2.7 Mammal and primate cortex and frontal cortex evolution: expansion of the six-layer mammalian cortex and granular layer four and initiating events.

References

1. Rose KD. *Beginning of the Origin of Mammals.* Johns Hopkins University Press, Baltimore, MD, 2006.

2. Fleagle JG. *Primate Adaptation and Evolution*, 3rd edn. Academic Press, Amsterdam, 2013.

3. Elston GN. Pyramidal cells of the frontal lobe: all the more spinous to think with. *J Neurosci*, 2000;20:1–4.

4. Churchland PS, Sejnowski TJ. *The Computational Brain.* MIT Press, Cambridge, MA, 1992.

5. Mackay S, Petrides M. Quantitative demonstration of comparable architectonic areas within the ventromedial and lateral orbital frontal cortex in the human and the macaque monkey brains. *Eur J Neurosci* 2010;32:1940–1950.

6. Estruch R, Ros E, Salas-Salvadó J, et al. Primary prevention of cardiovascular disease with a Mediterranean diet. *N Engl J Med*. 2013;368:1279–1290.

7. Hankey G. Role of nutrition in the risk and burden of stroke. *Stroke* 2017;48: 3168–3174.

8. Dal Zilio L, van Dinther Y, Gerya TV, Pranger CC. Seismic behavior of mountain belts controlled by plate convergence rate. *Earth Planet Sci Lett* 2018;482:81–92.

9. Fleagle JG. Identifying primate species. *Evol Anthropol* 2014;23(1):1.

10. Seiffert ER. Revised age estimates for the later Paleogene mammal faunas of Egypt and Oman. *Proc Natl Acad Sci USA* 2006;103(13):5000–5005.

11. Isbell LA. *The Fruit, the Tree and the Serpent.* Harvard University Press, Cambridge, MA, 2009.

12. Martin RD. Combing the primate record. *Nature* 2003;422:390–391.

13. Seyfarth RM, Cheney DL. The evolution of language from social cognition. *Curr Opin Neurobiol* 2014;28:5–9.

14. Bradley RS. *Paleoclimatology. Reconstructing Climates of the Quaternary*, 3rd edn. Elsevier, Amsterdam, 2015.

15. Stow D. *Vanished Ocean: How Tethys Reshaped the World.* Oxford University Press, Oxford, 2010.

16. Passingham RE, Wise SP. *The Neurobiology of the Prefrontal Cortex.* Oxford University Press, Oxford, 2012.

17. Schultz S, Nelson E, Dunbar RIM. Hominin cognitive evolution: identifying patterns and processes in the fossil and archaeological record. *Phil Trans R Soc B* 2012;367:2130–2140.

18. Kuhlbrodt T, Griesel A, Montoya M, et al. On the driving processes of the Atlantic meridional overturning circulation. *Rev Geophys* 2007;45:RG2001.

19. Raymo ME, Ruddimen WF, Froelich PN. Influence of the Late Cenozoic mountain building on ocean geochemical cycles. *Geology* 1988;16:649–653.

20. Yoshida K, Saito N, Iriki A, Isoda M. Representation of others' action by neurons in monkey medial frontal cortex. *Curr Biol* 2011;21:249–253.

21. Elston GN, Benavides-Piccione R, Elston A, et al. Specializations of the granular prefrontal cortex of primates: implications for cognitive processing. *Anat Record A Discov Mol Cell Evol Biol* 2009;288A:26–35.

22. Hughes A. The topography of vision in mammals of contrasting life style: comparative optics and retinal organization. In: Crescitelli F (ed.), *The Visual System of Vertebrates*, Springer, New York, 1977.

23. Ross CF. The tarsier fovea, functionless vestige or nocturnal adaptation? In: Ross CF, Kay RF, *Anthropoid Origins.* Kluwer Academic/Plenum, New York, 2004.

24. Hoffmann JN, Montag AG, Dominy NJ. Meisser corpuscles and somatosensory acuity: the prehensile appendages of primates and elephants. *Anat Record A Discov Mol Cell Evol Biol* 2004;281:1138–1147.

25. Begun D. *The Real Planet of the Apes.* Princeton University Press, Princeton, NJ, 2016.

26. Vrba ES, Denton GH, Partridge TC, Buckle LH. *Paleoclimate and Evolution with Emphasis on Human Origins.* Yale University Press, New Haven, CT, 1995.

27. Nishihara H, Satta Y, Nikaido M et al. A retroposon analysis of Afrotherian phylogeny. *Mol Biol Evol* 2005;22:1823–1833.

28. Jones JH. Primates and the evolution of long, slow life histories *Curr Biol* 2011;21:R708–R717.

29. Nengo I, Trafforeau P, Gilbert CC, et al. New infant cranium from the African Miocene sheds light on ape evolution. *Nature* 2017;548:169–174.

30. Montgomery D. *Seashore Man and African Eve. An Exploration of Evolution in Africa,* 2nd edn. Lulu, Raleigh, NC, 2008.

31. Johnson SE. Life history and the competitive environment: trajectories of growth, maturation and reproductive output among chacma baboons. *Am J Phys Anthropol* 2003;120(1):83–98.

32. Coppens Y. East Side Story: the origin of humankind. *Scientific American* 1994;May:88–95.

33. Tobias PV. The Daryll Ford Memorial Lecture. University College London, Department of Anthropology, November 4, 1995.

34. Tobias PV. Revisiting water and hominin evolution. In: Vaneechoutte M, Kuliukas A, Verhaegen M (eds.), *Was Man More Aquatic in the Past? Fifty Years after Alister Hardy.* Bentham Science Publications, eBook, 2011.

35. Hardy A. Was man more aquatic in the past? *New Scientist* 1960;March 17:642–645.

36. Morgan E, Verhaegen M. In the beginning was the water. *New Scientist,* 1986;1498:62–63.

37. Morgan E. *The Scars of Evolution.* Souveni, London, 1990.

38. Verhaegen M. The aquatic ape evolves: common misconceptions and unproven assumptions about the so-called aquatic ape hypothesis. *Hum Evol* 2013;28:237–266.

39. Verhaegen M. Origin of hominid bipedalism. *Nature* 1987;325:305–306.

40. Bramble DM, Lieberman DE. Endurance running and the evolution of *Homo. Nature* 2004;432:345–352.

41. Niemitz C. The evolution of the upright posture and gait: a review and a new synthesis. *Naturwissenschaften* 2010;97:241–263.

42. Machnicki AL, Spurlock LB, Strier LB, et al. First steps of bipedality in hominids: evidence from the atelid and proconsulid pelvis. *Peer J* 2016. doi: 10.7717/peerj.1521.

43. Crompton RH, Vereecke EE, Thorpe SKS. Locomotion and posture from the common hominoid ancestor to fully modern hominins, with special reference to the last common panin/hominin ancestor. *J Anat* 2008;212:501–543.

44. Doran DM, McNeilage A, Greer D, et al. Western lowland gorilla diet and resource availability: new evidence, cross-site comparisons, and reflections on indirect sampling methods. *Am J Primatol* 2002;58:91–116.

45. MacLatchy L, Gebo D, Kityo R, Pilbeam D. Postcranial functional morphology of *Morotopithecus bishop*, with implications for the evolution of modern ape locomotion. *J Hum Evol* 2000;39:159–183.

46. Preuschoft H. Mechanisms for the acquisition of habitual bipedality: are there biomechanical reasons for the acquisition of upright bipedal posture? *Anat* 2004;204(5):363–384.

47. Williams MF. Morphological evidence of marine adaptations in human kidneys. *Medical Hypotheses* 2006;66:247–257.

48. Joordens JC, Dupont-Nivet G, Feibel G, et al. Improved age control on early *Homo* fossils from the Upper Burgi Member at Koobi Fora, Kenya. *J Hum Evol* 2013;65(6):731–745.

49. Verhaegen M, Munro S. Pachyosteosclerosis suggests archaic *Homo* frequently collected sessile littoral foods. *Homo* 2011;62:237–247.

50. Zhang Z, Ramstein G, Schuster M, et al. Aridification of the Sahara Desert caused by Tethys Sea shrinkage during the late Miocene. *Nature*. 2014;513(7518):401–404.

51. La Lumiere LP. Evolution of human bipedalism: a hypothesis about where it happened. *Phil Trans R Soc Lond B* 1981;292:103–107.

52. Mohr P. *Mapping of the Major Structures of the African Rift System.* Smithsonian Institution, Cambridge, MA, 1974.

53. Mohr P. AFAR. *Annu Rev Earth Planet Sci* 1978;6:145–172.

54. Mayr E, O'Hara RJ. The biogeographic evidence supporting the Pleistocene forest refuge hypothesis. *Evolution* 1986;40(1):55–67.

55. Johanson DC, Taieb M. Plio-Pleistocene hominid discoveries in Hadar, Ethiopia. *Nature* 1976;260(5549):293–297.

56. Farke AA. Evolution and functional morphology of the frontal sinuses in Bovidae (Mammalia: Artiodactyla), and implications for the evolution of cranial pneumaticity. *Zool J Linn Soc* 2010;159:988–1014.

57. Langdon JH. Umbrella hypotheses and parsimony in human evolution: a critique of the aquatic ape hypothesis. *J Hum Evol* 1997;33:479–494.

58. Reed KE. Early hominid evolution and ecological change through the African Plio-Pleistocene. *J Hum Evol*, 1997;32:289–322.

59. Schagatay E. Human breath-hold diving ability suggests a selective pressure for diving during human evolution. In: Vaneechoutte M, Kuliukas A, Verhaegen M (eds.), *Was Man More Aquatic in the Past? Fifty Years after Alister Hardy.* Bentham Science Publications, eBook, 2011.

60. Verhaegen M, Puech PF. Hominid lifestyle and diet reconsidered: paleo-environmental and comparative data. *Hum Evol*, 2000;15:175–186.

61. Verhaegen M, Puech PF, Munro S. Aquarboreal ancestors? *Trends Ecol Evol*, 2002;17:212–217.

62. Will M, Parkington JE, Kandel AW, Conard NJ. Coastal adaptations and the Middle Stone Age lithic assemblages from Hoedjiespunt 1 in the Western Cape, South Africa. *J Hum Evol*, 2013;64:518–537.

63. Benveniste RE, Todaro GJ. Evolution of type C viral genes: evidence for an Asian origin of man. *Nature* 1976;261:101–108.

64. Watanabe S, Kang DH, Feng L, et al. Uric acid, hominoid evolution, and the pathogenesis of salt-sensitivity. *Hypertension* 2002;40:355–360.

65. Eaton SB, Konner M. Paleolithic nutrition: a consideration of its nature and current implications. *N Engl J Med* 1985;312:283–289.

66. Dehghan A, van Hoek M, Sijbrands EJ, Hofman A, Witteman JC. High serum uric acid as a novel risk factor for type 2 diabetes mellitus. *Diabetes Care* 2007;31:361–362.

67. Boyko EJ, de Courten M, Zimmet PZ, et al. Features of the metabolic syndrome predict higher risk of diabetes and impaired glucose tolerance: a prospective study in Mauritius. *Diabetes Care* 2000;23:1242–1248.

68. Carnethon MR, Fortmann SP, Palaniappan L, et al. Risk factors for progression to incident hyperinsulinemia: the atherosclerosis risk in communities study, 1987–1998. *Am J Epidemiol* 2003;158:1058–1067.

69. Masuo K, Kawaguchi H, Mikami H, Ogihara T, Tuck ML. Serum uric acid and plasma norepinephrine concentrations predict subsequent weight gain and blood pressure elevation. *Hypertension* 2003;42:474–480.

70. Havel PJ. Dietary fructose: implications for dysregulation of energy homeostasis and lipid/carbohydrate metabolism. *Nutr Rev* 2005;63:133–157.

71. Bray GA, Nielsen SJ, Popkin BM. Consumption of high-fructose corn syrup in beverages may play a role in the epidemic of obesity. *Am J Clin Nutr* 2004;79:537–543.

72. Brown CM, Dulloo AG, Yepuri G, Montani JP. Fructose ingestion acutely elevates blood pressure in healthy young humans. *Am J Physiol* 2008;294:R730–737.

73. Ouyang X, Cirillo P, Sautin Y, et al. Fructose consumption as a risk factor for non-alcoholic fatty liver disease. *J Hepatol* 2008;48:993–999.

74. Ames BN, Cathcart R, Schwiers E, Hochstein P. Uric acid provides an antioxidant defense in humans against oxidant- and radical-caused aging and cancer: a hypothesis. *Proc Natl Acad Sci USA* 1981;78:6858–6862.

75. Pickford M. Palaeoenvironments and hominoid evolution. *Z Morphol Anthropol* 2002;83:337–348.

76. Johnson R, Sautin YY, Oliver WJ, et al. Lessons from comparative physiology: could uric acid represent a physiologic alarm signal gone awry in Western society? *J Comp Physiol B* 2009;179(1):67–76.

77. Darwin, C. *The Variation of Animals and Plants under Domestication*, John Murray, London, 1868.

78. Crawford MA, Broadhurst CL, Guest M, et al. A quantum theory for the irreplaceable role of docosahexanoic acid in neural signaling throughout evolution. *Prostaglandins Leukot Essent Fatty Acids* 2013;88:5–13.

79. Cunnane SC Stewart KM (eds.). *Human Brain Evolution: The Influence of Freshwater and Marine Food Resources.* Wiley-Blackwell Hoboken, NJ, 2010.

80. Crawford MA. Long chain polyunsaturated fatty acids in human brain evolution. In: Cunnane SC, Stewart KM (eds.), *Human Brain Evolution: The Influence of Freshwater and Marine Food Resources.* Wiley-Blackwell, Hoboken, NJ, 2010.

81. Jablonka E, Lamb MJ. Précis of evolution in four dimensions. *Behav Brain Sci* 2007;30(4):353–365.

82. Shabel AB. Brain size in carnivoran mammals that forage at the land–water ecotone with implications for robust australopithecine paleobiology. In: Cunnane SC, Stewart KM (eds.), *Human Brain Evolution: The Influence of Freshwater and Marine Food Resources.* Wiley-Blackwell, Hoboken, NJ, 2010.

83. Ralls K, Fiorelli P, Gish S. Vocalizations and vocal mimicry in captive harbor seals *Phoca vitulina. Can J Zool* 1985;63:1050–1056.

84. Scott BH, Mishkin M, Yin P. Monkeys have a limited form of short term memory in audition. *Proc Natl Acad Sci USA* 2012;109:12237–12241.

85. Ravignani A, Fitch WT, Hanke FD, et al. What pinnipeds have to say about human speech, music and the evolution of rhythm. *Front Neurosci* 2016;10:1–9.

Exponential White Matter Growth and Major Fiber Tract Systems Assembly

Even more profound than the brain size and gray matter increase is the remarkable surge in white matter fiber tract proliferation in the human lineage. During this phase, the major fiber tracts we measure and monitor today were formed. Specific examples include the extensive frontopontocerebellar (bipedality), frontoparietal (working memory) circuitry among mammals and Miocene apes, the mirror neuron tracts (copying actions, imitations, praxis), and the uncinate fasciculus (sociality, empathy). In addition, circuit modulators, the ascending neurotransmitter circuits, became repurposed. Eventually some of these circuits became exapted further into the so-called acquired cultural circuits.

The burgeoning brain size increases during human evolution included not only regional brain size increases, but also an even more impressive evolution of the cortical networks. In particular, the prefrontal cortex connectivity with respect to other brain regions may be viewed as a major driver of the human mind and cognition [1]. The hallmark of the human brain and frontal function and dysfunction is the human connectome. The average human brain contains $\sim 2 \times 10^{11}$ neurons, $\sim 1 \times 10^{12}$ glial cells, and 400 miles (700 km) of blood vessels. Perhaps the most striking vital statistic is the $\sim 100\,000$ miles (160 000 km) of axons (nerve fibers) comprising the neuropil. A most remarkable and defining feature of the human brain in comparison to the primate brain is the dramatic escalation in the neuropil (interwoven dendrites, axons, glial cells) and consequently connectivity in and at a microscopic level in association with granular cortical areas [2,3].

Frontal Lobe White Matter Tracts and Connectivity

The progressive increase in brain size is principally due to burgeoning frontal lobe white matter tracts and their connectivity. Volumetric data of white and gray matter frontal and non-frontal lobes determined in 18 anthropoid species concluded that a hyperscaling of neocortex and frontal lobe compared to the rest of the brain can be ascribed principally to frontal white matter. In addition, changes in frontal (but not non-frontal) white matter volume impact changes in other parts of the brain, such as subcortical structures like the basal ganglia, that are integral to executive control. These observations imply a central role for frontal lobe white matter and its hyperscaling with respect to brain size and upgraded neural structural connectivity in anthropoids. The hyperscaling of the frontal lobes with respect to the rest of the brain appears to be largely the effect of white matter; the volume of frontal white matter imparts 33.8 percent of the variation in size with respect to the rest of the brain. Volume changes in non-frontal

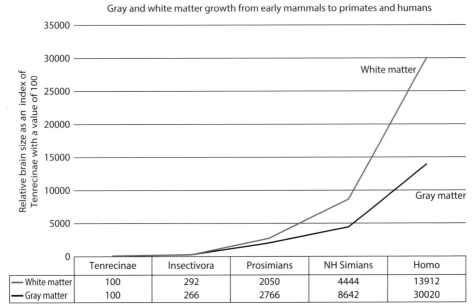

Gray and white matter growth from early mammals to primates and humans

	Tenrecinae	Insectivora	Prosimians	NH Simians	Homo
White matter	100	292	2050	4444	13912
Gray matter	100	266	2766	8642	30020

Early mammals to humans

Figure 3.1 The profound allometric volume increase of white matter proliferation in *Homo sapiens* compared to primates and mammals. Comparison in the figure is made to primates, non-human simians, prosimians, Insectivora and the stem mammals here represented by the extant Tenrecinae, the Madagascar hedgehog. The Tenrecinae are regarded as representing stem Insectivora with relatively primitive brain morphology. The size of the various brain components is referred to the Tenrecinae base of 100 on the y-axis.

Source: Figure compiled from the data of Stephan H, Baron G, Frahm H. *Comparative Brain Research in Mammals, vol. 1, Insectivora,* Springer, New York, 1991.

white matter, in comparison, are able to explain a mere 6.9 percent after controlling for frontal lobe size. From primate and human studies, it can be deduced that frontal white matter is the primary component contributing to increased brain size, with an observed hyperscaling of 4:3 white to gray matter of the frontal lobe versus non-frontal lobe. Hence, the frontal lobe hyperscales with respect to the rest of the brain [4]. The profound white matter connectivity expansion was already evident when examining progression indices. A progression index is a method of comparison that computes how many times larger a specific brain component is in a species compared to the identical brain component in hypothetical Tenrecinae, controlled for body size. The progression indices of forebrain white matter as compared to the visual area for basal insectivores (Tenrecinae, Madagascar hedgehogs), prosimians, simians, and humans are depicted in Figure 3.1 [2,5].

The Brain as a Connectome

Macroscopic Hardwired Tracts

The frontal lobes may be regarded as being chiefly concerned with motor action or deliberate non-action in the face of environmental or internal stimuli. In addition, the integration of behavior over time is one of the principal frontal lobe functions. During frontal lobe evolution there was progressive refinement of the major motor pathway for precision movements, the pyramidal tract. This initially mediated motor movements, later speech, and then, subsequently in evolution, behaviors related to cognitive and emotional processing. In a challenging environment, optimal responses or decisions depend on a flexible circuitry that can draw on the full range of sensory input and data, as well as triaging priorities to allow for the most appropriate responses. The substrate of such behavioral responses in the human brain has been forged within a progressively more complex circuitry that can be imaged by diffusion tensor imaging with three-dimensional color-coded directional specificity. The major tracts of the present-day cerebral network systems or human connectome include the following:

1. frontal subcortical circuits (the circuit comprises of cortex, basal nuclei, thalamus, cortex):
   a. dorsolateral prefrontal
   b. anterior cingulate
   c. orbitofrontal (medial)
   d. orbitofrontal (lateral)
   e. motor circuit (premotor area)
   f. oculomotor circuit (frontal eye fields)
   g. inferotemporal
   h. posterior parietal to prefrontal
2. superior longitudinal fasciculus
3. inferior longitudinal fasciculus
4. superior occipitofrontal fasciculus
5. perpendicular fasciculus
6. uncinate fasciculus
7. arcuate fasciculus
8. corpus callosum
9. cingulum
10. fornix
11. frontopontocerebellar circuit.

Neurochemical Tracts

The ascending neurochemical-based networks act in concert with the aforementioned major cerebral fasciculi. The fast-acting excitatory (glutaminergic) and inhibitory (GABA) amino acid neurotransmitters represent the major neurochemical cerebral systems. These are in turn modulated by several slower-acting (mostly G-protein linked) neurotransmitters with extensive projects. These neurotransmitter-based circuits serve to coordinate many networks in response to stimuli or threats. Currently, eight different neuro-modulatory tracts are recognized, including the tri-monoamine-based dopaminergic, serotonergic and noradrenergic. Others include acetylcholine, histamine, orexin, and oxytocin/vasopressin, all with their nuclei of origin in the brainstem, basal forebrain, or hypothalamus, and from which the extensive cortical matrix emanates (Figure 3.2) [6,7].

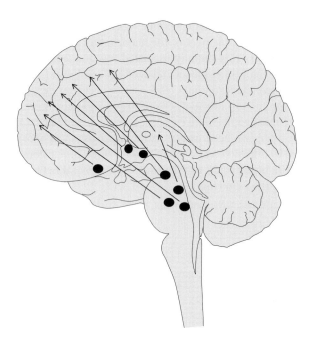

Figure 3.2 Neurotransmitter or connectional fingerprints are a function of the ascending neurotransmitter systems: acetylcholine, noradrenaline, serotonin, dopamine, histamine, orexin, vasopressin, and oxytocin.

Neurophysiological Frontal Functional Systems

Clinical frontal lobe presentations can be bewildering, with typically more than two dozen differing presentations described. Even more enigmatic, they may often be covert and even "silent" [8]. However, when grouping them according to their evolutionary development, a sensible categorization can be appreciated, as discussed below.

The Eight Frontal Subcortical Networks

All frontal subcortical networks share a similar basic circuit anatomy that extends through the components as follows: cortex–caudate–globus pallidus–thalamus–cortex. Impairment in any of these circuits after the cortex of origin mediate well-recognized frontal clinical syndromes (Figure 3.3):

- Motor: premotor (BA 6) motor circuit (BA 4) for striated muscle movement of the face, arms, and legs.
- Oculomotor: external ocular eye movements mediated by the frontal eye field (BA 8), third, fourth, and sixth cranial nerves and conjugate eye movement centers in the pons and midbrain.
- Dorsolateral prefrontal cortex (DLPFC) circuit: mediates dysexecutive syndrome and incurs deficits that affect the temporal organization of information, working memory, and multitasking.
- Anterior cingulate circuit: mediates the motivation for behaviors; impairments result in a range of disorders from akinetic mutism to abulias, alexithymias, and apathy [9,10].

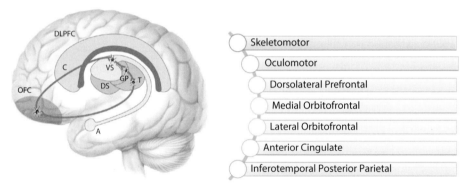

Figure 3.3 The frontal subcortical circuits: all have in common the cortex–striatum–thalamus–cortex. OFC = orbitofrontal cortex, DLPFC = dorsolateral prefrontal cortex, C = corpus callosum, DS = dorsal striatum; VS = ventral striatum; GP = globus pallidus; T = thalamus; A = amygdala.

- The orbitofrontal (OFC) circuitry includes the cortical component of the limbic system, which integrates emotional and social behaviors into a behavioral output. Lesions here cause disinhibitory syndromes [11]. The medial OFC circuitry specifically mediates empathy and socially appropriate deportment. Not infrequently, profound personality change in the context of normal cognitive functions is evident which leads to profound medical management dilemmas. Various forms of field-dependent behavior and loss of autonomy from environmental influences cause presentations of imitation behavior, echopraxia, utilization behavior, and environmental-dependency syndromes. These may be the dominant clinical syndromes, especially in acute frontal syndromes as with stroke. The medial OFC circuitry is concerned with the emotional valence of events, which influence the strength of an episodic memory or engram. In addition, alterations of autonomic and endocrine functions may be associated with medial OFC lesions [12]. Lateral OFC circuitry compromise may present with the spectrum of obsessive compulsive disorders, depression, irritability, and mood disorders, as well as field-dependent behaviors. The obsessive compulsive disorder spectrum includes obsessions (intrusive urges or thoughts), compulsions (repetitive, ritualistic activities that may be cognitive or physical in nature), Gille del la Tourette's syndrome, pathological gambling, kleptomania, risk-seeking behavior, and body dysmorphic disorder [13].
- Inferotemporal subcortical circuit impairment may be associated with visual hallucinations, visual discrimination, and visual scanning deficits and psychosis [14].
- The posterior parietal (BA 7) to prefrontal region (BA 46) mediates visual stimuli significance and consequently influences visuospatial processing [13].
- The extensive frontoparietal group – such as the superior longitudinal fasciculi, inferior longitudinal fasciculi, superior occipitofrontal fasciculus, and arcuate fasciculi – are tracts that subserve working memory, the mirror neuron system, and language (Figure 3.4). Representative clinical syndromes include multitasking problems, field-dependent behaviors, dysexecutive syndrome, dysmemory, and dysnomias.

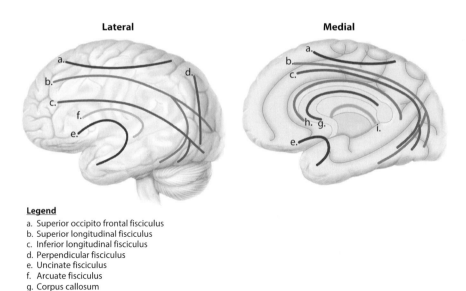

Legend
a. Superior occipito frontal fisciculus
b. Superior longitudinal fisciculus
c. Inferior longitudinal fisciculus
d. Perpendicular fisciculus
e. Uncinate fisciculus
f. Arcuate fisciculus
g. Corpus callosum
h. Cingulum
i. Fornix

Figure 3.4 The major cerebral fiber tracts.

- The uncinate fasciculus (UF) links the inferior frontal lobes with the anterior temporal lobes and is an evolutionarily more recent circuit among primates which imparts social, emotional, and episodic memory adeptness. The UF is one of the long-range association fiber tracts that is particularly relatively enlarged among humans compared to our closet primate cousins (Figure 3.5). From a clinical point of view, the UF has a special vulnerability in the setting of traumatic brain injury (TBI), frontotemporal dementia, and a number of neuropsychiatric syndromes. Of particular relevance is that it matures remarkably late, well into the third and even fourth decade [15]. The three principal disorders associated with UF impairment include social deportment disorders, emotional conduct disorders and episodic dysmemory. In addition, a number of neuropsychiatric syndromes associated with UF impairment include anxiety disorders, schizophrenia, and antisocial personality disorder. Less frequent syndromes include seizure disorders, specific epileptic syndromes including uncinate fits (olfactory hallucinations, gustatory hallucinations, dreamy states), the Klüver–Bücy syndrome, emotional arousal syndromes, involuntary orofacial movements, and content-specific delusions (delusional misidentification syndromes: DMIS) such as Capgras syndrome and reduplicative paramnesias. The DMIS spectrum of disorders have been attributed to the severance of circuits between limbic areas and facial processing areas mediating emotionality in response to facial percepts. People with Capgras syndrome, for example, are able to correctly identify a familiar individual by their facial features, but devoid of the usual emotions normally associated, which leads them to conclude the person is someone else. UF function is disrupted in people experiencing DMIS [16]. The principal functions of the UF are the linking of memory, social, and emotional processing, and mediation of mnemonic associations over time [17].

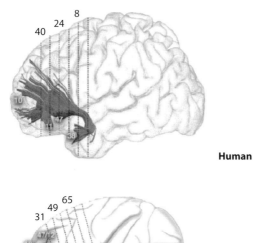

Figure 3.5 Uncinate fasciculus evolution: comparative analysis of human and macaque. *Source:* Thiebaut de Schotten M, Dell'Acqua F, Valabregue R, Catani M. Monkey to human comparative anatomy of the frontal lobe association tracts. *Cortex* 2012;48:82–96. Reproduced with permission from Elsevier.

Human

Macaque

- Frontopontocerebellar circuit: several clinical neurological syndromes are attributable to pathology of the cerebellum or the tracts that connect it to the frontal lobe via the pons and thalamus. Examples include cerebellar cognitive affective, cerebellar, and cognitive dysmetria (problems with coordinating mental activity) syndrome, with examples of disorders of this circuitry usually caused by stroke but also with schizophrenia and inherited ataxia syndromes [18]. Gait disorders such as gait ataxia, gait apraxia, and frontal lobe ataxia may be directly related to cerebellar pathology or related fiber tracts [19]. Neuroimaging advances by MRI diffusion tension imaging nowadays allow imaging of this extensive tract that can be associated with a number of frontal syndromes, such as executive dysfunction, but may also precipitate behavioral abnormalities even though the lesion is remote, in the posterior fossa. Ascending neurotransmitter-based systems mediate "state-dependent" conditions such as arousal, learning, and attention disorders, with either deficiency or excess of one or several neurotransmitters encountered in clinical conditions. Attention, working memory, and executive function are dependent on these monoaminergic systems, and deficiencies in these lead to impairments in these functions, such as in Parkinson's disease (dopamine-deficiency state). Neurotransmitter perturbations may also occur with excessive activity, such as with the neuroleptic malignant syndrome, the cholinergic toxidrome, serotonin toxidrome, and malignant hyperpyrexia.

The Frontoparietal Group

There is archeological evidence that humans' enhanced working memory attained a hypothetical stage 7 in comparison to a chimpanzee's stage 2 [20,21] (Figure 3.6). Wynn and

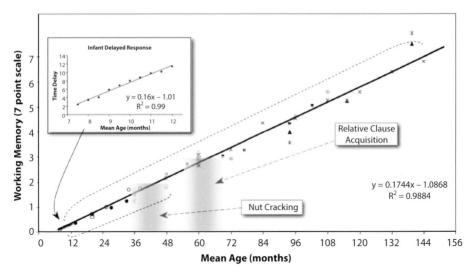

Figure 3.6 Working memory trajectory in humans, graded 7 compared to *Pan paniscus,* bonobo chimpanzee, graded at level 2. The upper dashed line represents the growth trajectory for modern human working memory and the lower dashed line for *Pan*, developing at similar rates. Working memory level 2 develops at about 3–4 years of age in humans and continues to develop for about 7 years (144 months) in humans, whereas in *Pan* it stabilizes at level 2 as per the meta-analyses from the listed datasets.

Source: Read D. Working memory: a cognitive limit to non-human primate recursive thinking prior to hominid evolution. *Evol Psychol* 2008;6(4):676–714. Reproduced with permission of SAGE Publishing Inc.

Coolidge speculated that "enhanced WM capacity powered the appearance of the modern mind" [22]. Although stone tools may be associated with evidence of human modernity, they are regarded mainly as circuits mediating procedural and long-term memory processes. Reliable weapons (projectile tools, spears, hafting, traps, snares, bows, arrows), foraging, relying on external storage devices (e.g., Blombos cave engravings of ~70 kya) are associated with executive function and higher-level working memory capacity. In addition, these required response inhibitions are mediated by executive processes for empowering delayed gratification. Enhanced working memory or an upgrade from stage 6 to 7 is presumed to have occurred ~50 kya, with the development of abstract thoughts, improved behavioral flexibility, and creativity and theory of mind (TOM) [24]. Direct neuronal cell recordings have established that DLPFC (BA 46/9) neurons fire during the delay period between stimulus and motor response, supporting the cellular basis of maintenance of information. The mid-DLPFC represents the frontal lobe monitoring component by tracking relevant stimuli of information as the basis of working memory, also termed the epoptic process [23]. Online type of maintenance of information by the working memory circuitry also depends on posterior cortical association areas, including the superior temporal gyrus for auditory representations and the anterior inferotemporal cortex for object representations (Figure 3.7). The maintenance of information for further processing, or working memory, differs from the process of active retrieval of memory traces, a function of the mid-ventrolateral PFC (VLPFC) [24,25]. The posterior parietal

Working memory hubs

1. Epopticprocess: Mid-dorsolateralprefrontal cortex monitors information

2. Manipulation of information: Posterior parietal region around the intra-parietal sulcus

3. Both regions interact with the superior temporal region, the multimodal sensory integration area

Principal fiber tracts subserving working memory

A. Superior longitudinal fasciculus

B. Middle longitudinal fasciculus

C. Extreme capsule

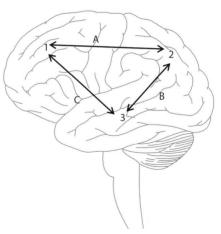

Figure 3.7 A fundamental and cardinal function of the frontal lobes is working memory.

region also processes the ability to manipulate information – for example, arithmetic and mental rotation of objects. The mid-dorsal lateral prefrontal cortex (MDLPFC) or BA 46 axons target layers I–III of the intraparietal sulcus in support of the modulatory role of the MDLPFC on parietal processing, also termed the epoptic process [26,27].

The Frontopontocerebellar Circuit

According to neuro-archeological evidence, the modern human brain size was achieved by ~200 kya. However, modern cerebellum size was achieved by a mere ~28 kya, associated with recent escalations in corticocerebellar connectivity, particularly the prefrontal cortex component, during the Late Pleistocene period (Figure 3.8) [28]. In both humans and chimpanzees there was increased prefrontal involvement in the frontocerebellar system, which progressed further within the human lineage and not in the chimpanzee lineage. This may have played a role in the involvement of the frontocerebellar circuit, with subsequent tool use and vocal articulatory elaboration (Figure 3.9). The expansion of the cerebellum in human cognitive evolution has been relatively underestimated. With a 45 percent increase in cerebellar size as we move from monkeys to apes and a further increase in hominins, the cerebellum, with four times more neurons than the cortex (69 billion neurons versus 15 billion), clearly must have key processing abilities and functions. The evolutionary trajectory of the frontocerebellar systems that have been primarily concerned with motor learning over 46 million years of primate evolution have been studied, comparing evolution of the frontal motor cortex, prefrontal cortex, and posterior cerebellar hemispheres. These studies reveal an increasing role for frontocerebellar systems among primates after they diverged from monkeys 30 million years earlier. Thereafter a further change occurred in this frontocerebellar system, with an increased role for the prefrontal cortex with respect to the frontal motor cortex in the hominin lineage since the divergence from the common ancestors with chimpanzees (~10 mya). Yet further changes occurred in the human lineage ~6 mya, and as recently as ~28 kya [29,30]. A possible scenario, given the previously cited biogeographic and paleo-climatological events, is that the forging of the prefrontopontocerebellar tracts in association with bipedal emergence may have occurred in the Late Miocene period in

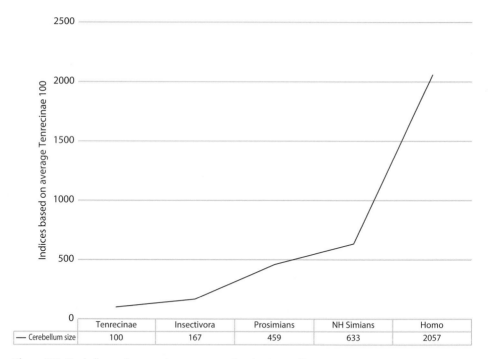

	Tenrecinae	Insectivora	Prosimians	NH Simians	Homo
— Cerebellum size	100	167	459	633	2057

Figure 3.8 Cerebellum enlargement across mammals, primates, and humans.
Source: compiled from the data of Stephan H, Baron G, Frahm H. Comparative Brain Research in Mammals, volume 1, Insectivora, Springer, New York, 1991.

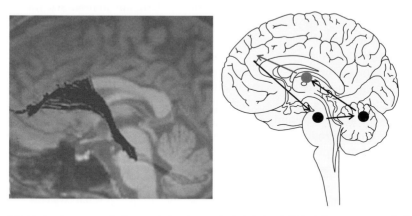

Figure 3.9 Modern human cerebellum evolution occurred relatively late (~28 kya). Frontopontocerebellar circuit imaged by MRI-DTI tractography (left) and schematic diagram (right).
Source: Kamali A, Kramer LA, Frye RE, Butler IJ, Hasan KM. Diffusion tensor tractography of the human brain cortico-ponto-cerebellar pathways: a quantitative preliminary study. *J Magn Reson Imaging* 2010;32:809–817. Reproduced with permission of John Wiley and Sons.

the Afar basin and Danakil Island. The inland sea basin had existed in Afar 7 mya to 70 kya, and lineages included in these events included the australopithecines at 4.2–2.0 mya and the robust australopithecines who ventured into open savannahs from whom we are not descended. The expanding corticocerebellar functions are likely to have been concerned with the evolution of human speech, tool-making and tool use. The cerebellar contributions to improved cognitive efficiency and as a component of working memory were the likely mechanisms [28].

Working memory is a key cognitive function that underlies most other cerebral cognitive processes, akin to a computer's processor that drives the operating system. Verbal working memory and the cerebellum may have been instrumental in language evolution, initially as inner speech with the verbal working memory holding information such as vocal sounds and later letters, words, and objects in phonological storage for several seconds to allow processing. Working memory expansion, speech, and language evolution were probably coupled. The phonological loop enabled storage and rehearsal during sound processing, which involved speech areas of the cortex as well as the lateral cerebellum. The phonological loop was probably gradually added to the initial form of working memory, the visuospatial working memory component [31]. Evolutionary repurposed circuitry mediates reading and arithmetic associated with these relatively recent cultural inventions. Mathematics, reading, and art were sculpted on existing primate brain circuitry. Dehaene posited that a boost of what is termed "conscious neuronal workspace" permitted a repurposing of this neuronal circuitry that has been termed the neuronal recycling hypothesis [32]. In humans and macaques, the temporal lobe areas associated with object identification reside in the inferior occipitotemporal region (BA 37) used for visual object identification for about ten million years [33]. This area was then exapted for reading, becoming the "brain's letterbox." Microelectrode recordings show that neurons in the intraparietal sulcus and prefrontal cortex respond and convey numerosity in monkeys. This supports numerosity being subserved by a parietofrontal network [34]. The horizontal component of the intraparietal sulcus, for example, is activated only when numbers are visualized and not when viewing colors or letters. Arithmetic skills have also been linked to the anterior component of the superior longitudinal fasciculus [35].

Brain Network Organization

Brain volume is limited by the laws of physics. As larger organisms also have larger brains, which also have more synapses per neuron, there is a disproportionate increase of white matter increase over gray matter increase in large brains. As larger brains are metabolically more expensive, various configurations have been deployed to circumvent these engineering challenges. One is sulcogyral folding of the cerebral cortex, which minimizes axonal projection distances. Most of the brain's metabolic cost is incurred through the process of maintaining electrochemical gradients across neuronal membranes, supporting signaling. Human brain networks exist as a balance between two extremes of wiring potential. At one extreme is the random topology model, which is configured so that each node is connected to a minimum of two or more other nodes. The disadvantage is the high wiring energy cost as a consequence of the increased number of long-distance connections. At the other extreme is the lattice topology, which is configured to minimize cost but has the disadvantage of less global integration, which is the substrate for information processing. Present-day human brain networks are instead configured for achieving maximal network efficiency that in turn allows optimal integrative processing by employing clusters of lattice-like short-distance connections as well as long-distance higher-cost components linking individual connector hubs. With neurological illnesses, in particular the cognitive impairment components tend to impact the most high-value hub components of the networks. These are the nodes or hubs that are most critical for integrative processing and therefore adaptive behavior (Figure 3.10) [36].

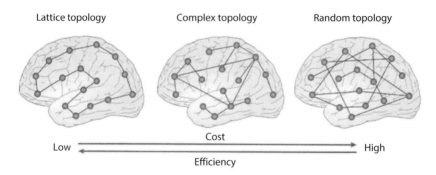

Figure 3.10 Brain network organization.
Reproduced by permission from Springer Nature from *Bullmore E, Sporns O. The economy of brain network organization. Nat Rev Neurosci 2012;13:*336–349.

It is at the connectomal level that nature and nurture meet. An animal's experiences reconnect and alter neuronal firing rates through the mechanisms of reweighting, rewiring, reconnecting, and regeneration, but genes shape connectomes as well [37].

The large-scale cerebral networks recognized at a functional level include:

- default mode network (DMN);
- salience network;
- executive (left and right) network;
- motor and visual networks.

For example, the brain regions affected in Alzheimer's disease (AD) fit neatly over a map of the areas that define the DMN. The DMN circuit includes the medial parietal area, medial prefrontal area, lateral parietal area, and lateral temporal cortex. In addition to AD, there are altered connections among brain cells in the DMN of patients with depression and schizophrenia [38]. Functional network disruption in the degenerative dementias can be assessed by functional MRI resting-state network scanning and diffusion tensor imaging scanning. Connectivity imaging disruption has been noted with the DMN in AD, the salience network in frontotemporal lobe dementia, and basal ganglia–thalamocortical loop disruption in Parkinson's and Lewy body dementia [39].

It is not surprising, therefore, that the efficiency of the resting-state network patterns becomes a predictor of cognitive performance. Our intellectual performance is ultimately related to how efficiently our brains integrate the information between many brain regions [40]. However, there is an important and optimistic message in that the disrupted energy metabolism and consequent neuronal circuit dysfunction results in the cognitive impairment of dementias such as AD. The current epidemic of global disorders of obesity, diabetes mellitus, and metabolic syndrome and obesity are closely linked to AD and cognitive aging. Animal and human studies are prolific, with data that indicate that lifestyle alterations, by improving global energy metabolism and therefore cerebral metabolism, are effective in preventing and potentially even reversing cognitive impairment, brain atrophy, and dementia. Network dysfunction occurs in parallel with metabolic dysfunction during cognitive aging and AD [41].

Table 3.1 Understanding frontal network presentations in the context of their evolutionary heritage aids insight and understanding

Principal circuits	Cognitive domains/ deficits	Clinical syndromes	Geological/ climate	Time
Frontopontocerebellar	Executive dysfunction	Tremor, ataxia, biped	Danakil	7–5 mya?
Frontoparietal group	Language, working memory, FDB	Apraxias	Arboreal	?
Frontal subcortical circuits	Dysexecutive, disinhibition, abulia	Parkinsonism	?	?
Uncinate fasciculus group	Social and emotional syndromes	FTD, KB syndrome	Late	?
Ascending neurotransmitter	Inattention, arousal, dysmemory	Sleep disorders	?	?
Evolutionary repurposed	Arithmetic, reading, writing problems	?	?	5–3 kya

From a physiological point of view, consciousness may be viewed as an emergent property (expressed by the whole but not the constituent parts) of the brain. Consciousness is such a cognitive process and emerges or is immanent in the brain's network complexity. Potential cerebral candidates for consciousness include the following:

- The 40 Hz hypothesis: cortical neurons firing rhythmically every 20–30 microseconds.
- Layer Five pyramidal cells: the principal cortical neurons, comprising three-quarters of cortical neurons.
- The claustrum: a sheet of neurons in the subcortical region crucial for awareness for the percepts of vision, sound, and touch. The claustrum function is thought to be responsible for rapidly integrating diverse neuronal information (cognitive, perception, action) from distinct cortical and subcortical regions. The claustrum is in an ideal position to integrate the most diverse kinds of information that underlie conscious perception, cognition, and action [42].

In summary, the approximate sequence of events of building the human brain circuitry was (Table 3.1):

1. frontoparietal: working memory, praxis, language;
2. frontopontocerebellar: bipedality, reaching, coordination;
3. prefrontopontocerebellar: cognitive fine tuning?;
4. frontal subcortical: eye movements, executive, volition, inhibition;
5. uncinate fasciculus: empathy, sociality, inhibition;
6. arcuate fasciculus: language.

Comparative Neuroanatomy: Are Animal Brains Bigger and More Complex than Ours?

Orcas (*Orcinus orca*), the supreme ocean creatures, have been around for about six million years, while *Homo sapiens* have existed a mere 200 000 years. Although focusing on orcas, they belong to cetaceans, which includes whales, dolphins, and porpoises, all of whom have a brain with a cortical thickness that is relatively thin compared to primates and humans. The gyrification or degree of folding of their cortices is, however, very much increased. This extensive folding swells the amount of total cortical nerve tissue for information processing for thought, language, and memory, as well as allowing transmission and handling of more data and faster processing. The gyrification index (GI) for humans is 2.2, for bottlenose dolphins is 5.62, and for *Orcinus orca* is 5.7. This is very significant for brain-processing capacity; Green et al. have found a positive correlation with gyrification and working memory even after allowance was made for surface area of the cortex [43]. Part of the reason may have been these animals' need for auditory processing in view of their sixth sense of echolocation (we have only five) and using their large brains to "see" underwater. They are able to construct mental representations and pictures using echolocation (we have linguistic elaboration) and are able to go back and forth between vision and echolocation and integrate the information. They also have what has been termed the paralimbic system, the function of which remains uncertain but may serve the function of possible navigation and spatial memory functions as well as, most importantly, emotional intelligence. In support of the latter is their highly developed amygdala that mediates emotional learning and long-term memory formation. In addition, their insula cortex is very elaborate, which is the brain structure integral to social cognition, self-awareness, attention, and focus [44]. The "blackfish" brain or the long-finned pilot whale (*Globicephalamelas*) brain has the highest neuronal count in the animal kingdom, with 37.29×10^9 neurons, almost twice as many as humans, and 127×10 glial cells. Their high glial to neuronal ratio and decreased density is particularly notable, a sign of complex brains [45].

In general, the enlarged cetacean cingulate and insular cortices, and elevated glial cell to neuron ratio, relates to advanced cognitive functions – in particular, social awareness, judgment, and intuition. The high glial cell to neuron ratio is found in complex brains that enable swift communication and synaptic efficiency. The higher cortical functions reported to date with cetacean brains are impressive. Delphinidae *Laegorhynchus albirostris* has an encephalization quotient (EQ) of 6.32 [46], whereas humans average 7. Studies have been mostly performed in bottlenose (BN) dolphins, orcas, and sperm and humpback whales. In brief these have included the following.

Executive Function

Bottlenose (BN) dolphins are able to recognize themselves in a mirror, demonstrate awareness of their own behavior, as well as metacognition (awareness of own knowledge states) [47]. BN dolphins have demonstrated understanding of symbolic depictions of items and events and can spontaneously learn sound and paired event associations. Dolphins have an expansive behavioral and vocal mimicry whereby they are able to comprehend the significance of human gestures, pointing, and eye gaze. They have the capability of a mental representation of their body and to compare it to another, including humans with the tail improvising for the human legs, for example (Figure 3.11). Dolphins have even demonstrated comprehension of symbolic references to items that are visually absent.

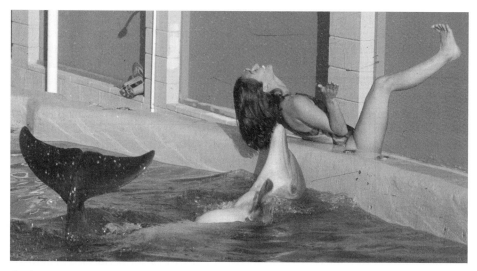

Figure 3.11 Imitation behavior is a critical ability for social learning. Dolphin imitation behavior, improvising the tail for the human leg.
Source: Marino L, Connor RC, Fordyce RE, et al. Cetaceans have complex brains for complex cognition. *PLoS Biol* 2007;5(5):e139.

Language

Bottlenose dolphins have semantic capability, as evidenced by their ability to comprehend symbolism or an artificial language via their own auditory and visual symbols.
A basic syntax capability has also been described, whereby changing the order of symbolic "words" changes the message. Learning and decoding of information has also been
described as being achieved through inference as opposed to direct instruction.

Memory-Related Functions

In addition to their understanding of symbolic representations related to items or events,
termed declarative knowledge, BN dolphins also appear to demonstrate basic mechanical
understanding of objects. This translates into their ability to manipulate objects and is
consistent with procedural knowledge and memory.

Tool Use

Closely related are the reports of tool use by BN dolphins, demonstrated by their ability
to manipulate sponges to explore crevices that may harbor prey. These abilities have also
been transmitted to their conspecifics, an example of cultural transference.

Social Complexity

Perhaps most impressive is the social culture and learning in terms of foraging and learning dialects among cetaceans. In addition, both group alliances and alliances of alliances
have been described. Most cetaceans studied (BN dolphins, orcas, sperm whales, humpback whales) display multiculturalism, referring to different cultural groups abiding
within the same habitats. The cultural learning of these varied behaviors has been documented both through imitation or motor mimicry, and more impressively through direct

instruction or pedagogy. The example cited by Marino et al. is that of orca calves being "instructed" by their mothers in beaching maneuvers to facilitate capturing seals [48]. Equally remarkable is the unique discovery of BN dolphins' individual identity, each having their own signature whistle [49]. Another feature that relates to cerebral complexity and enhanced working memory is the cerebellum, which is relatively larger in cetaceans compared to primates or humans [50]. Unprecedented is the lack of violence among cetaceans, including against humans, their tolerance for other cultures (multiculturalism) in their environment, and high demand for sociality. The latter even extends to taking on human companions in the absence of their own. This was well depicted in Neiwert's book describing the story of Luna, the orca residing in Nootka Sound, Vancouver Island, who replaced his pod family with humans [51].

Summary

Understanding the cerebral network evolution from which we inherited many distributed complex networks is becoming increasingly important from a clinical diagnostic and treatment point of view today. Assessing network integrity can be performed in both the spatial and temporal domains. Spatial-based imaging by fMRI can provide up to a 2–3 mm resolution, magnetoencephalography (MEG) and electroencephalography (EEG) are able to distinguish at a 5–30 mm resolution and diffusion tensor imaging (DTI) at a 3–6 mm resolution. In the temporal domains, fMRI allows resolutions within seconds and electrophysiological measurements within milliseconds. Similar to the "omics" networks at a cellular level (genomics, proteomics, lipidomics), at the mesoscale and macroscale level imaging the cerebral connectome has helped earlier diagnosis of most of our most common neurological and psychiatric conditions encountered today. These have yielded new diagnostic tools where none were available before, such as diagnosis of depression by MRI-based intrinsic connectivity analysis (ICN) or resting-state networks (RSN). Improved accuracy in diagnosis in TBI has been realized by DTI as well as RSN. In epilepsy, the network-based approach termed epileptomics has improved our understanding of seizure diagnosis and propagation and influenced treatment approaches. Functional MRI resting-state network and DTI have contributed profoundly to our connectomal understanding of diseases. With focal epilepsy, this has prompted our view of it being more of a system-level condition, with implications for epilepsy surgery decision-making [52,53]. Furthermore, the human connectome and its interaction with other complex systems and how they interact with other parts of the body, such as metabolomics and the human microbiome, are becoming increasingly relevant in understanding disease and therapies. Understanding the cause of phantom limb pain and the observation that the cerebral networks of the amputated limb remain preserved in the brain has empowered us with therapies for these conditions. Preservation of hand movement representation in the sensorimotor areas of the brain persists in amputees, for example [54].

References

1. Semendeferi K, Lu A, Schenker N, Damasio H. Humans and great apes share a large frontal cortex. *Nature Neurosci* 2002;5:272–276.

2. Zilles K. Evolution of the human brain and comparative cyto and receptor

architecture. In Dehaene S, Duhamel JR, Hauser MD, Rizzolatti G (eds.), *From Monkey Brain to Human Brain*. MIT Press, Cambridge, MA, 2005.

3. Elston GN, Benavides-Piccione R, Elston A, et al. Specializations of the

granular prefrontal cortex of primates: implications for cognitive processing. *Anat Record A Discov Mol Cell Evol Biol* 2006;288A:26–35.

4. Smaers JB, Schleicher A, Zilles K, Vinicius L. Frontal white matter volume is associated with brain enlargement and higher structural connectivity in anthropoid primates. *PLoS One* 2010;5:1–6.

5. Stephan H, Baron G, Frahm H. *Comparative Brain Research in Mammals*, vol. 1, *Insectivora*. Springer, New York, 1991.

6. Brady ST, Siegel GJ, Albers RW, Price DL (eds.), *Basic Neurochemistry: Principles of Molecular, Cellular and Medical Neurobiology*, 8th edn. Academic Press, Amsterdam, 2012.

7. Nestler EJ, Hyman SE, Malenka RC. *Molecular Neuropharmacology: A Foundation for Clinical Neuroscience*. McGraw-Hill, New York, 2009.

8. Stuss DT, Floden D, Alexander MP, Levine B, Katz D. Stroop performance in focal lesion patients: dissociation of process and frontal lobe lesion location. *Neuropsychologica* 2001;39:771–786.

9. Fesenmeier JT, Kuzniecky R, Garcia JH. Akinetic mutism caused by bilateral anterior cerebral tuberculous obliterative arteritis. *Neurology* 1990;40:1005–1006.

10. Bogousslavsky J, Regli F. Anterior cerebral artery territory infarction in the Lausanne stroke registry. *Arch Neurol* 1990;47:144–150.

11. Chow TW, Cummings JL. Frontal subcortical circuits. In: Miller B, Cummings JL (eds.), *The Human Frontal Lobes*. The Guilford Press, New York, 2009.

12. Berthier ML, Kulisevsky J, Gironell A, Heras JA. Obsessive compulsive disorders associated with brain lesions: clinical phenomenology, cognitive function and anatomic correlates. *Neurology* 1996;47:353–361.

13. Yeterian EH, Pandya DN. Striatal connections of the parietal association cortices in rhesus monkeys. *J Comp Neurol* 1993;332:175–197.

14. Lichter DG, Cummings JL. *Frontal Subcortical Circuits in Psychiatric and Neurological Disorders*. The Guilford Press, New York, 2001.

15. Seo JP, Kim OL, Kim SH, et al. Neural injury of uncinate fasciculus in patients with diffuse axonal injury. *Neurorehabilitation* 2012;30:323–328.

16. Hirstein W, Ramachandran VS. Capgras syndrome: a novel probe for understanding the neural representation of the identity and familiarity of persons. *Proc R Soc B* 1997;264:437–444.

17. Von Der Heide R, Skipper LM, Kobusicky E, Olsen IR. Dissecting the uncinate fasciculus: disorders, controversies and a hypothesis. *Brain* 2013;136:1692–1707.

18. Ramnani N. The primate cortico-cerebellar system: anatomy and function. *Nat Rev Neurosci* 2006;7:511–522.

19. Thompson PD. Frontal lobe ataxia. *Handb Clin Neurol* 2012;103:619–622.

20. Read D, van der Leeuw S. Biology is only part of the story. In: Renfrew C, Frith C, Malafouris L (eds.), *The Sapient Mind*. Oxford University Press, Oxford, 2009.

21. Read D. Working memory: a cognitive limit to nonhuman primate recursive thinking prior to hominid evolution? *Cog Sci Proceedings* 2006:2674–2679.

22. Coolidge FL, Wynn T. *The Rise of Homo Sapiens*. Wiley Blackwell, New York, 2009.

23. Petrides M. Dissociable roles of the mid dorsolateral prefrontal cortex and anterior inferotemporal cortex in visual working memory. *J Neurosci* 2000;20:7496–7503.

24. Champod AS, Petrides M. Dissociation within the frontoparietal network in verbal working memory: a parametric functional magnetic resonance imaging study. *J Neurosci Res* 2010;30:3849–3856.

25. Champod AS, Petrides M. Dissociable roles of the posterior parietal and the prefrontal cortex in manipulation and monitoring process. *PNAS* 2007;104:14837–14842.

26. Medalla M, Barbas H. Diversity of laminar connections linking periarcuate and lateral intraparietal areas depends

on cortical structure. *Eur J Neurosci* 2006;23:161–179.

27. Petrides M. The mid-dorsolateral prefrontal-parietal network and the epoptic process. In: Stuss DT, Knight RT (eds.), *Principles of Frontal Lobe Function.* Oxford University Press, Oxford, 2012.

28. Weaver, AH. Reciprocal evolution of the cerebellum and neocortex in fossil humans. *PNAS* 2005;102:3576–3580.

29. Smaers JB, Steele J, Case CR, Amunts K. Laterality and the evolution of the prefronto-cerebellar system in anthropoids. *Ann NY Acad Sci* 2014;1288:59–69.

30. Barton RA, Venditti C. Rapid evolution of the cerebellum in humans and other great apes. *Curr Biol* 2014;24:2440–2444.

31. Koziol LF, Budding D, Andreasen N, et al. Consensus paper: the cerebellum's role in movement and cognition. *Cerebellum* 2014;13(1):151–177.

32. Dehaene S. *Reading in the Brain.* Penguin, New York, 2009.

33. Tarkiainen A, Cornelissen PL, Salmelin R. Dynamics of visual feature analysis and object level processing in face versus letter-string perception. *Brain* 2002;125:1125–1136.

34. Nieder A, Miller EK. A parieto-frontal network for visual numerical information in the monkey. *PNAS* 2004;101:7457–7462.

35. Tsang JM, Dougherty RF, Deutsch GK, Wandell BA, Ben-Shachar M. Frontoparietal white matter diffusion properties predict mental arithmetic skills in children. *PNAS* 2009;106:22546–22551.

36. Bullmore E, Sporns O. The economy of brain network organization. *Nat Rev Neurosci* 2012;13:336–349.

37. Seug S. *Connectome.* Houghton Mifflin Harcourt, Boston, MA, 2012.

38. Zeng KK, Shen H, Wang L, et al. Identifying major depression using whole brain functional connectivity: a multivariate pattern analysis. *Brain* 2012;135:1498–1507.

39. Pievani M, De Haan W, Wu T, Seeley WW, Frisoni GB. Functional network disruption in the degenerative dementias. *Lancet Neurol* 2011;10:829–843.

40. Van den Heuvel MP, Stam CJ, Kahn RS, Hulshoff Pol HE. Efficiency of functional brain networks and intellectual performance. *J Neurosci* 2009;29:7619–7624.

41. Kapogiannis D, Mattson MP. Disrupted energy metabolism and neuronal circuit dysfunction in cognitive impairment and Alzheimer's disease. *Lancet Neurol* 2011;10:187–198.

42. Crick FC, Koch C. What is the function of the claustrum? *Philos Trans R Soc Lond B Biol Sci* 2005;360:1271–1279.

43. Green S, Blackmon K, Thesen T, et al. Parieto-frontal gyrification and working memory in healthy adults. *Brain Imaging Behav* 2017. doi: 10.1007/s11682-017-9696-9.

44. Wright A, Scadeng M, Stec D, et al. Neuroanatomy of the killer whale (*Orcinus orca*): a magnetic resonance imaging investigation of structure with insights on function and evolution. *Brain Struct Funct* 2016. doi: 10.1007/s00429-016-1225-x.

45. Mortensen HS, Pakkenberg B, Dam M, et al. Quantitative relationships in delphinid neocortex. *Front Neuroanat* 2014. doi: 10.3389/fnana.2014.00132.

46. Manger PR. An examination of cetacean brain structure with a novel hypothesis of the evolution of a big brain. *Biol Rev* 2006;81:293–338.

47. Smith JD. The uncertain response in the bottlenosed dolphin (*Tursiops truncatus*). *J Exp Psychol* 1995;124:391–408.

48. Marino L, Conner R, Fordyce R, et al. Cetaceans have complex brains for complex cognition. *PLoS Biology* 2007. doi: 10.1371/journal.pbio.0050139.g002.

49. King SL, Janik VM. Bottlenose dolphins can use learned vocal labels to address each other. *PNAS* 2013;110:13216–13221.

50. Marino L, Rilling JK, Lin SK, Ridgway SH. Relative volume of the cerebellum

in dolphins and comparison with anthropoid primates. *Brain Behav Evol* 2000;56:204–211.

51. Neiwert D. *Of Orcas and Men: What Killer Whales Can Teach Us.* Overlook, New York, 2015.

52. Bernasconi A. Connectome based models of the epileptogenic network: a step towards epileptomics? *Brain* 2017;140:2525–2527.

53. Besson P, Brandt SK, Proxi T, et al. Anatomic consistencies across epilepsies: a stereotactic-EEG informed high resolution structural connectivity study. *Brain* 2017;140:2639–2652.

54. Burrmijn MLCM, Pereboom IPL, Vansteensel MJ, et al. Preservation of hand movement representation in the sensorimotor areas of amputees. *Brain* 2017;140:3166–3178.

Cellular and Molecular Changes

The development of the fourth cortical layer, also called the granular cortex, of the six-layer mammalian cortex enabled profound increases in connectivity. Pyramidal cells became the principal cells of the mammalian and primate cortex. Supercells developed, called spindle cells (or von Economo cells) as well as fork cells in the frontal lobe polar cortex, unique among social animals, including humans. These "social cells" are part of the frontopolar cortex and the insula, and are regarded as the apex of human cognition. Synaptic complexity increased and the supporting cells, astrocytes, became intricately involved in listening and modulating neurons, forming astroglial networks.

The Connectome Unraveled

From its inception over 150 years ago, clinical neurology intimated that the human brain had a network configuration, and hinted at the connectomal concept. Charcot had a localization approach in diametric opposition to that of Brown-Sequard, who emphasized the extensive connectivity of the brain, which resulted in a dispute as early as 1875 [1]. Brown-Sequard had already noted the concept of remote effects of lesions that he used in support of extensive connectivity that would later be formulated by von Monakow as diaschisis. Further support comes from Lieberman's observations that subcortical damage is invariable and a required component of aphasia, rather than cortical damage in Broca's area, again underscoring the network concept [2].

The most decisive confirmation comes from the study of Crossley et al., who investigated hub networks with diffusion tensor imaging (DTI) and gray matter volume meta-analysis studies. The most extensively connected hub nodes of the cerebral networks, due to their long-distance connections, have relatively high metabolic demands and represent the neurological substrate subserving network integration and in turn appropriate behavioral responses. Because of the high metabolic demands, these hubs become more prone to the consequences of metabolic diseases, vascular disease, and neurodegenerative disease. Hence, most brain disorders demonstrate impairment of these so-called high-value hubs. With upgraded metabolism, oxidative stress occurs, which is a consequence of increased neuronal spiking and overall synaptic activity [3]. Hence, metabolic injury preferentially affects the "hotspots" of the human connectome. In their study of 26 different brain disorders, the most significant involvement of the high-value hubs was included among the most common neurological conditions: migraine, Alzheimer's disease, frontotemporal lobe dementia, temporal lobe epilepsy, juvenile myoclonic epilepsy, traumatic brain injury (TBI), post-traumatic stress disorder (PTSD), schizophrenia,

Asperger's syndrome, and progressive supranuclear palsy [4,5]. Intrinsic network imaging has also been shown to be the most sensitive diagnostic tool in diagnosis of traditionally neuroimaging-negative syndromes such as TBI, schizophrenia, depression, and epilepsy, as well as yielding improved insights into the pathophysiology and monitoring of brain disorders [3,6,7]. The effects of discreet pathology, such as due to a stroke, for example, may therefore ramify much more widely along specific brain circuits. A hub distribution effect may also occur, such as has been reported in people with TBI and multiple sclerosis, for example. In TBI, a hub redistribution effect emanating from brain regions such as the fusiform gyrus and precuneus has been observed, and may be regarded as a potential neuroimaging signature signal of network reorganization in these syndromes [8,9]. Another example of the emerging use of network imaging is resting-state network imaging in aiding recovery prediction in vegetative state and minimally conscious conditions [10]. An emerging network imaging observation is that in a majority of brain illnesses, the pattern of hub failure presents clinically with cognitive compromise within the domains of executive function, attention, and working memory [11]. From an evolutionary perspective, the most recent brain expansion region, the parietal lobe precuneal area, involved with "networking" the brain, can be viewed as having predisposed modern humans to neurodegenerative diseases such as Alzheimer's disease and frontotemporal lobe disorders [12].

The complexity is of course not limited to neural systems. Neuronal complex networks interact with the complex metabolic, immune, genetic, and social networks, all of which also interact with each other. Much emphasis is placed in the neuroarcheological literature on the threefold increase in human brain volume in comparison to extant great apes. However, this upstages the much more dramatic expansion in the neuropil and brain connectivity, glial cell proliferation, and the cortical granular layer and synaptic complexity escalation that provides higher "bandwidth." The current brain hardware vital statistics comprise ~100 billion neurons, approximately 6–10-fold more glial cells (about one trillion), and 700 km of blood vessels. The majority of the energy used by the brain is attributed to action potentials and synaptic activity, but perhaps the most mind-boggling statistic is the 150 000 km (long enough to encircle the Earth four times) of nerve fibers, the basis of the human connectome (Table 4.1).

Notably, non-conscious activity uses most of the energy and is the dominant brain activity. Even willed movement is initially non-conscious, with the readiness potential preceding awareness of the movement by one second – and up to eight seconds – prior in the frontopolar cortex. Hence, so-called free will actually has a significant, initial, non-conscious component [16].

Brain Processing Dimensions in 3D Space and Time

Astroglial Networks or Gliotransmission

Glial cells enabled mammals increasing speed of reaction and more complex brain functions. As animals became more complex, there was an increase in the glial cell to neuron ratio. Astrocytic processes are intimately associated with synapses and blood vessels and form the blood–brain barrier, as well as controlling potassium homeostasis and the uptake of cellular waste after brain insults. Astrocytes have receptors for the principal neurotransmitters (glutamate and GABA), hence the name tripartite synapse [17].

Table 4.1 Brain vital statistics

Brain	
Neurons	10^{11} (100 billion)
Glia	10^{12} (1 trillion)
Synapses	10^{15} (1 quadrillion)
Connectome	150 000 km of axons
Blood vessels	700 km
One mm³ brain comprises	
Neurons	50 000
Synapses	50×10^6
Dendrites	150 m
Axons	100 m
All our cells	10^{13} (10 trillion)
Microbiome	
Microbes	2×10^{14} (200 trillion)
Microbiome	1.5 kg
Neurophysiology	
Human sensory systems receive	~11 million bits of information per second
Conscious mind processing capability	~16–50 bits per second
Conscious activity	~5 percent of all cognition
Non-conscious activity	~95 percent of processing
Neurochemistry, energy consumption	
Action potentials energy	47 percent
Postsynaptic processing	34 percent
Resting neuronal potential	13 percent
Glutamate recycling	3 percent

Source: data from [13–15].

The increased ratio of glial cells to neurons observed in animal brains went further in humans, with a glial cell to neuron ratio of about 6:1 (~85 percent versus 15 percent). In humans there are more glial cells in the prefrontal cortex than there are in any other animals apart from cetaceans. Certain parts of tertiary association areas such as the inferior parietal cortex may be cytologically different. For example, Einstein's brain revealed a twofold increase in glial cell to neuron ratio in the inferior parietal lobule, compared to the human norm established from 11 male controls [18]. Nansen speculated that glial cells may be a factor in superior intellectual ability. Anatomical dissection of Einstein's brain revealed that the left inferior parietal lobe was also larger than the right, and the right superior parietal lobe larger than the left, together with expanded prefrontal cortices (compared to 25 human control brains). Interestingly, these brain components increased in size during hominin evolution and also showed considerable reorganization [19].

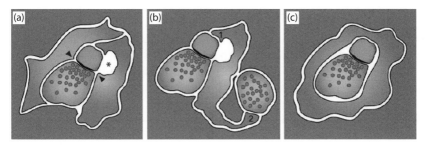

Figure 4.1 Microglial processes in health and disease: quadripartite rather than tripartite. A synapse between an axon terminal (blue) and dendritic spine (pink) contacted by an astrocyte (green) and microglial cell (taupe). Engulfment by a microglial process of an intact synapse between an axon terminal and a dendritic spine. This supports a microglial phagocytosis (ingestion) of synapse components that may be relevant to plasticity in the brain.
Source: Tremblay ME, Majewska AK. A role for microglia in synaptic plasticity? *Commun Integr Biol* 2011;4:220–222. Reproduced with permission of Taylor & Francis Ltd, www.tandfonline.com

Astrocyte Complexity and the Concept of the Glioneuronal Unit

Glial cells form astroglial networks and communicate with neurons and capillaries through the tripartite synapse [20]. In essence, they eavesdrop on neuronal signaling and have their own neurotransmitter receptors, which allows glia to furnish the brain with additional dimensions in information processing. A single astrocyte can envelop and influence approximately two million synapses and incorporate large groups of synapses and neurons into functional units [21].

This provides a prodigious increase in flexibility and power of information processing over and above synaptic strength modification of individual synapses within neural circuits. The expansive domains of operation of glia through chemical cellular transmission diffuses widely and can transgress the hardwired tracts of neuronal connections. This enables a more global scale of information processing compared to the point-to-point synapse-based neuronal systems. A useful analogy is to think of this as "the brain's special kind of internet system." Furthermore, the global glial communication networks also coordinate immunological, hormonal, and vascular networks.

In the study of mice by Tremblay et al., sensory experience was seen to alter the microglial–synaptic interactions. They interpreted these results as implying that microglia, in addition to their known role in immune surveillance in the brain, may play an active role in bestowing experience-dependent alteration of synapses as well as elimination of some synapses as part of their function in health. These functions contribute to learning and memory. These findings indicate a more complex arrangement than the tripartite synapses, involving the neuron, the glial cell, and capillary. With the addition of the microglial component often intricately associated with the tripartite synapses, a more appropriate term would be the quadripartite synapse (Figure 4.1) [22].

The glial to neuron cell ratio in humans is 1.65 compared to *Pan troglodytes'* 1.20 in layer two/three of the prefrontal cortex. Axon length increases accompanying brain enlargement and the concomitant energy required to fire a spike increased, therefore consuming more ATP by a factor of 3.3 in humans compared to rats [23]. Hence glia proliferate to support the increased metabolic demand of larger cortices in humans and the neurons with long-range axons are more susceptible to neurodegeneration and dementia [24].

Astrocytic Complexity of the Human Brain

Several different astrocyte subtypes have been discovered in the human brain thus far. These include human protoplasmic astrocytes (HPA), human intralaminar astrocytes (HIA), human polarized astrocytes (HPoA), and human fibrous astrocytes (HFA). The HPA are the most abundant and reside in layers 2–6, can monitor five microcapillaries, and have a large number of gap junctions composed of connexin that link processes within the cell. Comparative data between humans and rodent HPA are notable for the human cell having an approximate tenfold increase in processes radiating from the HPA cell, a feature that allows these cells to modulate approximately two million synapses. The HIA cells are thought to be specific to primates, occur in layer one of the cortex, which lacks neurons, and have exceptionally long, often unbranched extensions that traverse the cortex, usually terminating in layers three and four. The HPoA reside in the deeper part of the cortex, with processes containing numerous varicosities. The HFA occur in the white matter and have less glial fibrillary acidic protein (GFAP) containing processes and are thought to have primarily metabolic support functions (Figure 4.2).

Functions of astrocytes therefore include vascular effects, with blood flow regulation and blood–brain barrier maintenance, water and ion homeostasis, neurotransmitter production and removal, stem cell proliferation, and determination of synaptic number. Astrocytic domains have been identified in areas known to have a lot of synapses, such as the hippocampus, underscoring their role as synaptic transmission modulators. Astrocytes can also discern neuronal activity that may induce the release of gliotransmitters. This neurochemical interaction has created an additional dimension of communication involved in the processing of what has been termed "activity independent of synaptic transmission." Through these astrocytes and the increasing complexity and formation of the glioneuronal functional unit, integration of and control over larger sets of contiguous synaptic sets are possible. In this fashion, the glioneuronal functional unit augmented the human brain's processing power to surpass most, if not all other species [25].

Hence, increased connectivity has occurred at a cellular or molecular level as well as at a connectomal level. Glial cells are increasingly being implicated in almost all neurological disorders, including, stroke, dementia, migraine, and epilepsy by way of mechanisms involved with blood flow regulation, cell signaling, oxidative stress, inflammation, and apoptosis [26].

Cerebral Networks, Cellular Evolution and Cortical Expansion

These three elements – cerebral networks, cellular evolution, and cortical expansion – cannot be separated. For example, parietal lobe proclivity for expansion in modern humans, by becoming more globular (klinorhynchy) [27], permitted greater interconnectivity between the major cerebral lobes. The parietal lobes have a key role in visuospatial integration, including what Bruner has termed "imagined space," which he postulated as a future role for conceptual thinking and language development. Volumetric changes involved the superior parietal lobes, intraparietal sulcus (IPS), and upper gyri of the lower parietal lobe, as per predictions gleaned from endocast data. The enlargement of the IPS (superior to BA 7) is particularly important with regard to human evolution as this region has been found to be important in symbolic numerical processing and in decoding the intentions, actions, and ultimate goals of conspecifics. MRI-based structural studies by Bruner et al. comparing medial parietal lobes between humans and chimpanzees

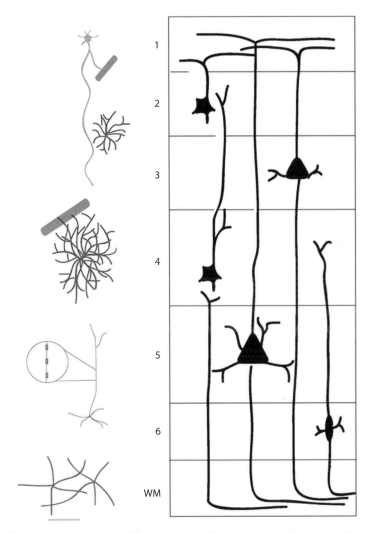

Figure 4.2 The human brain has many different astrocytes. Human astrocyte subtypes: Layer 1, interlaminar astrocytes send fibers widely within the cortex. Layers 2 and 3, protoplasmic astrocytes; some are associated with capillaries and neurons. Polarized astrocytes in layers 5 and 6. Layer 6, fibrous astrocytes are located in the white matter.

Source: Oberheim NA, Wang X, Goldman S, Nedergaard M. Astrocytic complexity distinguishes the human brain. *Trends Neurosci* 2006:10:547–553. Reproduced with permission from Elsevier.

revealed that the principal spatial difference was due to a significant prominent enlargement of the precuneus among humans. The precuneus is a key hub of cerebral networks, including the default mode network as well as visuospatial integration. These findings have been interpreted as one of the distinctive human neural specializations that were involved in our cognitive evolution. In agreement with several other converging lines of evidence, the approximate 150 000-year dating of the precuneal expansion is similar to the ~200 000-year modern human evolution time frame [28]. In summary, major changes at a macro- and microscale can be appreciated (Table 4.2).

Table 4.2 Neuroarcheologically based changes of brain size and reorganization in human evolution

Macroscale	Frontopolar cortex (BA 10) enlarged
	Inferior frontal (BA 13) size decreased
	Temporal lobe increased in size
	Amygdala basolateral nucleus increased in size
	Lunate sulcus moves more posteriorly with reduction in primary visual cortex
	Petalias left occipital, right frontal (cerebral torque)
Microscale	Progressive frontoparietal sensorimotor integration (working memory, mirror neuron circuitry)
	Neuropil less dense, particularly of prefrontal cortex and parietal lobes

Histological Architectural Changes of the Neuropil

Within the frontal lobes, the neuropil (axons, dendrites, space between neurons and glial cells) is decreased in human BA 10 (frontopolar cortex; FPC) relative to other primates as well as being twice as large in terms of brain volume compared to other great apes (1.2 percent in humans versus 0.46–0.74 percent in great apes). BA 13 is relatively reduced in overall size in humans [29,30]. Within BA 10 in "social animals," spindle cells (von Economo cells) are present in layer Vb in both FPC, frontoinsular and anterior cingulate cortex; this includes humans, African great apes, elephants, and cetaceans, in which they are about 30 percent more populous in the right hemisphere. They are regarded as having a key role in social and emotional processing, a higher cortical function that arose millions of years prior to language [31]. In addition to the spindle cells, fork cells are found in the frontoinsular regions; these are both correlated with higher-order cognition, including social emotion and self-consciousness [32]. The regions containing spindle cells connect with the FPC, the insular cortex, the amygdala, and the septum. In addition, the spindle cells and accompanying fork cells express neurmedin B, gastrin, and bombesin peptides, which mediate satiety signaling. These neurochemical findings have helped explain the impaired satiety signaling in people with frontotemporal lobe dementia in whom early loss of spindle cells and fork cells occurs, with later frontotemporal atrophy (Figure 4.3) [33].

The BA 10 neuronal density counts in cubic millimeters in humans are approximately half those of chimpanzees (human BA 10 is ~32 000, chimpanzee is ~60 000; BA 13 neurons per cubic millimeter counts are ~30 000 in humans and 43 000 in chimpanzees). This increase in the human neuropil is interpreted as being related to the heightened connectivity with other tertiary association cortical areas [34]. Relative temporal lobe enlargement, white matter increase, and the ratio of the gyral white matter to core white matter is also a human feature compared to other hominoids. Specifically, the gyral to core white matter ratio represents short association fiber tracts, related to increased interconnectivity [35]. Also within the anterior temporal lobe, the amygdala (basal, lateral, accessory nuclei) evolved with enlargement of the lateral nucleus. This again is reflective of white matter fiber tract proliferation of the more basic unimodal sensory aspects (vision, hearing) with polymodal sensory processing [36].

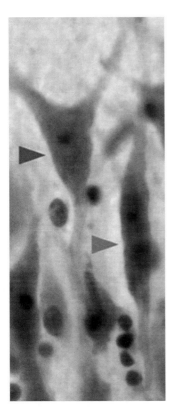

Figure 4.3 Spindle cells/von Economo cells (right arrow head) and fork cells (left arrow head) in the human frontal lobes (frontoinsular region).

Source: Kim EJ, Sidhu M, Gaus SE, et al. Selective frontoinsular von Economo neuron and fork cell loss in early behavioral variant frontotemporal dementia. *Cerebral Cortex* 2012;22:251–259, by permission of Oxford University Press.

Mosaic Systems and Brain Reorganization

The differential expansion of several brain regions such as the temporal lobes, amygdaloid complex, and inferior parietal lobes reflects brain reorganization in a coordinated fashion – termed mosaic evolution. This concept again underscores the importance of conceptualizing the brain network evolution and that evolutionary pressures acted on neural networks rather than on specific neural structures alone [37]. Anatomical volumetric increases in key hubs for social behavior, such as the limbic region of the frontal cortex and amygdaloid complex, occurred in conjunction with network reorganization. This also involved other networks and cortical and subcortical regions such as the orbitofrontal cortex, frontoinsular cortex, and temporal polar cortex, all of which are implicated in social and emotional processing. The temporal polar cortex also has important functions in language processing [38]. These evolutionary changes all are representative of mosaic reorganization in human evolution [39].

The Mosaic Cognitive Evolution

Imitation behavior abilities are a feature of primates and have been implicated in the cultural evolution of hominoids. Imitation behavior circuitry has visual, auditory, and tactile dimensions, and also has "mosaic" characteristics as it involves parietal, temporal, frontal, and cerebellar cortices and was likened by Subiaul to "an all purpose learning mechanism." The circuit includes both chemical and anatomical elements. Evolution of advanced memory, attention, language and tool use are postulated to be the result of this mosaic ensemble of this imitation facility, the substrate being the mirror neuron circuitry [40].

Evolution of Neurotransmitter Systems

The fundamental neuronal signaling transmitter systems include the rapid excitatory glutamate and inhibitory GABA networks with cellular ion channel communication that allows rapidity of response measured in microseconds. A slower-acting neuromodulatory signaling system includes the dopamine (DA), norepinephrine (NE), serotonin (5-HT), histamine (H), orexin (O), and acetylcholine (Ach) networks that disseminate more diffuse and longer responses acting through the G-protein cascade cellular systems. Passinghim et al. have proposed that the melding of both anatomically based and physiologically based connectional and behavioral fingerprints underscore brain connectivity evolution as a whole. A particular connectional fingerprint may therefore provide insights of a particular brain region's function [41]. These neurotransmitter systems modulate the various higher cortical functions and may be a biological marker in some neurodegenerative disease in which specific deficits occur, such as Ach in Alzheimer's disease, serotonin in FTD, and dopamine in Parkinson's disease. These modulatory effects likely made humans more prone to neuropsychiatric diseases, including schizophrenia, autism, and bipolar disease, which are unique to humans [42].

Dopamine

Among the eight frontal subcortical circuits, DA is considered the predominant neurotransmitter, with DA and Ach the principal neurotransmitters in the left hemisphere and serotonin and NE the predominant right hemisphere neurotransmitter system [43]. There may have been unique events whereby DA became a key factor in the unfolding of human intelligence. During the climatological events of East African aridity, heat management, and hyperthermia (including so-called heat stroke), DA may have been a critical factor in survival for the emergent bipedalists, the partially savannah dwelling australopithecines and the later *Homo erectus* [44]. The DA effect of lowering body temperature would have been a major advantage for early hominoids in better tolerating hyperthermia. The theory of chase hunting and catching savannah animals, by literally running them down until they overheated and succumbed to chase myopathy would be in support of this DA hypothesis [45,46]. Further evolutionary expansion of the dopaminergic systems would have been favored also by an upsurge in calcium metabolism consequent to prolonged aerobic activity and the increased dopamine precursor, tyrosine, in turn augmented by the increased meat in the diet in the period of 2–3 mya [47]. From a clinical point of view, many of the core frontal functions – cognitive flexibility, working memory, abstract reasoning, motor planning – became largely regulated by dopamine [41]. In addition, dopamine-blocking drugs (haloperidol, quetiapine, risperidone) may induce malignant hyperthermia and neuroleptic malignant syndromes, both with elevated temperature. These syndromes may therefore be interpreted from an evolutionary perspective and a consequence of the exaption of DA as the principal neurotransmitter of our developing brains.

DA has a modulatory effect of signal-to-noise ratio on PFC G-protein associated receptors on spines and dendritic shafts of the excitatory glutaminergic pyramidal neurons as well as dendrites of the inhibitory GABA-ergic neurons [48]. Through these mechanisms,

DA plays a role in the regulation of working memory, language, and executive functions. In support of these observations, both humans and the great apes have a network of DA input to all cerebral cortical areas. Measurement of cortical DA innervation and axon density may be determined by tyrosine hydroxylase immune-reactivity analysis. This is in direct contradistinction to the DA-sparse innervation features of rodents [49]. In humans there is also a distinct regional DA-ergic distribution, which is most expansive in layers one, five and six of the association cortices [50]. Another human feature in comparison to the great apes is a generalized increased DA input to prefrontal cortical regions. The dopaminergic human evolution hypothesis in human evolution infers that the DA expansion was a critically important factor in human abilities of tool-making and subsequently global exploration, as well as more recent cultural and scientific advances [41]. On the flip side, DA evolutionary theory may be associated with the handicaps of the manifold hyperdopaminergic syndromes, including bipolar disease, autism, schizophrenia, and attention deficit hyperactivity disorders [42].

Serotonin

There is an overall increase in the cortical serotonergic efferent networks among hominoids and humans compared to other mammals, which are relayed by at least 14 G-protein-related receptors as well as one ion channel receptor. The orbitofrontal cortex serotonin-related circuitry has been associated with regulation of inhibition, self-control, and emotional regulation [51]. Important in the modulation of not only inhibition but also memory and learning, these processes occur through the activity of receptor stimulation on pyramidal cells, dendritic shafts, and interneurons [52].

Acetylcholine

Acetylcholine also modulates working memory, cognitive flexibility, and learning, mediated through five muscarinic receptors (M1–M5), all of which are G-protein linked and nicotinic receptors that are ligand-gated ion channels. In turn, these mediate excitatory and inhibitory influences on pyramidal cells and GABA interneurons. Among humans and great apes, varicosities exist on Ach axons that are thought to be related to cortical plasticity, with a phenotypic expression of advanced attributes including innovative tool manufacture, social learning, and self-awareness [53,54].

Molecular Connectivity and Increasing Complexity of Neurons

Synapses pre-dated neuronal evolution, and synaptic complexity arose before neurons [55]. Synaptic scaffolding evolution was likely the first step in upgrading vertebrate complexity, with postulated mechanisms being genome duplication about 550 mya. Genome duplications were a mechanism for phenotypic innovation among earlier life forms such as plants, fungi, and vertebrates. Another postulated mechanism is the upgrading of postsynaptic genes and signaling proteins in early vertebrates, which occurred prior to any brain expansion among these early animals. Support for this premise comes from genes that support elementary learning mechanisms related to Dlg genes. The conservation of Dlg2 function for over 100 million years and its role in cognition, in both mice and humans, with their genetic common ancestor divergence ~90 mya underscores the importance of signaling proteins and synapses. During this period a 1000-fold difference in brain size occurred [56].

Pyramidal cells make up approximately 70 percent of the cortical neurons. Among primates, they are more spinous in the frontal lobes. In humans, the pyramidal cells of the granular prefrontal cortex are more spinous than in the baboon and vervet monkey by a factor of three and ~70 percent more spinous in comparison to those in the macaque [57].

Evolution of Higher Bandwidth Synapses in Humans

Information processing and storage in the human brain is dependent on pyramidal cell firing, synaptic transmission, and the plasticity of neuronal circuitry. Compared to rodent brains, human pyramidal cell information transfer is greater by a factor of 4–9-fold, with frequencies measured in the beta and gamma range. Sensory synaptic features that process temporal data were also conveyed at wider bandwidth in humans compared to rodents. A human feature of "fast recovering synapses" augments the information transfer during spike trains. Human pyramidal cells also have the capability of encoding higher synaptic information quantities. Together, these and probably other features have enabled human cerebral microcircuits to transmit information at overall "wider bandwidths" in comparison to the rodent microcircuitry [58].

Brief Genetic Insights into Human Evolution

DNA differences are miniscule between modern humans and Neanderthals, our closest extinct relative, with our genome 99.8 percent the same. Even with chimpanzees, our closest extant relative, our genomes differ by a mere 1 percent. Within these small differences some features are explained, such as the mutation pertaining to melanocortin 1 receptor gene coding for pale skin and red hair, and a gene related to language development, the FOXP2 gene which is common to modern humans and Neanderthals but does not occur in the chimpanzee. The mechanisms of switching certain genes on or off by epigenetic mechanisms explains more of our differences. Epigenetic mechanisms, including methylation, may repress or silence genes, as with HOXD in humans that was concerned with limb development. With over 500–1000 mitochondria in each of our cells, mitochondrial genetics has also been very illuminating in explaining genetic origins differences [59]. Arguably the most dramatic mitochondrial genetic story was that of Cann and Wilson, pointing to our common origins in Africa dating to ~150 kya – what has been popularized as Mitochondrial Eve [60]. Later confirmatory findings with the Y chromosome by Underhill and Cavalli-Sforza – sometimes referred to as Y chromosome Adam – pointed to a similar date supporting the genetic bottleneck triggered by a presumed environmental catastrophe that simultaneously affected both genetic mechanisms [61]. Among modern humans, base-pair variation is approximately 1 in 1000, translating into a 99.9 percent genetic congruence, which differs in many other animals, including the chimpanzee, with threefold more variance than in modern humans. The mitochondrial DNA and Y chromosome studies were important in that they pointed to the common human ancestor, to an exceedingly brief 150 kya, which is pithy in an evolutionary sense. The time period is too short for an appreciable amount of variation through mutation to have occurred, and the variation noted to date has not been correlated with race. If the basis of race were to be skin color, the white skin under the fur of chimpanzees and the relatively pale skin of the oldest clan on the planet, the San, counter such a basis. Skin color is of course entirely based on the latitude of one's residence, which influences the amount of melanin made in the skin in response to UV light, which controls how much vitamin D_3 is made [62]. In agreement with Watson, that as no significant genetic differences have been noted in people discerned as different "races," the evolutionary biological reasoning follows that societies might consider excluding such categorization altogether [59].

Despite these caveats, there have been impressive "genetic engineering" feats such as the CRISPR (clustered regularly interspaced short palindromic repeats) methodologies. Termed a kind of gene editing tool, a customized RNA molecule is used that incorporates a bacterial nuclease such as Cas, which singles out a DNA sequence, usually a mutation, and restores it with a mending patch [63].

Epigenetic Mechanisms and Evolution of the Mind

In addition to genetic drivers, various epigenetic-based mechanisms shaped evolution and the human mind. Epigenetic "switches" affect gene regulation as well as behavior and are mostly reversible. This is nowadays generally regarded as the process linking nature and nurture in the evolution of biological systems. Epigenetics incurs a change in gene expression without altering DNA sequences. Furthermore, transgenerational epigenetics is a process that can extend beyond a person's lifetime, such as may occur from a parent to their children. The neurobiological mechanisms are via DNA methylation, histone acetylation, and micro-RNA interference [64]. Epigenetics interject additional sources of variation among biological systems. The process of evolution can proceed through the epigenetic arena of hereditary mechanisms in the absence of genetic sequence alteration. Epigenetic variation also occurs at a much higher rate and is more responsive to environmental factors, such as climate and nutritional drivers, that may induce several epigenetic variations simultaneously. Together the higher-frequency generation of epigenetic mechanisms and that the change is more likely to be appropriate, in terms of adaptiveness, result in a more rapid adaptation by the organism.

Among the different epigenetic mechanisms are included memory of gene activity (one cell has genes turned on another has the genes turned off) and structural inheritance. In the latter the architecture of the cell rather than gene activity mediates the effect – an example being prion proteins. These have an abnormal three-dimensional configuration causing fatal diseases such as Creutzfeldt–Jakob and mad cow disease. Chromatin-marking systems affect the relationship of DNA with its associated histone protein. DNA is entwined around the histone protein; methylation by adding methyl (CH_3) groups and acetylation, for example, may slacken the chromatin structure rendering it more liable to be transcribed. Another mechanism is gene silencing. Small, interfering RNA molecules termed siRNAs may silence genes, with one mechanism being the Dicer enzyme that severs RNA into pieces. These can then be amplified, suppress messenger RNA (mRNA), and can migrate between cells within the body. The siRNA can also be associated with the gene from which it was derived and form enduring stable methylation or chromatin marks that can be transmitted to succeeding cell generations.

One of the roles that the RNAi system accomplishes is a type of cellular immune system. This is a type of intracellular defense mechanism for cells against viruses and so-called genomic parasites, also termed jumping genes or transposons, both of which generally generate double-stranded RNA. MicroRNAs (miRNA) are able to selectively inactivate genes by incorporating them into cells, and provide revolutionary tools for combating viral diseases – HIV and poliovirus being recent examples.

Behavioral inheritance may be transmitted to the offspring by substances impacting behavior, imitation-type learning, and social learning that is not imitative. An example of substances steering behavior include food preferences acquired through smell and taste characteristics of the mother while in the womb and later during breastfeeding. Imitative learning can be vocal or motor. Vocal imitative learning is common among birds, dolphins, primates, and rodents. Motor imitative learning is much rarer in these species and more common among humans.

Symbolic behavior refers to the processing of information and transfer of information, which is likely unique to humans, prompting Ernst Cassirer to refer to humans as "symbolic animals" [65]. He conceived of a neural system that, between receiving information and effecting action, has a third component that he referred to as the symbolic system. Jablonka and Lamb have proposed that genetic and even epigenetics are not the only drivers of evolution, but include the behavioral and symbolic systems and that evolution occurs in four dimensions [66].

Our Superior Information Processing and Working Memory Functions

The evolutionary history of our brain, literally honed by fire, ice, and environmental adversity, has endowed us with our 1350 cc brain, commonly referred to as the most intricate entity within our known universe. Our relatively large brain – with its expansive connectome measuring ~150 000 km of fibers – requires disproportionate amounts of energy. The downside is that an "Achilles heel" condition has made us prone to human-specific conditions such as degenerative (Alzheimer's, frontotemporal dementias) and developmental (schizophrenia, autism) disease. With larger brains also come more synapses per neuron and disproportionately more fiber tracts, which become metabolically more extortionate. The majority of the energetic costs are incurred by synaptic signaling and maintaining neuronal electrochemical gradients.

Endeavors to correlate degrees of animal and human intelligence with absolute and relative brain size, corrected for body size, have yielded large inconsistencies. Often regarded as the most intelligent mammals, primates and humans do not have the largest brains in absolute or relative terms. At the present time, perhaps the most accurate manner for deciphering the relation between degrees of intelligence and brain traits among mammals may be achieved by the combination of several factors. These include the overall number of cortical neurons, interneuronal distance, neuron packing density, and axon conduction velocity. These are traits that correlate with information-processing capacity (IPC), which may be seen as a marker or surrogate of general intelligence. Although the pinnacle of known IPCs is generally considered to be the human IPC, with great apes and elephants next, the IPC of cetaceans and pinnipeds is probably even higher. Cetacean brain macro- and microanatomy components differ in several respects from humans. In a similar sense, corvid and psittacid birds also have differing anatomical features to humans by having relatively small and densely packed pallial neurons and more numerous neurons, notwithstanding their particularly small brain volumes. These features may explain their superior intelligence. Referred to as an intelligence amplifier, language evolution, with its syntactical and grammatical elements in humans, may well have occurred in an analogous manner among songbirds and psittacids, termed "convergent evolution" [67].

The Importance of Information Acquisition and its Method

Information acquisition, as well as the method of acquisition, is a key evolutionary attainment by humans. Although it has been conjectured that we might well be at both the physical and physiological limits of brain size and processing speed, this remains debatable. The fundamental impediments include basic physics laws and interneuronal communication capacity [68]. The importance of these tenets are the observations that intellectual performance and functional brain network efficiency are correlated. Resting-state connectivity, as for example the default mode network efficiency, is predictive of cognitive potential. In essence, overall intellectual performance is correlated with how efficiently our brains integrate and assimilate information from several different brain regions [69]. This has important evolution-based consequences. The more rapidly a specific type of environmental information can be processed by an animal as a function of time, the higher is the chance of survival or success of a chosen course of action. This is also dependent on how rapidly information processing can occur with respect to consulting laid down long-term memory stores that may influence decision-making with regard to a particular challenge.

It should therefore come as no surprise that we have an inherent drive for knowledge acquisition. The impelling link with the hedonic reward circuitry of the brain underscores the importance of this attribute. For example, reading is a widespread leisure activity that may be reflective of this drive within us [70]. The manner of acquiring information, though, is also important. Merely perusing novelty information, as is common with surfing the web and other electronic means, leads to diversive curiosity. Integrating knowledge with that which is already present in the brain is termed epistemic knowledge, which is fueled by curiosity. This process involves more expansive brain circuitry that is engaged and transmodally available [71,72]. It may be obvious that with more knowledge and information, as we have in our current environment, the more likely we are to make a more beneficial decision. Astrophysical, geological, climatological, and biological factors forged our brains and bodies in a specific manner. We are predestined to conform to this legacy and live our lives accordingly.

References

1. Brown-Sequard CE. Séance du 18 decembre. *CR Soc Biol* 1875;424.

2. Lieberman P. Synapses, language and being human. *Science* 2013;342:944–945.

3. Saxena S, Caroni P. Selective neuronal vulnerability in neurodegenerative disease: from stressor thresholds to degeneration. *Neuron* 2011;71:35–48.

4. Crossley NA, Mechelli A, Scott J, et al. The hubs of the human connectome are generally implicated in the anatomy of brain disorders. *Brain* 2014;137:2382–2395.

5. Liu X, Li G, Xiong S, et al. Hierarchical alteration of brain structural and functional networks in female migraine sufferers. *PLoS One* 2012;7:e51250.

6. Buckner RL, Sepulchre J, Talukdar T, et al. Cortical hubs revealed by intrinsic functional connectivity: mapping, assessment of stability and relation to Alzheimer's disease. *J Neurosci* 2009;29:1860–1873.

7. Seeley WW, Menon V, Schatzberg AF, et al. Dissociable intrinsic connectivity networks for salience processing and executive control. *J Neurosci* 2007;27:2349–2356.

8. Han K, MacDonald CL, Johnson AM, et al. Disrupted modular organization

of resting state cortical functional connectivity in US military personnel following concussive "mild" blast related traumatic brain injury. *Neuroimage* 2014;84:76–96.

9. Achard S, Delon-Martin C, Vértes PE, et al. Hubs of brain functional networks are radically reorganized in comatose patients. *PNAS* 2012;109:20608–20613.

10. Rosanova M, Gosseries O, Casarotto S, et al. Recovery of cortical effective connectivity and recovery of consciousness in vegetative patients. *Brain* 2012;135:1308–1320.

11. Stam CJ. Modern network science of neurological disorders. *Nat Rev Neurosci* 2014;15:683–695.

12. Bruner E, Jacobs HI. Alzheimer's disease: the downside of a highly evolved parietal lobe? *J Alzheimers Dis* 2013;35(2):227–240.

13. Attwell D, Laughlin SB. An energy budget for signaling in the grey matter of the brain. *J Cereb Blood Flow Metab* 2001;21:1133–1145.

14. Zimmerman M. The nervous system in the context of information theory. In Schmidt RF, Thews G (eds.), *Human Physiology*. Springer, Berlin, 1989.

15. Hassin RR, Uleman JS, Bargh JA. *The New Unconscious*. Oxford University Press, Oxford, 2005.

16. Libet B, Gleason CA, Wright EW, Pearl DK. Time of conscious intention to act in relation to onset of cerebral activity (readiness potential): the unconscious initiation of a freely voluntary act. *Brain* 1983;106:623–642.

17. Squire L, Berg D, Bloom FE, et al. Gliotransmission. In *Fundamental Neuroscience*. Elsevier, Amsterdam, 2012.

18. Diamond MC, Scheibel AB, Murphy GM Jr, Harvey T. On the brain of a scientist: Albert Einstein. *Exp Neurol* 1985;88(1):198–204.

19. Falk D. New information about Albert Einstein's brain. *Front Evol Neurosci* 2009;1:3.

20. Oberheim NA, Takano T, Han X, et al. Uniquely hominid features of adult human astrocytes. *J Neurosci* 2009;29(10):3276.

21. Han X, Chen M, Wang F, et al. Forebrain engraftment by human glial progenitor cells enhances synaptic plasticity and learning in adult mice. *Cell Stem Cell* 2013;12:342–353.

22. Tremblay ME, Lowery AL, Majewska AK. Microglial interactions with synapses are modulated by visual experience. *Commun Integr Biol* 2011;4:220–222.

23. Lennie P. The cost of cortical computation. *Curr Biol* 2003;13:493–497.

24. Sherwood CC, Stimpson CD, Raghanti MA, et al. Evolution of increased glia–neuron ratios in the human frontal cortex. *PNAS* 2006;103:13606–13611.

25. Oberheim NA, Wang X, Goldman S, Nedergaard M. Astrocyte complexity distinguishes the human brain. *Trends Neurosci* 2006;29:547–553.

26. Ricci G, Volpi L, Pasquali L, Petrozzi L, Siciliano G. Astrocyte–neuron interactions in neurological disorders. *J Biol Phys* 2009;35:317–336.

27. Arnold WH, von Zieten P, Schmidt E. Measurements of postnatal growth of the skull of *Pan troglodytes verus* using lateral cephalograms. *Anthropol Anz* 2003;61:190–132.

28. Bruner E, Preuss TM, Chen X, Rilling JK. Evidence for expansion of the precuneus in human evolution. *Brain Struct Funct* 2017;222(2):1053–1060.

29. Semendeferi K, Armstrong E, Schleicher A, Zilles K, Van Hoesen GW. Limbic frontal cortex in hominoids: a comparative study of area 13. *Am J Phys Anthropol* 1998;106:129–155.

30. Semendeferi K, Armstrong E, Schleicher A, Zilles K, Van Hoesen GW. Prefrontal cortex in humans and apes: a comparative study of area 10. *Am J Phys Anthropol* 2001;114:224–241.

31. Hof PR, Mufson EJ, Morrison JH. Human orbitofrontal cortex: cytoarchitecture and quantitative immuno-histochemical

parcellation. *J Comp Neurol* 1995;359: 48–68.

32. Kim EJ, Sidhu M, Gaus SE, et al. Selective frontoinsular von Economo neuron and fork cell loss in early behavioral variant frontotemporal dementia. *Cerebral Cortex* 2012;22:251–259.

33. Allman JM, Tetreault NA, Hakeem AY, Park S. The von Economo neurons in apes and humans. *Am J Hum Biol* 2011;23(1):5–21.

34. Hof PR, Van Der Gucht E. Structure of the cerebral cortex of the humpback whale, *Megaptera novaeangeliae. Anat Record A Discov Mol Cell Evol Biol* 2007;290:1–31.

35. Schenker N, Desgouttes AM, Semendeferi K. Neural connectivity and cortical substrates of cognition in hominoids. *J Hum Evol* 2005;49:547–569.

36. Schumann C, Amaral DG. Stereological estimation of the number of neurons in the human amygdaloid complex. *J Comp Neurol* 2005;491:320–329.

37. Barton RA, Aggleton JP, Grenyer R. Evolutionary coherence of the mammalian amygdala. *Proc Biol Sci* 2003;270:539–543.

38. Brothers L. The social brain: a project for integrating primate behavior and neurophysiology in a new domain. *Concepts Neurosci* 1990;1:27–51.

39. Bargar N, Stefanacci L, Semendeferi K. A comparative volumetric analysis of amygdaloid complex and basolateral division in the human and ape brain. *Am J Phys Anthropol* 2007;134:392–403.

40. Subiaul F. Mosaic cognitive evolution: the case of imitation behavior. In: Broadfield D, Yuan M, Schick K, Toth N (eds.), *The Human Brain Evolving.* Stone Age Institute Press, Gosport, IN, 2010.

41. Passinghim RE, Stephan KE, Kotter R. The anatomical basis of functional localization in the cortex. *Nat Rev Neurosci* 2002;3:606–616.

42. Willamson PC, Allman JM. *The Human Illnesses: Neuropsychiatric Disorders and the Nature of the Human Brain.* Oxford University Press, Oxford, 2011.

43. Previc FH. Dopamine and the origin of human intelligence. *Brain Cogn* 1999;41:299–350.

44. Coppens Y. East Side Story: the origin of humankind. *Scientific American,* May 1994: 88–95.

45. Bortz WM II. Physical exercise as an evolutionary force. *J Hum Evol* 1985;14:145–155.

46. Carrier DR. The energetic paradox of human running and hominid evolution. *Curr Anthropol* 1984;25:483–495.

47. Leonard WR, Robertson MS. Comparative primate energetics and hominid evolution. *Am J Phys Anthropol* 1997;102:265–281.

48. Raghanti MA, Stimpson CD, Erwien JM, Hof PR, Sherwood CC. Cortical dopaminergic innervation of the frontal cortex: differences among humans, chimpanzees and macaque monkeys. *Neuroscience* 2008;155:203–220.

49. Berger B, Gaspar P, Verney C. Dopaminergic innervation of the cerebral cortex: unexpected differences between rodents and primates. *Trends Neurosci* 1991;14:21–27.

50. Lewis DA, Melchitzky DS, Sesack SR, et al. Dopamine transporter immunoreactivity in monkey cerebral cortex: regional, laminar and ultrastructural organization. *J Comp Neurol* 2001;432:119–136.

51. Soubrie P. Reconciling the role of central serotonin neurons in human and animal behavior. *Behav Brain Sci* 1986;9:319–364.

52. Jakab RL, Goldman Rakic PS. Segregation of serotonin 5HT 2A and 5HT 3 receptors in inhibitory circuits in the primate cerebral cortex. *J Comp Neurol* 2000;417:337–348.

53. Sarter M, Parikh V. Choline transporters, cholinergic transmission and cognition. *Nat Rev Neurosci* 2005;6:48–56.

54. Levin ED, Simon BB. Nicotinic acetylcholine involvement in cognitive function in animals. *Psychopharmacology* 1998;138:217–230.

55. Ryan TJ, Grant SGN. The origin and evolution of synapses. *Nat Rev Neurosci* 2009;10:701–712.

56. Nithianandharajah J, Komiyama NH, McKechanie A, et al. Synaptic scaffold evolution generated components of vertebrate cognitive complexity. *Nat Neurosci* 2013;16(1):16–24.

57. Elston GN, Benavides-Piccione R, Elston A, et al. Specializations of the granular prefrontal cortex of primates: implications for cognitive processing. *Anat Record A Discov Mol Cell Evol Biol* 2006;288A:26–35.

58. Testa-Silva G, Verhoog MG, Linaro D, et al. High bandwidth synaptic communication and frequency tracking in human neocortex. *PLoS Biology* 2014;12(11):e1002007.

59. Watson J. *DNA: The Story of the Genetic Revolution*. Knopf, New York, 2017.

60. Cann RL, Brown WM, Wilson AC. Evolution of human mitochondrial DNA: a preliminary report. *Prog Clin Biol Res* 1982;103:157–165.

61. Underhill PA, Shen P, Lin AA, et al. Y chromosome sequence variation and the history of human populations. *Nat Genet* 2000;26:358–361.

62. Crawford NG, Kelly DE, Hansen EG, et al. Loci associated with skin pigmentation identified in African populations. *Science* 2017. doi: 10.1126/science.aan8433.

63. Jinek M, Chylinski K, Fonfara I, et al. A programmable dual-RNA-guided DNA endonuclease in adaptive bacterial immunity. *Science* 2012;337:816–821.

64. Carey N. *The Epigenetics Revolution.* Columbia University Press, New York, 2012.

65. Cassirer E. *Essay on Man.* Yale University Press, New Haven, CT, 1944.

66. Jablonka E, Lamb MJ. *Evolution in Four Dimensions.* MIT Press, Cambridge MA, 2014.

67. Dicke U, Roth G. Neuronal factors determining high intelligence. *Philos Trans R Soc Lond B Biol Sci* 2016;371(1685):20150180.

68. Fox D. The limits of intelligence. *Scientific American* July 2011:36–43.

69. Van den Heuvel MP, Stam CJ, Kahn RS, Hulshoff Pol HE. Efficiency of functional brain networks and intellectual performance. *J Neurosci* 2009;29:7619–7624.

70. Kringelbach MI, Vuust P, Geake J. The pleasure of reading. *Interdiscip Sci Rev* 2008;33:321–333.

71. Berlyne DE. Uncertainty and epistemic curiosity. *Br J Psychol* 1962;53:27–34.

72. Leslie I. *Curious: The Desire to Know and Why your Future Depends on It.* Basic Books, New York, 2014.

The Core Frontal Systems

Chapter 5

Primate tree living honed sensorimotor locomotor abilities and the expansive frontoparietal networks. Based on these large-scale networks, the major cognitive abilities such as working memory capability and the mirror neuron system were forged over time. Other critical networks developed during primate and human frontal lobe development, such as the inhibitory systems that brake the mirror neuron copying systems. The mirror neuron system enabled a theory of mind capability important in social interactions from which mentalizing and empathy evolved. By about 500 kya, the frontal lobes had reached the modern size, as exemplified by southern African *Homo heidelbergensis*, Saldahna man and Kabwe man.

Overall frontal lobe size increases in mammalian species from rodents upwards, increasing further in size in species such as cats and dogs and becoming largest among primates and hominoids. The increase, however, is in an allometric (the study of body size increase and shape or biological scaling) manner [1]. Although the overall frontal lobe size is not proportionally greater in humans when compared to the great apes, the region termed the prefrontal cortex is relatively larger compared to other primates.

However, the frontopolar cortex (BA 10) is proportionally larger and the BA 13 is proportionally smaller in humans compared to apes [2]. In humans, the frontal lobes occupy ~37–39 percent of the cerebral cortical area and are connected reciprocally to all other brain regions [3,4]. Other important differences in human brains with respect to other mammals include hemispheric asymmetry and what has been termed cerebral torque, wherein the right frontal and left occipital are enlarged (petalias). In addition, connectivity reorganization, neuropil reorganization, and progressive sophistication of neurotransmitters and receptors continued in our lineage [5]. Granular prefrontal cortical areas appeared among early primates ~65 mya. Microscopically, the proliferation of the granular cortex is defined by the appearance of the distinctive layer four of the cerebral cortex association areas of the prefrontal, temporal and parietal cortices and is regarded as a defining characteristic of *Homo sapiens*. Specifically, the prefrontal granular cortex expanded within humans and is key for executive function abilities. The granular layer four receives largely afferents from the thalamus and is the place where extensive intracortical connectivity occurs. Furthermore, human prefrontal cortex (PFC) pyramidal cells have additional branching and greater spine density in comparison to temporal, occipital, and parietal cortices. The PFC layer three has been documented to have as many as 61 spines per 10 μm. In comparison to the homologous macaque cortical region, the human layer three is 23-fold more spinous [1]. The tertiary association cortices of the PFC, parietal, and inferotemporal neuronal discharge activity from cells with numerous spines have been shown to be tonic rather than phasic discharge associated with primary cortical visual area V1, for example. Persistent firing of neurons in a so-called delay period between stimulus and activity is regarded as the neurobiological basis of holding a memory, sound, or activity by the PFC that can endure even when distractors are applied. Also termed working memory or working attention, this is seen to underlie core frontal functions, and the surge of pyramidal cell complexity and increase in spinous pyramidal cells occurred in the PFC during hominin evolution [6–8].

Passingham and Wise advanced a comprehensive treatise of primate frontal evolution with specific reference to the frontal cortical subcomponents having evolved in stages. This perhaps explains part of the phenomenon of frontal syndromes with fractionated frontal sub-syndromes. There may be a dissonance, for example, with markedly deficient social behavior while scoring normal on neuropsychological cognitive scores in people with frontotemporal lobe dementia syndromes, for example. The initial areas of development, as noted, were the granular caudal PFC and the frontal eye fields (BA 8) and orbital prefrontal cortical region (BA 11, 13, 14). Subsequent, additional prefrontal granular cortical areas developed, including the mid-lateral PFC (BA 46 and 9), the dorsomedial PFC (BA 12, 44, 45, and 47), the ventromedial PFC (BA 11, 13, 14, 25, and 32), and the polar PFC (BA 10) [9]. This occurred with the development of the internal granular layer (layer four) of the cerebral cortex in an approximate caudal to rostral (from the back to the front) progression. At a microscopic level this was associated with an increase in the density of cells occupying this stratum. When above a certain density threshold, it is termed granular as opposed to being agranular. This elaboration is associated with increased connectivity and expansion is seen to occur as one progresses from monkeys to humans [10]. The dorsal PFC, ventral PFC, and polar PFC allowed primates to use adaptive responses and advantages in relation to their major adversities, chiefly climate, food availability, and primate societal relationships. In essence, these frontal regions facilitated overall error reduction in their responses to their environmental challenges [11].

The prefrontal subcomponents have distinctive behavioral attributes, with the caudal PFC and frontal eye field (BA 8) regions promoting object search by virtue of harnessing attention and eye orientation, while the OPFC mediates designation of value to items. The caudal PFC/frontal eye field unit connects to both ventral and dorsal visual radiations from the posterior cortex, as well as to the brainstem motor eye movement nuclei, that form part of the cranial nerves 3, 4, and 6. The medial prefrontal cortex (MPFC) subserves action choice that is based on previous experiences and outcomes. Such behavior is mediated by hippocampal connections and amygdala for prior events, and connections to the medial premotor cortex for subsequent action. The MPFC allows choice and action independent of external sensory stimuli and differs from the OPFC, which enables action in response to external stimuli. The extensive dorsolateral prefrontal cortex (DLPFC) connections with the orbital prefrontal cortex (OPFC), premotor cortex, hippocampus, and posterior parietal cortex allows integration of all the preprocessed information from these and other prefrontal areas, for eventual action output via the premotor and motor cortices. Visual (inferior temporal) and acoustic (superior temporal) inputs relay into the ventrolateral prefrontal cortex (VLPFC) for decisions based on combined visual and acoustic sources [11]. The frontopolar cortex (FPC) (subregions 10 p frontal pole, 10 r and 10 m medially) is the most elaborated of all the PFC subcomponents in humans compared to extant apes, occupying the largest area at 28 000 mm³ with ~500 million neurons. Despite the neuron number, the neuronal density is relatively decreased. Furthermore, dendritic spines and density counts are higher compared to other PFC areas. Importantly, for developing humans, the FPC develops relatively late in life, often in the fourth decade as maturation of dendritic spines is protracted [12–14]. Metacognition or self-reflection is considered to be an important component of the FPC region. Other higher cortical function attributes of the FPC include episodic memory, multitasking, relational integration, self-referential evaluation, and introspection [15,16]. The net result of the sophisticated PFC subcomponent evolution was key for evolving hominoids, allowing fewer errors through imitation of others, engaging in mental time travel, and imaging actions before actual engagement of actions. Archeological evidence from several skulls, including the Bodo skull from Ethiopia (~600 kya), the Kabwe skull from Zambia (~300 kya), and Saldahna man from South Africa, shows that, although having large brow ridges, the slope of the inner frontal brain case is not significantly different from that of modern humans [17]. This implies that their frontal lobes had reached modern *Homo sapiens* size and shape by ~600–300 kya. This may be considered relatively early in the history of our evolution and long before the cultural evolution dated to 70–50 kya [18].

Ventral and Dorsal Premotor Cortices

Among earlier primates, the ventral premotor cortex (VPMC) connected to corticospinal projections to the seventh nerve facial nucleus and upper cervical spinal cord segments. These projections subserved facial motility; facial expression refined motor control of the mouth, head, and arm-reaching movements. The dorsal premotor cortex (DPMC) pre-supplementary motor area (pre-SMA) incorporated leg control [19]. Taken together these provided us with phenotype variations today including:

- working memory
- initiation
- disinhibition
- attention
- monitoring
- emotional control

Working Memory

Working memory is also referred to as short-term memory, measured in seconds to minutes and allowing mental processing of information such as occurs with manipulating numbers, constructing a sentence, or just mere thoughts. This differs from episodic memory, which is measured in minutes (episodic short term) to many years (episodic long term). Hence working memory has been likened to the brain's operating system that is integral to the core frontal lobe functions of attention, disinhibition, and initiation. The expansive working memory circuitry comprises a frontal, temporal, parietal, and subcortical network. A fundamental assignment of the PFC is working memory or the physiological process of monitoring information or items while engaging in further computation as the information is being held "online" [20,21]. The evolution of these abilities is relatively specific to primates; non-primate mammals seem either to lack this ability or have more rudimentary abilities in this regard.

Such statements, though, are prone to modification as rodents are able to learn the radial maze task, which suggests they have the ability to remember and monitor information at the same time. Several investigators in addition to Baddeley have come up with terms for these PFC processes. In addition to Baddeley's working memory [22], Dehaene's global workspace and Duncan's multiple-demand theories have been proposed [23]. These theories all define roles for both the PFC and posterior parietal cortex and that both cortical regions contribute to working memory.

Intraneuronal recordings have implicated the DLPFC (BA 46 and 9) activity during the delay period in support of the cellular basis of sustaining information for ultimate action planning. The monitoring component (such as tracking an important stimulus) of this process has been attributed to the mid-DLPFC and the posterior parietal regions. The posterior parietal area is involved with the further manipulation of the information being held online, also referred to as the epoptic process by Petrides [20]. The maintenance-of-information component of working memory circuitry is within the superior temporal gyrus for auditory information and the inferotemporal cortex for faces and items. The posterior parietal region, for example, contains circuitry permitting the processing of information required for arithmetic functions and mental rotation of objects (PFC BA 46 axons connecting to layers 1–3 of the intraparietal sulcus). The mid-DLPFC is required for monitoring information, during which time further processing or manipulation of such information is being done [24,25] (see Figure 3.7). The retrieval of memories is accomplished by the mid-ventrolateral PFC (VLPFC) and differs from maintenance of information of working memory [21,26].

The process of working memory evolution has been envisaged by Read and Diamond as on a scale of 1–7, with chimpanzees having acquired level 2 compared to modern humans at a level 7 working memory capacity [27,28] (see Figure 3.6). These studies of chimpanzee short-term memory capacity assigned a level 2, possibly 3, that was based on nut cracking, gestures, and object manipulation studies. Chimpanzees are able to coordinate manipulation of two objects or items (rarely three) by three years of age. Examples include Congo basic chimpanzees termite foraging with "fishing sticks." Human infant short-term working memory capacity growth trajectories differed markedly in comparison to those of chimpanzees in the 7–144 months age period. These studies corroborate archeological data of working memory capacity with the common ancestor of hominins (working memory level 7) and *Pan* (working memory level 2–3) [27].

Working Memory as a "Missing Link"

Working memory may be considered a "missing link" in early modern humans, sparking the cultural evolution of creativity, language, and visual art development. The elaboration of working memory evolution based on the extensive frontoparietal circuitry, and subsequently the advent of what has been termed by Wynne and Coolidge as enhanced working memory (EWM), may be regarded as a major cognitive watershed in human evolution. EWM evolved around 200 and 40 kya and will be elaborated on further in Chapter 6 [29]. Neuroplasticity capabilities and evolution of the tertiary association cortices would serve as the basis of more sophisticated human abilities such as advanced tool-making, visual art forms, and language, which included the component of recursion [30].

Working memory functions and manifestations of disorders are recognized in regard to multitasking, planning for the future, engaging in abstract thoughts, and retaining verbal and nonverbal information for further processing. Some of these are often referred to as executive functions, including sustained attention to allow the temporal organization of behavior. These may be summarized to involve task setting, task initiation, monitoring of the motor activity, the detection of possible errors, and the facilitation of self-regulation [31]. The neural circuitry that underlies these functions includes the frontal subcortical circuits: the left DLPFC (task setting), right DLPFC (monitoring and error detection), bilateral superior medial frontal circuits (initiation of the task), and medial orbital frontal cortex (OFC) (regulation of behavior) [32].

Initiation

The intention to act is perhaps easier to understand when deficient. Various terms such as abulia, lack of conation (Latin: conatus – natural tendency to strive toward or have directed effort), or cerebral torpor have been used. In clinical neurology, the spectrum of behaviors ranges from akinetic mutism to abulia, with lesser forms termed hypobulia, apathy, and alexithymia. These denote the various degrees from no movement to some movement. Alexithymia refers to an inability to identify and describe one's own emotions. Such syndromes may form part of any neurological disorder, most commonly after stroke and recognized with schizophrenia. In the latter, the avolitional component is a core feature, and anhedonia, asociality, and alogia are part of the clinical manifestations of the primary avolitional deficit [33]. Additionally, the loss of creativity, emotion, initiative, and curiosity may be manifest [34].

Abulia may underlie a number of behavioral disorders, including episodic dysmemory, which is in turn ascribed to inattention as well as impaired registration and poor retrieval, and self-neglect. In its severest form it can present as senile squalor syndrome. In addition, lack of empathy and emotional flatness represent distressing behaviors for family and friends, and ritualistic and stereotyped behavior may take the form of various repetitive activities such as feasting on the same foods, humming, foot tapping, grunting, clock watching, and punding (extended stereotyped, purposeless behaviors). The cause of abulia is important and may present with coma and akinetic mutism that are usually viewed as portending a grave prognosis. Indeed, that was the case with two examples, both young women with similar tegmentothalamic lesions, one with deep venous system thrombosis post-partum and the other secondary to viral encephalitis or *Mycoplasma pneumonia*. Both recovered well to complete functionality (Figure 5.1). Viral encephalitis causing transient coma, and tegmentothalamic lesions with good recovery, have also been reported several times by other investigators as due to different organisms [35].

Disinhibition

Disinhibition may manifest with impulsivity, socially inappropriate behavior, and abnormal eating behaviors, and affect the extensive mirror neuron network disruption, causing a wide array of field-dependent behaviors. The latter may be more elementary, such as imitation behavior, or more complex forms (discussed under the section on mirror neuron circuit disruption) [36].

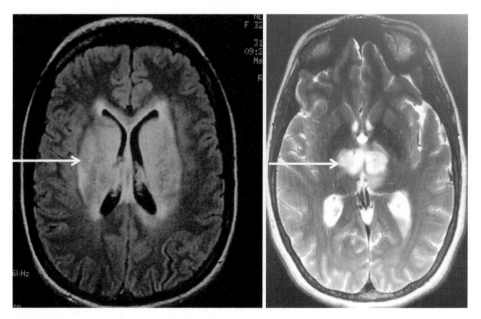

Figure 5.1 Athymhormia spectrum disorders: akinetic mutism, abulia, hypobulia, apathy. Two different processes causing coma and akinetic mutism in young women due to bilateral tegmentothalamic lesions. Akinetic mutism secondary to deep venous system thrombosis postpartum (arrows). Right image due to encephalitis presumed *Mycoplasma pneumonia* related (arrows). Both recovered to good functionality.

Attention

Attention is a fundamental brain function that is mediated by cerebral networks for alertness and arousal. Attention differs from working memory in that it allows a specific stimulus, whether sensory or cognitive in nature, to be given priority or preference over and above other competing stimuli. Working memory enables the maintenance of certain limited information for a few seconds to minutes, at most, for the further processing or manipulation of that retained information. Attention is commonly considered as one of the following:

- sustained attention: maintenance of consistent behavior in the context of repetitive or continuous activity;
- focused attention: responding to specific auditory, tactile, or visual stimuli;
- selective attention: maintenance of the behavioral response in the face of competing or distracting stimuli;
- divided attention: being able to respond concurrently to several tasks;
- alternating attention: the ability to vary the focus of attention and navigate between tasks, also termed mental flexibility [32,37].

Monitoring

Monitoring of intended actions is largely within the frontopolar cortex domain and will be discussed in more depth under the relevant section. Clinical syndromes seen when "monitoring" is impaired include perseveration and impersistence. Perseveration refers to the repetition of an action, response, or speech when the inciting stimulus has ceased or is no longer appropriate. Impersistence is a kind of opposite response and denotes an inability to sustain a specific movement, action, or speech function as per the request or instruction.

Emotional Control

Emotional control is mediated by the orbitofrontal cortex, medial frontal regions, and anterior temporal regions, which are the part of the neural network concerned with emotional responses, including both cognitive and affective empathy. The neurobiological emotional network proposed by Pessoa et al. has been expanded considerably to include these cortical areas in addition to the traditional components of the amygdala, hypothalamus, brainstem, hippocampus, septum, and anterior and posterior cingulate gyri [38,39].

Frontopolar Cortex

Situated in the most anterior part of the human brain, the frontopolar cortex (FPC) or Brodmann's area 10 is an example of one of relatively few brain areas that is strikingly enlarged, allometrically expanded, in humans in comparison to our closest extant primate relatives [40]. The FPC functions may be regarded as the most apical human cognitive abilities. The core abilities include the simultaneous consideration of several competing tasks or options in order to achieve the most favorable output selection. Another function of the FPC is in alternating between external and internally derived thoughts. These functions have been gleaned from functional magnetic resonance imaging research, as well as from frontal lobe clinical lesion studies [41,42].

Cognitive, Behavioral, and Motor Syndromes as Reflections of Evolutionary Connectomal Neurobiology

Cognitive, behavioral, and motor syndromes may be recognized that reflect the evolutionary connectomal neurobiology of the frontal lobes. In addition to the primary or core frontal functions of working memory – initiation, disinhibition, attention, monitoring, and emotional control – a myriad of secondary syndromes (phenotypic presentations) are recognized (Table 5.1). However, as a useful clinical simplification, the three principal frontal clinical syndromes and their related hubs within the frontosubcortical circuitry include dysexecutive disorder (dorsolateral prefrontal cortical hub), disinhibitory disorders (orbitoprefrontal cortical hub), and the abulia spectrum of disorders (mesial prefrontal and anterior cingulate hub).

Metacognition, the FPC (BA 10) and its Disorders

The largest architectonic region within the frontal lobes, the FPC, has the lowest neuronal density among the great apes, but is satiated with dendrites. Comparative neurobiological data are notable in that the right BA 10 contains ~254.4 million neurons in humans in comparison to ~8 million in gibbons [12]. In addition, all the principal projections to the FPC originate in tertiary association areas of the PFC, the parietal and temporal lobes.

The primate FPC developed a pivotal role in weighing the benefits of persistent exploitation of a current benefit source (such as food) in favor of new exploratory behavior for

Table 5.1 Secondary syndromes

Behavioral	Multiple disinhibition syndromes
	Field-dependent behavior syndromes
	Disinhibitory control syndromes
Cognitive	Executive dysfunction syndromes
	Multitasking impairment
	Motor sequencing impairments
	Motor dysphasia syndromes
Motor	Abulic spectrum of disorders
	Eye movement syndromes
	Obsessive and compulsive disorders
	Alien hand syndromes
Disconnection (hodological) syndromes	Emergent visual artistic proficiency
	Emergent musical artistic proficiency
	Cerebellar cognitive affective syndrome

potential other, improved alternative resources. A fundamental specialization of the primate FPC was concerned with addressing competing goals by monitoring both current and possible alternative goals and adjusting behaviors. The human FPC (lateral subdivision of BA 10) circuitry enabled the monitoring of diverse competing goals simultaneously, and the ability to transition between them. These cortical advancements allowed for the options of responding to environmental challenge by aborting the exploitation of a current food or reward source in favor of exploring new avenues and thereby rendering a survival advantage. The human FPC is also concerned with integrating abstract information, creativity, and social cognitive and emotional processes. The developing frontoparietal brain circuitry endowed primates and humans with a balance of posterior PFC-located exploitation-related impulses and FPC-centered exploratory drive that delegates a redistribution of resources away from the current task, which is an advantage when competing goals might be more beneficial due to a change in circumstances (Figure 5.2). Unsurprisingly, people with FPC-related lesions are often normal by cognitive testing but have significant impairments with regard to dealing with novel or open-ended situations and simply with managing day-to-day challenges [43].

An all-important FPC function involves the concepts of metacognition and introspection. As decision outcomes may be encoded in prefrontal and parietal cortical brain activity up to ten seconds before entering awareness, the concept of non-conscious components of free decisions in the human brain has emerged [44]. Research into the process of prospective judgments has been evaluated in terms of "feelings of knowing," and judgment of learning is used to refer to the estimation of how successful a person's recall is thought to be [45].

In addition to the FPC, white matter microstructure has also been shown to correlate with introspective ability, including the genu of the anterior corpus callosum (CC) with subdivision of the CC fibers connected with the anterior and orbital prefrontal cortex, showing that metacognition is dependent not only on anterior prefrontal gray matter, but also on reciprocal projections [46]. The neural signature of self-control also involves a veto function and final predictive check, which involves the anteromedian cortex and anterior insula [47].

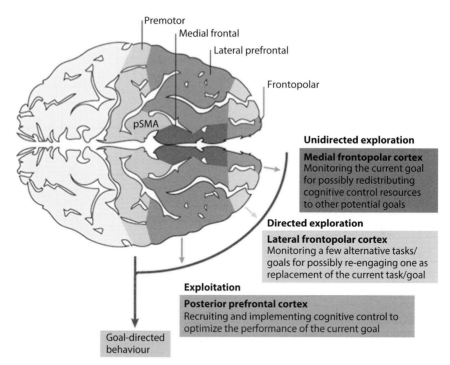

Figure 5.2 The principal frontal cortical subregions and functions.
Reproduced by permission from Springer Nature from Mansouri FA, Koechlin E, Rosa MGP, Buckley MJ. Managing competing goals: a key role for the frontopolar cortex. *Nat Rev Neurosci* 2017;18:645–657.

Interpersonal Cognition before Intrapersonal Cognitive Control

As cooperation became a central feature of the human way of life, with coordinated joint action and organized cooperative projects, a supra-personal system of cognitive control evolved. The cognitive processes for intrapersonal cognitive control are thought to have come second and arose as a development of the selection of a system of metacognition for interpersonally coordinated action. Shea et al. propose a two-part model: that of a cognitively lean, system 1 metacognition operating "implicitly" for the control of processes within one agent (intrapersonal cognitive control), which is common in many animals; and a cognitively rich system 2, or metacognition, thought to be unique to humans for controlling processes related to multiple agents, referred to as supra-personal cognitive control (Figure 5.3) [48].

Hence metacognition evolution can be viewed as a sequence of mirror neuron system elaborations, followed by evolution of metacognition for interpersonally coordinated action, then metacognition for intrapersonal cognitive control, and finally emotional intelligence.

A meta-analysis of action studies of healthy young adults revealed that episodic memory and retrieval of working memory were associated with lateral activations of the frontopolar region. In addition, other memory processes associated with FPC activity include retrieval verification, contextual recollection, source memory, and prospective memory. Studies concerned with mentalizing or paying attention to one's emotions or the mental

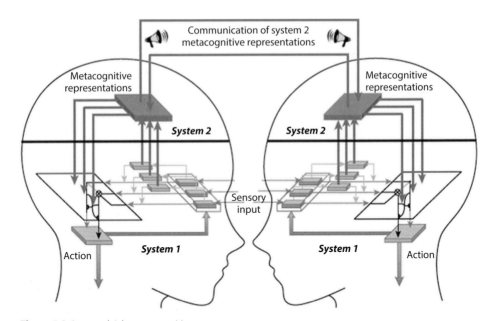

Figure 5.3 Lean and rich meta-cognitive systems.
Source: Shea N, Boldt A, Bang D, Yeung N, Heyes C, Frith CD. Suprapersonal cognitive control and metacognition. *Trends Cogn Sci* 2014;18:186–193. https://doi.org/10.1016/j.tics.2014.01.006 Reproduced under the CC BY 4.0 license https://creativecommons.org/licenses/by/4.0/

states of other people were associated with medial activations of the frontopolar region. The FPC is not interconnected with other cortical downstream areas as is the case with the prefrontal cortical areas. Its connections are limited to the supramodal PFC cortical areas, the anterior temporal cortex, and cingulate cortices. Furthermore, a hierarchy of function exists whereby the ventrolateral PFC (BA 12, 45, and 47) function is for the active retrieval of information from long-term storage sites, usually for one or several items of information. The dorsolateral PFC (BA 9 and 46) mediates the monitoring and manipulation of externally derived information. The third component, the overarching function of the FPC (BA 10), mediates the monitoring and manipulation of internally based information and processes internal states [15]. The other functions of the FPC include cognitive branching and multitasking – or holding information of a pending task, completing subtasks, or secondary goals. In this manner, cognitive branching is seen to enable what is termed multitasking. In addition, an important function is that of relational integration or the activity of several different external or internal processes and self-referential evaluation, important for generation of new strategies in the context of novel activities [49,50].

The pre-SMA is located between the PFC and motor areas, the SMA proper, and the primary motor cortex, and is a key structure engaged during voluntary action, transforming thoughts into actions. Transcranial magnetic stimulation studies have intimated that the pre-SMA function is in the preparation of entire movement sequences but also in suppressing automatic responses to environmental stimuli. Lesions in the pre-SMA cause hyper-responsiveness [51] and have been associated with utilization behavior (compulsive grasping of objects in the immediate environment) and anarchic hand syndrome (contralateral hand reacts automatically to a stimulus). These findings are important in understanding field-dependent behavior discussed below.

FDB Recognition for Diagnosis and Therapy

Field-dependent behavior (FDB) recognition is important to recognize for diagnostic and therapeutic reasons. The mirror neuron systems refer to an extensive frontoparietal network and a neurobiological substrate for several key higher cognitive function abilities, including theory of mind, learning by observation, language, and praxis. During primate evolution, the mirror neuron system circuitry became progressively more elaborate and complex; a seven-stage extended mirror neuron system hypothesis was proposed by Arbib. He suggested that stages 1–3 took place within primate evolution of grasping and simple imitation. From our last common ancestor (LCA) onwards to modern humans, presumably stages 4–7 evolved. The stages are:

1. grasping;
2. mirror system for grasping;
3. simple imitation (shared with chimpanzees but not macaques);
4. complex imitation (beyond chimpanzees);
5. protosign (key innovation; open repertoire);
6. protospeech (key innovation; neocortical vocal control via collateralization);
7. modern language [52].

A variety of frontal lobe lesions frequently cause FDB syndromes that have been attributed to a disruption or an uncoupling of the brain's mirror neuron system circuitry. The concept of theory of mind, our intentionalities, social cognition, and language are all integral to the MNS [53]. The diagnosis of FDB is especially important, because one of the consequences may be loss of personal autonomy of someone who appears on the surface quite normal, with relatively intact cognition and who may be actively employed. Lesion studies have revealed that the superior part of the SMA (BA 6 of the frontal lobes) is associated with what has been termed elementary forms of FDB. Examples include imitation behavior, very similar to echopraxia, as well as utilization behavior. The inferior parts of the frontal lobes, in particular the right orbitofrontal area, are involved when more complex FDB syndromes are recognized. Examples include environmental-dependency syndrome [54–56]. There may be a temporal component as well, with imitation behavior and utilization behavior predominating in the early period post-injury, such as acute stroke, whereas environmental-dependency syndrome tends to develop later in the course of the brain lesion [57–59]. Aside from the diagnostic importance, there are therapeutic implications integral to the mirror neuron system that may be advantageously exploited. For example, with severe motor deficits post-stroke, rehabilitation "action observation" techniques engage similar circuits to those that are actually involved with performing such an action. To date, differing variations of mirror visual feedback therapy have been shown to be effective in phantom limb pain, stroke, and some neuropsychiatric syndromes [60,61]. There is also evidence that gestural therapy in improving expressive aphasia is based on the rehabilitative aspects [62].

Language Evolution, Praxis, and Stone-Knapping Biface Technology

Archeological, present-day primate research, neuro-radiological functional imaging, and human clinical studies point to a convergence of the language networks, praxis networks, and tool use. It has therefore been theorized that brain praxis circuitry was involved with australopithecine-era stone knapping, that itself evolved from earlier flake-type tools to more advanced biface hand axes and laid the framework of the future language network. Both praxis and language also feature extensive left hemisphere networks. In addition, the early gestural type communication evident among extant primates today may be representative of an intervening stage between stone knapping and language evolution. Both feature action recognition as well as imitation elements [63]. The language and praxis networks similarly involve key hub regions within the superior temporal, ventral premotor and inferior temporal cortical areas, stressing the commonality in regard to functional processes. Clinical neurological support comes from the frequent co-occurrence of aphasias and apraxias accompanying left hemisphere lesions.

There is also a shared neural architecture of language and praxis in terms of lexicon, syntax, and semantics. Within Broca's area reside motor programs that also orchestrate speech-related muscles. The inferior parietal lobe is an area that links words and concepts in a cross-modal manner. The superior temporal area mediates meaning or semantics. These hubs are all linked via the mirror neuron system in a cross-modal fashion so that auditory (sounds), visual (images) and motor maps may all be conjoined. Other clinical observations, such as synkinesis in which movements of hands influence mouth movements, can occur with anteriorly located lesions. With posteriorly located lesions, synesthesia may similarly occur, wherein "crossed" responses to stimuli result. In brief, stimulation of one sensory pathway (sound) may lead to the involuntary experience within a second sensory pathway such as taste. It has been proposed that synkinesis might have been a mechanism through which gestural protolanguage gradually transformed into spoken language. The linking of these three key regions formed the underlying concept termed Synesthetic Bootstrapping Hypothesis of Ramachandran [64].

The neighboring supramarginal gyrus is involved with imitation of skilled and complex movements that are due to coordinated muscle and proprioception senses, with visual input. Earlier in primate evolution, this circuitry was critical for negotiating 30 m (100 foot) high forest canopies during the arboreal phase of primates. These requirements laid the cross-modal abstractions of the visual image of a branch, for example, and the required upper limb, hand, and arm proprioceptive and tactile muscle coordination. This hand–eye coordination allowed safe and efficient brachiation through the trees and formed the basic supramarginal gyrus (SMG) circuitry later exapted for human praxis. With damage often due to stroke, for example, a variety of apraxia syndromes may arise. These may also be regarded as forming part of the mirror neuron system and its defects. It has been proposed that a possible gene duplication of the SMG may have contributed to the formation of the angular gyrus (AG), which is part of the inferior parietal lobe (IPL). The IPL, in turn, became exapted for another cross-modal abstraction – namely, that used for the linking of concepts and word-objects. Lesion of the IPL may present with naming problems or anomias, as well as metaphor and proverb interpretation impairment [65].

Syntax or sentence construction has been viewed as a possible exaption of basic stone-knapping techniques by Stout et al. With the proposal that the stone tool, held in the right hand of the knapper corresponding to the subject, with the strike akin to the verb and hitting another stone referred to as the object held in the left hand. These activities may be likened to basic language syntax (subject–verb–object). Furthermore, it has been postulated that Broca's region, involved with motor programming for tool manufacture, may have been incurred as gene duplication during evolutionary development, with the duplicated region evolving a new syntactical area. This region was also connected to the IPL, primarily the SMG. From this circuitry, a hierarchichal, multimodal tool-assembly process was now possible. The duplicated region now involved with syntactic language ability became linked to the mirror neuron system circuitry, which included the superior temporal lobe semantic abilities, the IPL, and Broca's area [66].

Social and Emotional Circuitry Revealed by Disruption of the Uncinate Fasciculus

Disruption of the uncinate fasciculus (UF) due to relatively common diseases reveals features of the assembly of the social and emotional circuitry of the human brain. The UF is one of several large-scale human cerebral fiber tracts that have expanded dramatically in the course of hominin evolution, with arcuate fasciculus being another. The UF has extensive fiber tracts connecting the anterior temporal lobe and the orbitofrontal cortex (OFC), which has notable inhibitory control. A peculiar feature of this relatively expansive fiber tract is its proneness to shearing injury associated with traumatic brain injury (TBI), no matter where the impact of injury occurred on the brain case. Similarly, the inferior frontal lobe as well as the anterior temporal lobe are particularly prone to injury associated with TBI [67,68]. The UF is also impacted in several common neurological disorders such as stroke, frontotemporal lobe syndromes, and multiple sclerosis. Because this fiber tract and associated cortical regions of inferior frontal and anterior temporal lobe reach maturity as late as the third or fourth decades, this makes it uniquely vulnerable to a variety of neuropsychiatric conditions that preferentially affect the young adult population [69].

One of the principal UF functions is the mediation of choice in response to information acquired from social and emotional stimuli; it also has episodic memory functions. The anterior temporal pole hub for memory storage is specific for person-related memory, social memories, and theory of mind. Hence, delusional misidentification syndromes (DMISs) in which emotions and memory are disconnected is explainable. With Capgras syndrome, for example, a familiar person is viewed by the patient as a stranger despite the emotional reaction remaining intact. In a related but kind of opposite situation, Fregoli's syndrome involves a disruption of the tracts subserving face processing and the cortical areas for limbic-related emotive regions that allow the person to perceive a familiar face but to lack relevant emotional valence. The person so afflicted will therefore conclude that the "familiar" person is a stranger [70]. Other core UF functions include episodic memory processing, social, emotional, and linguistic functions. People with UF dysfunction also report schizophrenic-type symptoms, generalized anxiety, uncinate fits, and forme fruste-type Klüver–Bücy syndromes [71].

Syndromes

Geschwind-Gastaut Syndrome

"Silent brain lesions" is a term used, albeit less frequently, for inexplicable or absent syndromes when known lesions have affected certain brain regions, mostly involving the frontal lobes, temporal and right parietal areas. Geschwind-Gastaut Syndrome (GGS) is representative of relatively silent brain syndromes. This constitutes a constellation of signs

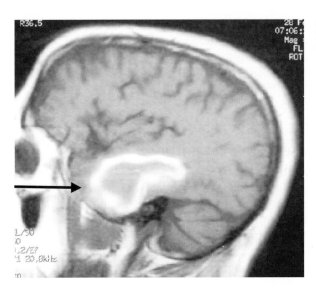

Figure 5.4 Geschwind-Gastaut Syndrome due to isolated right temporal lobe hemorrhage (arrow).

and symptoms typified by (1) a viscous personality, (2) metaphysical obsessions, and (3) altered physiological drives. The "viscous personality" is regarded as the principal component and includes over-inclusive verbal discourse, circumstantiality in speech, inordinately detailed information that is shared, and a peculiar prolongation of interpersonal discourse or encounters. In addition, hypergraphia (excessive writing), excessive drawing, or painting may be additional features. Metaphysical engrossments take the form of moral and intellectual preoccupations in philosophy and religion. Physiological alterations include hyposexuality, fear, or aggression [72]. The syndrome was first described in association with epileptic syndromes and subsequently due to temporal lobe brain hemorrhage affecting the uncinate fasciculus (Figure 5.4) [73]. This intriguing syndrome provides a remarkable perspective on the diverse functions of the temporal lobes and their association with the frontal lobes [74]. The cardinal components of this syndrome may be viewed as an unraveling of the recent human brain circuitry associated with the "cultural explosion" that archeological discoveries have associated with episodic memory enhancement, mental time travel, and ruminations about the afterlife [75].

Other clinical neurological syndromes, such as frontotemporal lobe dementia, yield additional insights into the diversity of human cognitive evolution, such as visual artistry and spiritual processing, by unraveling circuitry in this part of the brain due to various neurodegenerations. The two-way process whereby neuro-archeology and clinical neurosciences inform each other about brain evolution is again underscored by these observations.

Frontoparietal Fragmentation, the Visual Dorsal and Ventral Radiations, and Balint's Syndrome

Frontoparietal sensorimotor skills had evolved to the extent of basic stone knapping, yielding flakes, or lithic mode 1, also termed Oldowan technology, by 3.4 mya (Dikika,

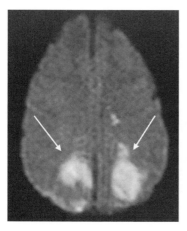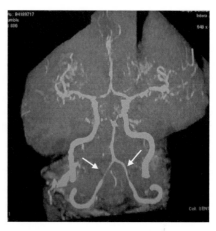

Figure 5.5 Dorsal and visual field disruption. Piecemeal vision (simultanagnosia), impaired pointing (optic ataxia) and eye gaze (optic apraxia). Balint's syndrome in a young pregnant woman with eclampsia causing bilateral posterior reversible brain lesions (left image arrows) and vasospasm (vessel narrowing) of intracranial arteries (right image arrows).

Ethiopia). Subsequently more sophisticated stone knapping allowed hand axes or biface tools, termed mode 2 or Archeulean, that required additional cognitive circuitry for processing visual object shaping and spatial coordinates [76]. Paleoneurological insights allow us to relate these to the two major visual radiations, the ventral radiation and dorsal stream, respectively. From extant primate studies to date, the coordination of these two activities was not within ape competence. The long-term procedural memory storage for these capabilities was possible by ~1.8 mya. The skills for constructing hand axes or biface technology requires the recruitment of the anterior intraparietal sulcus (IPS) and inferior frontal sulcus of the left hemisphere, both components of the mirror neuron system. This provides additional support for social learning being a crucial constituent in the acquisition of abilities required for biface technology [77].

Clinical neurological syndromes that may be seen as unraveling of both dorsal and ventral visual radiations come from posterior brain syndromes. Common neurological conditions that cause bilateral parietooccipital lesions include stroke, eclampsia, cerebral infarcts, and posterior reversible encephalopathy syndrome (PRES) (Figure 5.5). These processes cause an unraveling or fragmentation of the ventral and dorsal visual streams. These present with piecemeal vision (simultanagnosia), optic ataxia (impaired conjugate gaze direction), and optic apraxia (impaired visual guidance for object pointing). Although these may occur in isolation or two together, if all three coexist the syndrome is termed Balint's syndrome.

Alien Hand Syndrome

A relatively infrequent clinical syndrome termed alien hand or anarchic hand syndrome refers to either the hand or arm behaving autonomously. This may take the form of unintended object grabbing, unwittingly hitting a bed partner while asleep, or one hand may obstruct or interfere with the other hand while it is performing a particular action, such as lifting a fork to the mouth while eating. These are involuntary actions, occurring non-consciously and to some extent may be subsumed under the conditions discussed under "loss of sense of self disorders." Several different alien hand subtypes have been recognized, including, parietal, frontal, ictal, and corpus callosal. The parietal type presents with a withdrawal reaction from contact (parietal avoidance syndrome), whereas with the frontal-type grasping actions occur [60]. In the corpus callosal subtype an inter-manual disputation between hands occurs, with the two hands performing opposite actions, also termed diagnostic ideomotor apraxia. In epilepsy-associated alien hand or ictal alien hand, these syndromes may present transiently, usually with corpus callosal or mesial frontal damage. From a neurobiological and evolutionary point of view, fMRI studies have yielded insights that the primary motor cortex is relatively isolated from premotor cortical control, where motor programs are finalized. Rehabilitation measures have benefited from these insights, with measures for the frontal variant by placing objects in that hand to counter the tendency of grabbing and grasping [61,62,72].

Cerebellar Cognitive Affective Syndromes

With the substantiation of modern human capacities in terms of culture and brain size by ~200 kya, archeological endocast data indicate that the cerebellum achieved modern proportions as recently as ~28 kya. These findings may be attributed to the surge in cortico-cerebellar connectivity of the PFC that transpired during the latter part of the Pleistocene period, 2.5 mya to 12 kya). This circuitry has been attributed to improvement in cognitive efficiency, probably co-occurring with the development of EWM [78]. Clinical neurological evidence of disruption of this neurobiological evolutionary circuitry is represented by cerebellar cognitive dysmetria and cerebellar cognitive affective syndrome. This is further corroborated by neuroimaging findings that demonstrate fractional anisotropic impairment of these tracts in these syndromes as well as the findings of corticocerebellar, crossed diaschisis [79,80].

Remote Brain Effects of Lesions: Hodological Perspectives, Improved Behavior, and Hyperfunction

Frontal network syndromes may at times be due to remote effects of a disease process, termed diaschisis. This may take the form of either hypofunction (decreased function) or hyperfunction (increased function) of the network. In addition, the lesion itself may affect the underlying cortex, rendering it either hypo- or hyperfunctioning. Sometimes parts of the brain that have increased function result in dramatic syndromes such as a savant syndrome. Paradoxical functional facilitation was a hypothesis proposed by Kapur, wherein one brain area reverses an inhibitory influence on another area, with augmentation of function. For example, increased originality is facilitated by relative left hemisphere inhibition in the setting of an otherwise-intact right hemisphere [81]. Specific examples of these syndromes include:

- savant syndromes that may present with various forms, such as superlative talent in mathematics, visual art, music, or visuospatial ability. The acquisition may be acquired prodigiously, suddenly, or be of splinter talented subtypes [82];
- emergent artistic expertise associated with neurodegenerative disease such as frontotemporal dementia, Alzheimer's disease, or Parkinson's disease, but also seen with stroke, epilepsy, and migraine [83];

- literary artist aptitude associated with right temporal lobe impairment [84];
- content-specific delusion or DMIS, in association with right frontal stroke [85];
- visual imagery loss in the setting of dreaming [86];
- increased sense of humor, reported after right frontal lesions [87].

References

1. Elston GN. Cortex, cognition and the cell: new insights into the pyramidal neuron and prefrontal function. *Cerebral Cortex* 2003;13:1124–1138.

2. Passingham RE. The frontal cortex: does size matter? *Nat Neurosci* 2002;5:190–192.

3. Semendeferi K, Damasio H, Frank R, Van Hoesen GW. The evolution of frontal lobes: a volumetric analysis based on three dimensional reconstructions of magnetic resonance scans of human and ape brains. *J Hum Evol* 1997;32:375–388.

4. Semendeferi K, Lu A, Schenker N, Damasio H. Humans and apes share a large frontal cortex. *Nat Neurosci* 2002;5:272–276.

5. Holloway RL. The human brain evolving: a personal perspective. In: Broadfield D, Yuan M, Schick K, Toth N (eds.), *The Human Brain Evolving*. Stone Age Institute Press, Gosport, IN, 2010.

6. Fuster JM. *The Prefrontal Cortex: Anatomy, Physiology, and Neuropsychology of the Frontal Lobe*. Lippincott-Raven, Philadelphia, PA, 1997.

7. Elston GN, Benavides-Piccione R, Elston A et al. Specializations of the granular prefrontal cortex of primates: implications for cognitive processing. *Anat Record A Discov Mol Cell Evol Biol* 2006;288A:26–35.

8. Goldman-Rakic PS. The prefrontal landscape: implications for functional architecture for understanding human mentation and the central executive. *Phil Trans R Soc Lond Ser B* 1996;351:1445–1453.

9. Kaas JH, Stepniewska I. Evolution of posterior parietal cortex and parietal-frontal networks for specific actions in primates. *J Comp Neurol*. 2015. doi: 10.1002/cne.23838.

10. Mackey S, Petrides M. Quantitative demonstration of comparable cyto-architectonic areas within the ventromedial and lateral orbital frontal cortex in human and macaque monkey brains. *Eur J Neurosci* 2010;32:1940–1950.

11. Passingham RE, Wise SP. *The Neurobiology of the Prefrontal Cortex*. Oxford University Press, Oxford, 2012.

12. Semendeferi K, Armstrong E, Schleicher A, Zilles K, Van Hoesen GW. Prefrontal cortex in humans and apes: a comparative study of area 10. *Am J Phys Anthropol* 2001;114:224–241.

13. Jacobs B, Schall M, Prather M, et al. Regional dendritic and spine variation in human cerebral cortex: a quantitative Golgi study. *Cereb Cortex* 2001;11:558–571.

14. Ongur D, Ferry AT, Price JL. Architectonic subdivision of the human orbital and medial prefrontal cortex. *J Com Neurol* 2003;460:425–449.

15. Christoff K, Gabrieli JDE. The frontopolar cortex and human cognition: evidence for a rostrocaudal hierarchical organization within the human prefrontal cortex. *Psychobiology* 2000;28:168–186.

16. Tsujimoto S, Genovesio A, Weiss SP. Frontal pole cortex: encoding ends at the end of the endbrain. *Trends Cogn Sci* 2011;15:169–176.

17. Singer R. The Saldanha skull from Hopefield, South Africa. *Am J Phys Anthropol* 1954;12(3):345–362.

18. Bookstein F, Schaefter K, Prossinger H, et al. Comparing frontal cranial profiles in archaic and modern *Homo* by morphometric analysis. *Anat Record A Discov Mol Cell Evol Biol* 1999;257:217–224.

19. Nudo RJ, Masterton RB. Descending pathways to the spinal cord, IV: some

factors related to the amount of cortex devoted to the corticospinal tract. *J Comp Neurol* 1990;296:584–597.

20. Petrides M. Dissociable roles of the mid dorsolateral prefrontal cortex and anterior inferotemporal cortex in visual working memory. *J Neurosci* 2000;20:7496–7503.

21. Champod AS, Petrides M. Dissociable roles of the posterior parietal and the prefrontal cortex in manipulation and monitoring process. *PNAS* 2007;104:14837–14842.

22. Baddley A. Working memory: looking back and looking forward *Nat Rev Neurosi* 2003;4:829–839.

23. Dehaene S. *Reading in the Brain.* Penguin, New York, 2009.

24. Medalla M, Barbas H. Diversity of laminar connections linking periarcuate and lateral intraparietal areas depends on cortical structure. *Eur J Neurosci* 2006;23:161–179.

25. Petrides M. The mid-dorsolateral prefrontal-parietal network and the epoptic process. In: Stuss DT, Knight RT (eds.), *Principles of Frontal Lobe Function.* Oxford University Press, Oxford, 2012.

26. Champod AS, Petrides M. Dissociation within the frontoparietal network in verbal working memory: a parametric functional magnetic resonance imaging study. *J Neurosci* 2010;30:3849–3856.

27. Read D, van der Leeuw S. Biology is only part of the story. In: Renfrew C, Frith C, Malafouris L (eds.), *The Sapient Mind: Archeology Meets Neuroscience.* Oxford University Press, New York, 2009.

28. Diamond A, Doar B. The performance of human infants on a measure of frontal cortex function, the delayed response task. *Dev Psychobiol* 1989;22:271–294.

29. Wynn T, Balter M. Did working memory spark creative culture ? *Science* 2010;328:160–163.

30. Skoyles J. Evolution's "missing link": a hypothesis upon neural plasticity, prefrontal working memory and the origins of modern cognition. *Med Hypotheses* 1997;48:499–501.

31. Stuss DT. New approaches to prefrontal lobe testing. In: Miller B, Cummings JL (eds.), *The Human Frontal Lobes.* The Guilford Press, New York, 2009.

32. Stuss DT, Binns MA, Murphy KJ, Alexander MP. Dissociations within the anterior attentional system: effects of task complexity and irrelevant information on reaction time speech and accuracy. *Neuropsychologica* 2002;16:500–513.

33. Foussias G, Remington G. Negative symptoms in schizophrenia: avolition and Occam's razor. *Schizophrenia Bull* 2010;36:359–369.

34. Yung AR, McGorry PD. The prodromal phase of first episode psychosis: past and current conceptualizations. *Schizophrenia Bull* 1996;22:353–370.

35. Gerwig M, Kastrup O, Wanke I, Diener HC. Adult post-infectious thalamic encephalitis: acute onset and benign course. *Eur J Neurol* 2004;11:135–139.

36. Hoffmann M. The panoply of field dependent behavior in 1436 stroke patients: the mirror neuron system uncoupled and the consequences of loss of personal autonomy. *Neurocase* 2014;20(5):556–568.

37. Cicerone KD. Attention deficits and dual task demands after mild traumatic brain injury. *Brain Injury* 1996;10:79–89.

38. Pessoa L. On the relationship between emotion and cognition. *Nat Rev Neurosci* 2008;9:148–158.

39. Shamay-Tsoory SG, Tomer R, et al. Impairment in cognitive and affective empathy in patients with brain lesions: anatomical and cognitive correlates. *J Clin Exp Neuropsychol* 2004;26:1113–1127.

40. Semendeferi K, Barger N, Schenker N. *Brain Reorganization in Humans and Apes: The Human Brain Evolving.* Stone Age Institute Press, Gosport, IN, 2010.

41. Koechlin E, Hyafil A. Anterior prefrontal function and the limits of human decision making. *Science* 2007;318:594–598.

42. Burgess PW, Durmontheil I, Gilbert SJ. The gateway hypothesis of rostral

prefrontal cortex (area 10) function. *Trends Cogn Sci* 2007;11(7):290–298.

43. Mansouri FA, Koechlin E, Rosa MGP, Buckley MJ. Managing competing goals: a key role for the frontopolar cortex. *Nat Rev Neurosci* 2017;18:645–657.

44. Soon CS, Brass M, Heinze H-J, Haynes J-D. Unconscious determinants of free decisions in the human brain. *Nat Neurosci* 2008;11:543–545.

45. Fleming SM, Dolan RJ. Review: neural basis of metacognition. *Phil Trans R Soc B* 2012;367:1338–1349.

46. Fleming SM, Weil RS, Nagy Z, et al. Relating introspective accuracy to individual differences in brain structure. *Science* 2010;329:1541–1543.

47. Brass M, Haggard P. To do or not to do: the neural signature of self control. *J Neurosci* 1999;27:9141–9145.

48. Shea N, Boldt A, Bang D, et al. Suprapersonal cognitive control and metacognition. *Trends Cogn Sci* 2014;18:186–193.

49. Christoff K, Prabhakaran V, Dorfman J, et al. Rostrolateral prefrontal cortex involvement in relational integration during reasoning. *Neuroimage* 2001;14:1136–1149.

50. Prabhakaran V, Narayanan K, Zhao Z, Gabrieli JD. Integration of diverse information in working memory within the frontal lobe. *Nat Neurosci* 2000;3:85–90.

51. Fried I, Katz A, McCarthy G, et al. Functional organization of human supplementary motor cortex studied by electrical stimulation. *J Neurosci* 11;1991:3656–3666.

52. Arbib M. From mirror neurons to complex imitation in the evolution of language and tool use. *Ann Rev Anthropol* 2011;40:257–273.

53. Rumiati RI, Weiss PH, Tessari A, et al. Common and differential neural mechanisms supporting imitation of meaningful and meaningless actions. *J Cogn Neurosci* 2005;17:1420–1431.

54. Lhermitte F. Human autonomy and the frontal lobes. Part II: patient behavior in complex and social situations – the "environmental dependency syndrome." *Ann Neurol* 1986;19:335–343.

55. Besnard J, Allain P, Aubin G, et al. A contribution to the study of environmental dependency phenomena: the social hypothesis. *Neuropsychologia* 2011;49:3279–3294.

56. Bien N, Roebuck A, Goebel R, Sack AT. The brain's intention to imitate: the neurobiology of intentional versus automatic imitation. *Cerebral Cortex* 2009;19:2338–2351.

57. Ragno Paquier C, Assal F. A case of oral spelling behavior: another environmental dependency syndrome. *Cogn Behav Neurol* 2007;20:235–237.

58. Volle E, Beato R, Levy R, Dubois B. Forced collectionism after orbitofrontal damage. *Neurology* 2002;58:488–490.

59. Shin JS, Kim MS, Kim NS, et al. Excessive TV watching in patients with frontotemporal dementia. *Neurocase* 2012. doi: 10.1080/13554794.2012.701638.

60. Garrison KA, Winstein CJ, Aziz-Zadeh L. The mirror neuron system: a neural substrate for methods in stroke rehabilitation. *Neurorehabil Neural Repair* 2010;24:404–412.

61. Yavuzer G, Selles R, Sezer N, et al. Mirror therapy improves hand function in subacute stroke: a randomized controlled trial. *Arch Phys Med Rehabil* 2008;89:393–398.

62. Hanlon Brown RE, Brown JW, Gerstman LJ. Enhancement of naming in non-fluent aphasia through gesture. *Brain Lang* 1990;38:298–314.

63. Roby Brami A, Hermsdoerfer J, Roy AC, Jacobs S. A neuropsychological perspective on the link between language and praxis in modern humans. *Phil Trans R Soc B* 2012;367:144–160.

64. Ramachandran VS. *The Tell-Tale Brain.* W.W. Norton, New York, 2011.

65. McGeoch PD, Brang D, Ramachandran VS. Apraxia, metaphor and mirror neurons. *Med Hypotheses* 2007;69(6):1165–1168.

66. Stout D, Toth N, Schick K, Chaminade T. Neural correlates of Early Stone Age toolmaking: technology, language and cognition in human evolution. *Phil Trans R Soc B* 2008;363:1939–1949.

67. Seo JP, Kim OL, Kim SH, et al. Neural injury of uncinate fasciculus in patients with diffuse axonal injury. *NeuroRehabilitation* 2012;30:323–328.

68. Ewing-Cobbs L, Prasad MR. Outcome after abusive head injury. In: Jenny C (ed.), *Child Abuse and Neglect: Diagnosis, Treatment, and Evidence.* Elsevier Saunders, St. Louis, MO, 2011.

69. Paus T, Keshavan M, Giedd JN. Why do many psychiatric disorders emerge during adolescence? *Nat Rev Neurosci* 2008;9:947–957.

70. Hirstein W, Ramachandran VS. Capgras syndrome: a novel probe for understanding the neural representation of the identity and familiarity of persons. *Proc R Soc B* 1997;264:437–444.

71. Von Der Heide R, Skipper LM, Kobusicky E, Olsen IR. Dissecting the uncinate fasciculus: disorders, controversies and a hypothesis. *Brain* 2013;136:1692–1707.

72. Bear DM, Fedio P. Quantitative analysis of interictal behavior in temporal lobe epilepsy. *Arch Neurol* 1977;34:454.

73. Hoffmann M. Isolated right temporal lobe stroke patients present with Geschwind Gastaut syndrome, frontal network syndrome and delusional misidentification syndromes. *Behav Neurol* 2009;20:83–89.

74. Trimble M, Mendez MF, Cummings JL. Neuropsychiatric symptoms from the temporolimbic lobes. *J Neuropsychiatry Clin Neurosci* 1997;9:429–438.

75. Suddendorf T, Corballis M. The evolution of foresight: what is mental time travel and is it unique to humans. *Behav Brain Sci* 2007;30:299–313.

76. Stout D, Passingham R, Frith C, Apel J, Chaminade T. Technology, expertise and social cognition in human evolution. *Eur J Neurosci* 2011;33:1328–1338.

77. Wynn T. Archeology and cognitive evolution. *Behav Brain Sci* 2002;25:389–438.

78. Weaver AH. Reciprocal evolution of the cerebellum and neocortex in fossil humans. *PNAS* 2005;102:3576–3580.

79. Ramnani N. The primate cortico-cerebellar system: anatomy and function. *Nat Rev Neurosci* 2006;7:511–522.

80. Kamali A, Kramer LA, Frye RE, Butler IJ, Hasan KM. Diffusion tensor tractography of the human brain cortico-ponto-cerebellar pathways: a quantitative preliminary study. *J Magn Reson Imaging* 2010;32:809–817.

81. Kapur N. Paradoxical functional facilitation in brain behavior research: a critical review. *Brain* 1996;119:1775–1790.

82. Treffert DA. *Islands of Genius.* Jessica Kingsley Publishers, London, 2010.

83. Schott GD. Pictures as a neurological tool: lessons from enhanced and emergent artistry in brain disease. *Brain* 2012;135:1947–1963.

84. Miller B. *The Frontotemporal Lobe Dementias*, Oxford University Press, New York, 2013.

85. Christodoulou GN, Magariti M, Kontaxakis VP, Christodoulou NG. The delusion misidentification syndromes: strange, fascinating and instructive. *Curr Psychiatry Rep* 2009;11:185–189.

86. Peña-Casanova J, Roig-Rovira T, Bermudez A, Tolosa-Sarro E. Optic aphasia, optic apraxia and loss of dreaming. *Brain Lang* 1985;26:63–71.

87. Pell MD. Judging emotion and attitudes from prosody following brain damage. *Prog Brain Res* 2006;156:303–317.

Enhanced Working Memory

Working memory, the brain's "operating system" and basic to all other cognitive processes, was enhanced later in our history. The so-called enhanced working memory (EWM) systems may have been prompted by particularly severe climatic conditions during a time categorized by paleo-climatologists as Marine Isotope Stage 6 from about 190 kya. Unique environmental conditions limited a small group of surviving humans in southern Africa to a highly nutritious seafood and tuber diet. Epigenetic and genetic factors likely played a role too, and from archeological discoveries the concomitant parietal enlargement points to a substantial increase in brain interconnectivity. Following that, many more sophisticated tools and cultural artifacts were found and soon thereafter early man spread to the rest of the globe.

The Stages of Cognitive Evolution and "Out of Africa" Expeditions

The most ancient archeological hominin remains, namely that of *Sahelanthropus tchadensis*, were found in the Sahara Desert and australopithecine remains were found thousands of kilometers away in various parts of the East African Rift Valley and southern Africa. Geological and accompanying paleo-climatological events in East Africa together conjured up a complex topography associated with erratic climate conditions. Based on these findings, Maslin et al. proposed their Pulsed Climate Variability Hypothesis whereby the extended East African arid period was interspersed by brief, wet periods correlating with hominin brain growth, speciation, and Out of Africa dispersals [1]. Flaking of stone tools (Oldowan method) by hominins become evident in the archeological record in the period 3.4–2.5 mya. Experimental evidence by Morgan et al. postulated that perhaps limited imitation behavior in the initial stone tool manufacture by hominins was of a "low fidelity social transmission" capability. A ~1 million year stone flaking stasis ensued [2]. A proposal by Morgan et al. was that instruction through rudimentary protolanguage was the likely factor in precipitating the next stage leading to blades or biface (Archeulean) type technology [2]. It has also been surmised that cerebral reorganization occurred before an overall increase in brain size. These findings concur with the seven-stage extended mirror neuron system proposed by Arbib. In his model, stages 1–3 involved simple imitation procedures, within the chimpanzee's capabilities. At stage 4, more complex imitation, being a further evolution of this capability, permitted the next step to protosign or stage 5; thereafter came protospeech (stage 6) and finally modern language (stage 7) [3].

The technological advancements of biface technology were associated with the period of *Homo erectus* ~1.8 mya. During this period, coevolution factors such as the advent of ground sleep, which was associated with increased REM sleep and dreaming as well as slow-wave sleep, fire use, and consequently chemical food processing and ultimately sociality were all associated with a progressive increase in group size. These "first" hominins were bestowed with sufficient brain size and power to be successful in the first of three "Out of Africa" expeditions, initially reaching distant places such as modern-day China [4].

The next notable cognitive elaboration, represented by *Homo heidelbergensis* sporting a brain size ~1200 cc, almost that of modern humans, lived in the time period 800–200 kya. In Africa they were referred to as *Homo rhodensiensis*, while in Europe they were referred to as *Homo heidelbergensis*; these, in turn, gave rise to the Neanderthals in Europe as well as modern humans in Africa. Following additional marked climactic fluctuations with resultant erratic resources for early hominins, a number of different granular frontal cortex elaborations ensued. Together, these culminated in overall error reduction by early hominins in their challenging environment. Moreover, these additional granular PFC areas equipped these hominins for learning by imitation and the concept of mental time travel. The latter faculties allowed imagined action before engagement [5]. Further scrutiny of the *Homo rhodensiensis* skulls found in Bodo (Ethiopia), Kabwe (Zambia), and Saldanha (South Africa) revealed that the inner frontal brain cases did not differ significantly from those measured in modern human skulls. Together such data imply that modern human proportions of the frontal lobes had been attained, well before "cultural evolution," which occurred around 70–50 kya [6].

At this stage, a number of fundamental stages in human cognitive evolution may be expounded:

- progressive elaboration of sensorimotor/frontoparietal integration;
- bipedalism;
- progressive brain size increases;
- working memory enhancement;
- mirror neuron circuitry enhancement;
- dentate gyrus neurogenesis;
- autonoesis and mental time travel;
- elaboration of neural circuitry for higher-order cognition, including language, spirituality, and culture.

Archeological finds point to a gradual assembly of the modern human mind in Africa [7]. Wynn and Coolidge have gathered evidence from archeological remnants that support executive function and working memory upgrades. For example, traps and snares, as well as foraging systems (crop storage), support long-range future planning in temporal and spatial domains. Reliable weapons represented by bows and arrows, spears, as well as hafting (stone tool fitted to a shaft) indicate multicomponent sequencing and assembly abilities. Similarly, anticipating animal herd behavior and intervening by hunting and subsequent storage of meat are seen as evidence of more progressive working memory functions [8,9].

However, the limits of working memory capacity had inherent restrictions that were subsequently handled by external information storage apart from the brain, a kind of external hard drive. This allowed freeing up the episodic buffer component of working memory circuitry from holding information online and facilitated central executive component information processing [10–12]. The earliest archeological evidence for such externalization of information comes from artifacts from the Blombos cave in South

Africa. The engravings on artifacts with ocher, as well as marine shell and bone artifacts, have been dated as early 77 kya [13]. Further archeological findings in Germany, dated to ~32 kya, are represented by the Hohlenstein–Stadel Lionman, a therianthropic (human mythological ability to change or metamorphose into animals) figurine. The abstraction implied by the combination of a human and lion in one figure and its possible implications are seen as evidence for a more advanced or extended working memory capacity. Wynn and Coolidge interpreted this figurine as the earliest evidence for executive function and that the people who configured it may have done so to help satisfy their metaphysical or existential challenge [14]. The various artifactual finds point to the evolution of working memory capacity in the period 77–30 kya [15]. Tracing the expansion of working memory from an estimated level 6 within Neanderthals into the enhanced working memory level 7 of modern humans can be approximated by archeological finds and their extrapolation to cognitive abilities. These include engraved lines, numbers, and other external storage means gradually giving way to written storage in scrolls, later in books, and currently on computer disks and in cloud storage [16].

The following neurobiological elaborations presumably were the drivers of the enhancement of the subcomponents inherent in the expansive working memory circuitry. These components included the visuospatial sketchpad (innovation, modeling, and simulation of the future), phonologic storage capacity increases (facilitating modern language through syntax and recursion), and episodic buffer augmentation (creativity) [17,18]:

- genetic and/or epigenetic events [19];
- high-bandwidth synapse formation (precipitated by aquatic diet?) [20];
- gliotransmission and astroglial networks [21];
- augmentation of prefrontal inhibitory function (enhanced social interfacing) [22];
- prefrontal lobe connectivity, both internally and with other cortical areas [23];
- parietal lobe expansion and connectivity [24];
- cerebellar expansion [25].

Southern Africa Rendezvous for the Origins of the Modern Mind?

Do the relatively unique paleo-climatological and geological events in the period 200–100 kya help explain the sapient paradox? Although archeological evidence strongly favors anatomically modern humans (AMH) evolving in eastern Africa by 200 kya, the modern human mind may well have evolved in southern Africa. Renfrew drew specific attention to the approximately 150 000-year unexplained time lag separating AMHs and the emergence of the forging of the "modern mind" at about ~50 kya [26]. Archeological, genetic, and linguistic research all support these deductions. Intriguing evidence was provided by Marean et al. for enhanced cognition manifesting during environmental hardship, in turn due to prolonged and extreme cooling and aridity 164–75 kya. This was as a consequence of Marine Isotope stage 6 (195–123 kya) and Marine Isotope stage 5 (130–80 kya). Over 100 of these alternating warming and cooling stages have been identified within the last six million years and defined according to oxygen isotope stages derived from drilling of deep sea core samples.

In one of Marean's publications on the topic, "When the sea saved humanity," he speculated that possibly only a few thousand or perhaps a few hundred AMH managed to survive the catastrophic ice age conditions due to unique prevailing conditions along the extreme southern African coast [27]. Fortuitous caves adjacent to the coast, with multiple rocky outgrowths interspersed by intertidal pools that teemed with shellfish, crustaceans, and fish provided critical nutrients. These "condominiums by the sea" may have been extensive, as far north as the eastern South African coastline, with discovery of the Sibudu Cave 1500 km northwards in Kwa-Zulu Natal near Durban [28]. The unrivaled assemblage of docosahexaenoic acid (DHA) from fish and shellfish availability, high-quality protein provided by the temperate climate, the neighboring Agulhas current and adjacent land-based tubers providing complex carbohydrates, seemed to coincide with the substantiation of symbolic behavior. These archeological finds can be correlated with the formation of the modern mind, supported by the findings of bladelet stone technology and pigment use discovered in the caves next to the ocean at Pinnacle point and other sites [29].

The Middle Paleolithic has been deemed to have contained more remarkable conceptual advances than modern humans' blade technology and art of the Upper Paleolithic that occurred several hundred thousand years later. Hence, our African ancestors had the skills of language and symbolic representation long before their African exodus, estimated at 80 kya. To gain perspective on tool and blade technology, the following time frame by Opperman may be used as a guide;

1. pebble stone industry – Oldowan
2. biface industry – Archeulean
3. prepared core industry – Middle Stone Age
4. blade industries – Upper Paleolithic
5. microlithic industries – small flakes and blades, retouched and used in composite tools [30].

The prepared core technologies of the Middle Paleolithic associated with the emergence of *Homo helmei*, and not the Upper Paleolithic blade technologies, are regarded as the best markers for the global migration of modern humans. McBrearty and Brooks maintain that African Middle Stone Age (AMSA) modern human cognitive evolution commenced 250–300 kya. They regarded this period in Africa as more vigorous and enterprising from a cultural evolutionary point of view than its equivalent of the Middle Paleolithic period that transpired in Europe. Archeologically, the smart African blade tools were evident during the AMSA approximately 280 kya, whereas European blade tools emerged 40–50 kya, with the African blade tools therefore pre-dating modern humans by about 250 ky. Specifically, tools with stone points are found within a range of 250 000 years within various African sites, markedly longer in duration compared to Europe. Mode 5 technology or microliths also originated in Africa at the Mumba Rock Shelter in Tanzania 70 kya, considerably earlier than the European discoveries dated to only 8000 years ago. African art represented by the Apollo 11 cave in Namibia, as the oldest known art, dates to 40–60 kya and so also has greater antiquity, pre-dating the Chauvet cave art in France (Figure 6.1) [7,30].

With the importance of DHA and EPA as constituents of neurons and synapses, the evidence of extensive coastal, beachcombing, and aquatic foraging for shellfish and fishing activities may have been decisive to new behaviors ~150 kya. Evidence for beachcombing was discovered at the Klasiers River, South Africa and at Abdur, Eritrea on the Red Sea. The latter is of particular importance as this was the likely site of crossing over

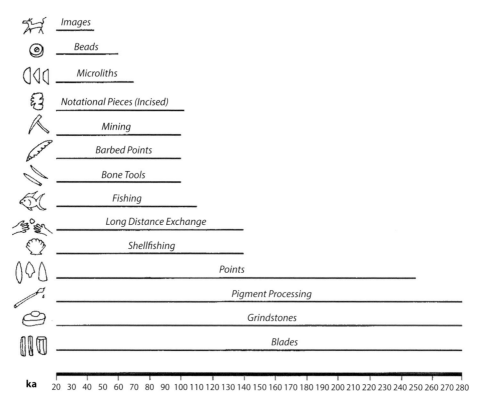

Figure 6.1 African Middle Paleolithic: artifacts and tools implicating modern behavior in Africa over the last ~300 000 years.

Source: McBrearty S, Brooks AS. The revolution that wasn't: a new interpretation of the origin of modern human behavior. *J Human Evol* 2000;39(5):453–563. Reproduced with permission from Academic Press.

to Arabia, with the ultimate destination being Australia. McBrearty and Brooks proposed that the transition from beachcombing to fishing took place within Africa by ~100 kya. Middle Stone Age tools and shellfish, as well as large African herbivore remains, have been found cluttered together from about 125 kya, during the last interglacial when there were sea-level changes.

During this period, archeological finds, such as the Skhul 5 skull, with a volume of 1520 cc (current human skull size averages 1350 cc), indicates we were bigger and more robust, with larger brain sizes, at ~125 kya (Figure 6.2). Since the time of African exodus, an overall diminution in size and reduction in robusticity occurred globally among all people, particularly within the last 100 ky, probably due to nutritional challenges as opposed to genetic factors. With farming, child and adult size decreased markedly, particularly in people eating rice without much animal protein, as in the Far East. McBrearty and Brooks have marshaled evidence that by this time both our physical and behavioral zenith had been reached by modern humans. For the first AMH, appearing by ~140 kya, evidence for half of the 14 proposed principal behavioral and cognitive competences (Figure 6.1) were already in place and behaviors were already present. During this time, cultural evolution superseded genetic evolution at least since 300 kya.

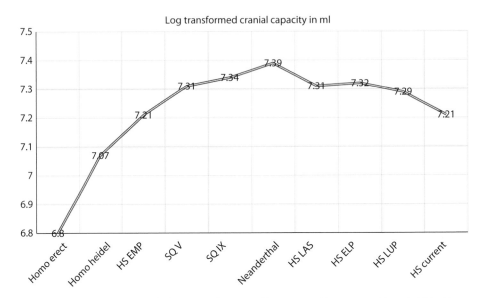

Figure 6.2 Cranial capacity over the last two million years. Homo erect – *Homo erectus*; Homo heidel – *Homo heidelbergensis*; HS – *Homo sapiens*; EMP – Early Middle Pleistocene; ELP – Early Late Pleistocene; SQ – Skhul Qafzeh; HS LAS – last archaic *Homo sapiens*; HS LUP – Late Upper Paleolithic.
Source: data from Johanson D, Edgar B. *From Lucy to Language*. Simon and Schuster, New York, 2006; Ruff CB, Trinkaus E, Holliday TW. Body mass and encephalization in Pleistocene *Homo*. *Nature* 1997;387:173–176.

Evolution of Africans, Asians, Australians, and Europeans

Europeans evolved last, after Africans, Asians and Australians; there were two kinds of Europeans and two early modern cultures in Europe. After the exodus from Africa ~80 kya into southern Arabia via the Gate of Grief, or Bab al Mandab, the eventual Europeans' ancestors marked time for tens of thousands of years in South Asia. The move from there was only possible at about 50 kya, during a warm moist phase associated with the greening of the Arabian Desert, similar to the Sahara Pump Theory greening of the Sahara Desert. The adjacent fertile crescent (modern-day Iran and Iraq) presented a corridor for migration in a north-west direction toward the region of modern-day Turkey and the Levant (eastern Mediterranean, north east Africa, western Asia). The other group of modern humans in South Asia were not affected by these restrictive conditions and these trail-blazing beachcombers followed the Indian Ocean coastline all the way to Southeast Asia and ultimately into Australia, where they arrived about 60 kya, thousands of years earlier than the colonization of Europe. In Oppenheimer's view, as the first non-African modern humans were Asians, geographically as well as genetically, Europeans are regarded as a side-branch development of the "Out of Africa" human migrations. The proposal for a South Asian origin for Europeans differs from a previously conventionally held view of the migrations taking the route from North Africa along the eastern Mediterranean and from there into Europe. There is meager evidence for this latter route and much stronger evidence coming from our maternal genetic tree of a 50 000-year-old South Asian origin for early Europeans. Their routing through the fertile crescent and avoidance of the Arabian and Libyan Deserts was only possible during a brief interstadial 55–65 kya as the fertile crescent was impenetrable for the last 100 000 years. The earliest modern cultures in Europe included the Aurignacian, dated to ~46 kya (first appearing in Bulgaria and Turkey) and the Gravettian, dated to ~21–30 kya. These AMHs with their new style of Aurignacian-type tools transitioned along the Danube River through the regions of modern-day Hungary westward, to Austria, and to the upper Danube at Geissenkösterle, Germany. Another branch had also migrated earlier, in a southerly direction from Austria to the present-day Riviera and to the Pyrenees and northern Spain by 38 kya [31].

Genetic and Linguistic Evidence

Among our 30 000 genes, recombination and mixing of small amounts of duplications and crossovers between maternal and paternal DNA genes occurs with each generation. However, two distinct parts of our DNA (mtDNA and the Y chromosome) do not recombine and hence these can be traced more easily through the generations. Mitochondrial DNA inheritance occurs along the female lineage, with males that receive it from their mother not being able to transmit to their children. All humans alive today have therefore inherited their mtDNA from one female alive around 200 kya. The mtDNA represents relative stability in comparison to changing DNA molecules, mediating inheritance characteristics. MtDNA point mutations do occur, but are rare – on average one mutation occurring per 1000 generations. Over a period of about 200 ky, we have each had 7–15 mutations on our own personal Eve record. We can see where certain mutations occurred, whether in Europe, Africa, or Asia. Because the mutations occur at a statistically consistent, though random, rate, we can approximate the time when they happened. We can now trace migrations of modern humans around the planet. The oldest changes in our mtDNA took place in Africa around 150–190 kya. Then new mutations appear in Asia about 60–80 kya. This tells us that modern humans evolved in Africa and that some migrated to Asia 80 kya. In an analogous fashion, the Y chromosome is only passed along the male lineage, with the unpaired Y chromosome having no role in the exchange of DNA and playing no part in the more indiscriminate exchange of DNA by the other somatic chromosomes. The Y chromosome can therefore also be tracked relatively untampered through each generation and traced back to our original paternal ancestor [32,33].

Further support comes from the molecular clock concept tied to the natural evolution of DNA sequences. The postulated "mitochondrial Eve" originating in Africa approximately 180 kya was associated with a population bottleneck and very low population density, a likely consequence of Marine Isotope stage 6 climatic effects. Thereafter, two modern surviving human populations groups are recognized, genetically dating to ~130 kya: the ancestral Khoe and San located in southern Africa, the other in eastern and central Africa. The oldest mtDNA haplogroups, L0d and L0k, are found in especially high frequencies in the Khoe–San groups of southern Africa around ~100 kya (Figure 6.3). These are also representative of the most penetrating mtDNA clades so far recorded among modern humans [34]. It has therefore been deduced that the L0 has a southern Africa origin, emerging from ancestral modern San and Khoe people. The evidence supports the L1 originating in central Africa and L2'6 in eastern Africa within the time frame of ~130 kya. The latter period also coincided with the extreme climate changes of cold and aridity that precipitated one of the African "megadroughts" related to both Marine Isotope stage 6 and Marine Isotope stage 5. Remarkably, during this period extensive archeological evidence of Middle Stone Age tools (termed mode 3), represented by flake tools originating from prepared cores, first appeared [35].

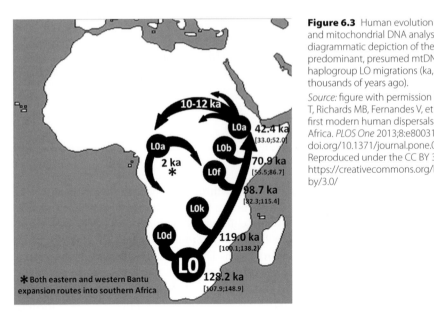

Figure 6.3 Human evolution and mitochondrial DNA analysis: diagrammatic depiction of the predominant, presumed mtDNA haplogroup L0 migrations (ka, thousands of years ago).

Source: figure with permission from Rito T, Richards MB, Fernandes V, et al. The first modern human dispersals across Africa. *PLOS One* 2013;8:e80031. https://doi.org/10.1371/journal.pone.0080031 Reproduced under the CC BY 3.0 https://creativecommons.org/licenses/by/3.0/

Linguistics provides corroborating support on the basis of click language analysis. Tishkoff et al. have surmised that the southern African San people are "the oldest population on Earth." Of the ~30 different click languages recognized within the southern African region, only the present-day hunter-gatherer Sandawe and eastern African Hadzabe people have click language [36]. On this basis, it has been assumed a migration occurred originally from the south-western African region into eastern Africa [37]. This premise is supported by genetic analysis, with modern human expansion from the eastern African region to all other parts of the world [34,38,39].

The Impact of Diet

Neurochemical Factors, DHA, Micronutrients, and Synaptic Bandwidth

Our association with DHA extends back ~600 million years, during which time no molecular changes took place. In contradistinction, profound genetic changes among animals were evident during this period of hundreds of millions of years. This prompted Crawford to expound that DHA was more important than DNA and it was DHA that dictated to DNA [40]. DHA availability has an important effect on brain size and connectivity, and has many synaptic regulatory effects. In addition, AMHs have high-bandwidth synapses in comparison to rodents, and dietary omega-3 fatty acids also have significant neural gene expression effects. When moving away from coastal and aquatic to terrestrial environments, the very low availability of DHA of the land-based food chain underscores the actuality of much smaller terrestrial mammalian brains while body sizes increased. This is in part due to mammals lacking specific enzymes essential for synthesis of omega-3 fatty acid precursors. DHA alone is not the only critical ingredient for optimal brain growth, however. Within marine and lacustrine environments, food, in addition to ample DHA, supplies specific and essential micronutrients including selenium, zinc, iodine, copper, and manganese, all of which oppose peroxidation and have been regarded as key factors in the surge of hominin brain size and intra-connectivity [41].

Furthermore, polyunsaturated fatty acids (PUFAs), especially DHA, regulate a number of critical brain processes. These include regulation of glial cell structure and function, neurogenesis, synaptic function, endothelial cells, and control of brain inflammation. Dietary PUFA deficiency has associations with numerous neurological and psychiatric syndromes, principally those of cognitive impairments and mood disorders. Proposed neurobiological mechanisms that are implicated include:

- cell signaling networks;
- regulation of membrane dynamics;
- synaptaminde-mediated synaptogenesis;
- receptor activation;
- modulation of brain endocannabinoids;
- neuronal growth and differentiation.

Additional brain health factors include the DHA-related anti-amyloidogenic effect mediated by neuroprotectin D1 (NPD1) and DHA-derived regulator and mediator of cerebral glucose uptake [42]. The remarkable and protean DHA neuronal, glial, and synaptic functions underscore the important role of DHA in the most prevalent neurological disease states such as stroke, dementia, depression, and attention deficit disorder, as well as migraine, myocardial infarction, and other organ systems. Omega-3 fatty acids have also been reported to have anti-nociceptive attributes that regulate pain-related processes, whereas omega-6 fatty acids have pro-nociceptive properties (leading to pain perception). Randomized trials have already shown significant effects in reducing chronic headaches by increasing omega-3 fatty acids and decreasing omega-6 fatty acids [43].

Diet as a Driver of Increased Brain Connectivity and Synaptic Bandwidth

The high-quality sea food and tuber diet that dominated during Marine Isotope stage 6 in southern Africa may have been a driver of the marked increase in brain connectivity and synaptic bandwidth. An overall increase in synaptic density can be traced from primates to humans, with ~2000–5600 synapses per neuron in monkey brains compared to ~6800–10 000 on average in human neurons. Within the prefrontal cortex, prefrontal pyramidal cells average ~15 100 spines, which is 72 percent more than the macaque [44,45]. Several factors can help in the determination of the timing of the AMH mind circuitry "modernization." With apparently modern frontal lobes already in place by 600–300 kya (Kabwe, Bodo, Saldahna Man skull data), the subsequent development of more extensive intracortical connectivity associated with higher synaptic bandwidth development seems to be a plausible explanation of the sapient paradox lag period of 200–50 kya [17].

Archeological Evidence of Increased Intra-connectivity

The parietal lobes and cerebellum enlarged, leading to increased intra-connectivity and the foundations of the modern human connectome and EWM. Parietal lobe globularization and expansion occurred relatively recently in human evolution ~150–100 kya. The

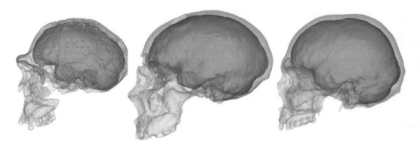

Figure 6.4 Frontoparietal geometric changes in early humans *Homo ergaster* (left), Neanderthal (middle), modern human (right).
Source: adapted from Bruner E, Manuel de la Cuétara J, Masters M, et al. Functional craniology and brain evolution: from paleontology to biomedicine. *Front Neuroanat* 2014. doi: 10.3389/fnana.2014.00019. Reproduced under the CC BY 3.0 license https://creativecommons.org/licenses/by/3.0/

enlargement had both vertical expansion as well as anterior widening components (see Figure 6.4). This results in a forward inclination of the facial skeleton in relation to the base of the skull or cranial base, termed klinorhynchy, a feature unique to AMH [46]. This was already noted in the cranial endocast features of skulls of Jebel Irhoud (Morocco ~150 kya) and Skhul V (Near East ~120 kya) [47]. These morphological attributes are consistent with an escalation of neural intra-connectivity [48]. The neurobiological parietal lobe capabilities of analysis and elaboration of sensory input, visuospatial working memory function, number, time, and space computations facilitated abilities such as the representation of the body within external and internal frames of reference. The parietal lobes also have cross-modal sensory proficiency that enabled language comprehension and metaphor interpretation. In addition to the key function of visuospatial working memory, other key functions included hand–eye coordination, motor planning, and three-dimensional spatial renditions [49,50]. Such abilities endowed AMH with superior geographical navigation, increased finger dexterity allowing more advanced tool-making, and ultimately manufacture of more intricate and reliable weapons. Numerosity developed, or the understanding of quantity by finger counting to an initial amount of five, as an intraparietal sulcus function. Some evidence for these comes from the French Cosquer Cave, where stencils dated to 27 kya are seen as representative of early numeric codes. Numerosity systems appear to be mostly decimal, less often quinary (5) and vegesimal (20), which has been interpreted as intriguing evidence that the human hands played a significant role [51].

Clinical neurological impairments that can be seen to reflect this development of the human brain are exemplified by Gerstmann's syndrome. A discrete lesion, usually stroke-related, in the left inferior parietal lobe induces abnormalities of calculation (acalculia), problems with finger identification (finger anomia), as well as a right and left disorientation and writing impairment (dysgraphia). Unless these specific deficits are tested for in the clinical setting, which is rarely done, the syndrome can be easily missed altogether (Figure 6.5).

The southern African Blombos Cave and Pinnacle Point archeological finds suggest that numerosity concepts may be older than 100 ky, as inferred by the strung-bead discoveries. These and other parietal functions, such as symbolism conceptualization, abstract thinking, language, and metaphor abilities, have their representation in the various

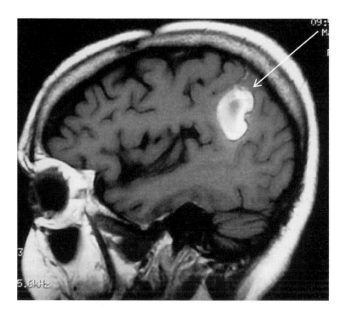

Figure 6.5 A very discreet isolated cortical hemorrhage in left angular gyrus (arrow), related to amyloid angiopathy causing Gerstmann's syndrome in a woman without any other neurological deficit.

figurines, ornaments, complex weaponry, and cave art typical of the Upper Paleolithic period from 50–10 kya. Other advanced AMH functions are centered in the superior parietal lobe, which includes the precuneus and intraparietal sulcus, associated with prospective memory function and numerosity. The precuneus and its connections are particularly noteworthy as this region has the highest metabolic activity in the brain, most evident in the resting state, and forms part of the all-important default mode network. The precuneus is currently regarded as a key hub region involved with the integration of diverse brain networks that mediate self-consciousness and autobiographical memory functions [52,53].

At least by archeological dating methods, cerebellum enlargement occurred even later at 35–11 kya. From a neurobiological perspective the AMH cerebellum to cortex ratio was significantly greater in comparison to Neanderthals. Other notable changes included a relatively higher neuronal density: of the brain's ~100 billion neurons, 70–80 percent are in the cerebellum. All major cerebral cortical regions project via the pons to the cerebellum in a reciprocal manner back to the cortical regions. Specifically, the extensive connectivity with the frontal lobes via the frontopontocerebellar tracts was associated with particular enlargements within the cerebellum, including the dentate cerebellar nuclei. Connections to 14 different cerebral cortical areas have been reported, which have been implicated in the promotion of cortical efficiency. From a physiological point of view, cerebellar function is associated with the precise timing of neural responses and enhancement of the processing of cognitive, motor, and sensory signaling. The pervasive working memory circuitry includes cerebellar components and is thought to fine-tune and improve efficiency in both motor and cognitive processes [54]. Other capabilities attributed to the cerebellum were involvement in emotional processing, a critical human attribute that evolved in response to the increasingly more complex social challenges and complexities among AMH [23]. Together these refinements of brain information processing would have been particularly advantageous to AMH of the Upper Paleolithic period. Vandervert et al. have also proposed that the cortical–cerebellar–cortical reciprocal circuitry may have been crucial to the neurobiological foundations of innovation creativity [55].

The Abrupt Florescence of Modern Behavior and Capacity for Culture ~50 kya

With the exception of apex predators, to which group the hominins did not belong, all animals have evolved differing solutions to their particular predation challenges. The primate's formula included color vision as their major sensing of the environment, and sociality, existing within a group. Support for the latter comes from Dunbar's social brain hypothesis (SBH) that indicates a correlation of increasing brain size with increasing group size. As the primate group size increased further, fission–fusion group behaviors and geographical dispersion of the groups developed. Social complexities progressively increased with expanding numbers of interacting dyads and triads within the group [56]. What has been termed a "virtual group member" had to be considered with the dispersion of the groups and the accompanying social dynamics. These requirements were thought to have further increased the cognitive load in the evolution of earlier primate brains [57]. The specific brain circuitry deployed to deal with the progressively increasing social complexity included the emotional circuitry for nurturing social bonds. Although social grooming evolved from tactile, face-to-face events, emotions were fostered and mediated by oxytocin release with enhancement of bonding. Other brain circuitry that became "upgraded" included mind reading, mentalizing or theory of mind (TOM), and the mirror neuron-based system and its related grades of intentionalities (graded from 1–5). As a group, mammals in general have first-order intentionality, second-order intentionality within chimpanzees and presumably australopithecines, as this would suffice for basic stone tool manufacture, with Neanderthals having fourth-order and AMH fifth-order intentionality [58]. The later evolution of social emotions such as remorse, shame, greed, and guilt that differ from the primary emotions of fear, anger, happiness, and sadness evolved. As group size enlarged, a change from tactile grooming to vocal grooming was achieved by virtue of early protolanguage, the coevolution of controlled fire use, and musicality. Hence communication with a considerably larger group of individuals emerged as opposed to the one-on-one method afforded by tactile grooming. Musicality, with its emotive features, presumably evolved in a similar fashion to infant-directed speech (IDS). The chanting and dance associated with musicality that preceded language may have been an "emotion amplifier" in social contexts. Both increasing population sizes and emotions were considered critical elements in the formation of strong bonds. These in turn required more advanced mind reading or TOM, with populations becoming more dispersed in time and place, which placed demands on social interaction [59].

Settlement in higher latitudes, primarily in Eurasia, presented seasonality and variable day/night challenges, as well as unpredictable food sources. With increased dispersion, AMH networks were mitigated by social bonding. The smaller Neanderthal network size in contrast to AMH demanded less "cultural scaffolding" for social network maintenance, as speculated by Pearce et al. [60]. Seasonality and extreme winters selected for larger brain size in primates, birds, and our hominin lineage. The progressive encephalization and behavioral adaptations of hominin speciation in general were linked in turn to the orbitally induced paleo-climatological fluctuations, but with a differential effect imposed by higher-latitude dwelling [58,61]. Both Neanderthals and AMH had the largest brain sizes of any hominins except those dating to 100–120 kya. Some notable differences included the Neanderthal's larger orbits, associated with larger occipital lobes, attributed to decreased light exposure as well as having larger bodies in comparison to AMH. The neural implications were that more neural "real estate" was dedicated to the visual and somatic functions due to their large bodies, related to higher meat and protein diets [62,63]. Therefore, it may be deduced that AMH overall had relatively larger brains when standardized for the loss incurred by visual and somatic area neural dedication. AMH, on the other hand, had larger parietal lobes, which in turn augmented connectivity, some of which was required for social brain performance. Social brain circuitry and competence, especially orbitofrontal cortex size, has been correlated to mind reading and levels of intentionality, and competed with areas deployed for somatic systems and those required for the major organ systems [64].

Higher-latitude AMH fissioned into more groups in comparison to Neanderthals, with the average number in a group being 152 versus 106. Network maintenance in the context of geographical dispersion was challenged and to some extent circumvented by periodic assemblages, as well as artifacts and gift exchanges that were used as proxies for personal or face-to-face meetings, termed the Visual Display Hypothesis, and the notion of cultural scaffolding [65]. The more expansive and more interconnected AMH groups in turn incited innovations, which led to a so-called "ratchet effect" of knowledge accumulation that was progressively and continuously improved upon, instead of intermittently fizzling out as it may have done with the Neanderthals [66]. Notwithstanding these observations, there is a considerable body of evidence favoring strong dietary implications. Neanderthals were terrestrial, not marine or aquatic based (at least until ~40 kya). In general, animals inhabiting the littoral zone such as pinnipeds and otters, as well as the robust australopithecines (see the durophage ecotone model discussed in Chapter 2) were afforded a diet that promoted elevated working memory, as has been noted in comparing pinniped working memory capacity to primate working memory capacity. A littoral zone diet has other micronutrients that are required for synaptic efficiency. The Neanderthals had no parietal bulge, a less interconnected brain, were less social, lived in smaller groups, and had no formal language, but presumably they sang and danced – hence the "Singing Neanderthals" theory proposed by Mithen [67]. In addition to their larger visual cortices, they had smaller orbitofrontal cortices and smaller anterior temporal lobes, implying sociality was less developed than in AMH. The AMH represented by Cro Magnons were capable of making harpoons and other weapons used for fishing, and their habitats were coastal, lacustrine, and riverine. It was probably no mystery that the art of the French caves was found next to the Ardèche River, and the musical instruments and Venus figurines were found next to major river systems such as the Danube. An impactful hypothesis, the Danube Kulturpumpe (Danube Corridor) model, suggests this was a vital route for people and their ideas, and posited that the Swabian Jura in southwest Germany became a region where pivotal behavioral developments emerged, such as symbolic and mythical behavior, music, and figurative art about 40–45 kya. Arguably, one of the most compelling artifacts ever found, the Hohlenstein–Stadel figurine, "The Lionman," dated to 40–35 kya may be the oldest evidence for modern executive function (Figure 6.6) [14]. From the Swabian Jura sites such as Hohle Fels, Hohlenstein–Stadel, Geissenklösterle, and Vogelherd, these subsequently spread to other parts of present-day Europe [68,69].

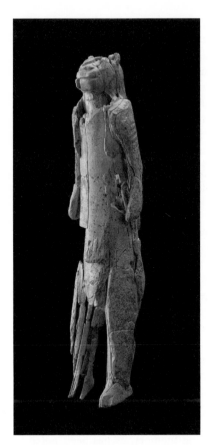

Figure 6.6 The mythical Hohlenstein–Stadel figurine: "Lion Man." Early evidence of modern executive function. *Source:* photo Yvonne Mühleis © State Office for Cultural Heritage Baden-Wuerttemberg/Museum Ulm, Germany; located in the Ulmer Museum, Stadt Ulm, Germany.

The Neanderthals ultimately became extinct by ~39 kya, with the last vestiges of habitat in present-day coastal Spain and perhaps as recently as 24 kya in Asia [70]. It may be surmised that they were less flexible and also had less adaptable brains when environmental, climactic, solar storms, volcanism, and magnetic reversals challenged their way of life [71].

References

1. Maslin MA, Shultz S, Trauth MH. A synthesis of the theories and concepts of early human evolution. *Phil Trans R Soc B* 2015 370:20140064.

2. Morgan TJ, Uomini NT, Rendell LE, et al. Experimental evidence for the co-evolution of hominin tool-making teaching and language. *Nat Commun* 2015;6:6029. doi: 10.1038/ncomms7029.

3. Arbib, M. From mirror neurons to complex imitation in the evolution of

language and tool use. *Ann Rev Antropol* 2011;40:257–273.

4. Klein RG. *The Human Career*, 3rd edn. University of Chicago Press, London, 2009.

5. Rowe JB, Owen AM, Johnsrude IS, Passingham RE. Imaging the mental components of a planning task. *Neuropsychologia* 2001;39:315–327.

6. Bookstein F, Schaefter K, Prossinger H, et al. Comparing frontal cranial profiles in archaic and modern *Homo*

by morphometric analysis. *Anat Record A Discov Mol Cell Evol Biol* 1999;257:217–224.

7. McBrearty S, Brooks AS. The revolution that wasn't: a new interpretation of the origin of modern human behavior. *J Hum Evol.* 2000;39, 453–563.

8. Coolidge FL, Wynn T. *The Rise of Homo Sapiens.* Oxford University Press, Oxford, 2018.

9. Wynn T. Archeology and cognitive evolution. *Behav Brain Sci* 2002;25:389–438.

10. Petrides M. Dissociable roles of the mid dorsolateral prefrontal cortex and anterior inferotemporal cortex in visual working memory. *J Neurosci* 2000;20:7496–7503.

11. Champod AS, Petrides M. Dissociation within the frontoparietal network in verbal working memory: a parametric functional magnetic resonance imaging study. *J Neurosci* 2010;30:3849–3856.

12. Champod AS, Petrides M. Dissociable roles of the posterior parietal and the prefrontal cortex in manipulation and monitoring process. *PNAS* 2007;104:14837–14842.

13. Mourre V, Villa P, Henshilwood CS. Early use of pressure flaking on lithic artifacts at Blombos Cave, South Africa. *Science.* 2010;330(6004):659–662.

14. Wynn T, Coolidge FI. The implications of the working memory model for the evolution of modern cognition. *Int J Evol Biol* 2011. doi: 10.4061/2011/741357.

15. Wynn T, Balter M. Did working memory spark creative culture ? *Science* 2010;328:160–163.

16. Eren MI, Lycett SJ. Why Levallois? A morphometric comparison of experimental "preferential" Levallois flakes versus debitage flakes. *PLoS One* 2012;7(1):e29273. doi: 10.1371/journal.pone.0029273.

17. Addis DR, Wond AT, Schacter DL. Remembering the past and imagining the future: common and distinct neural substrates during event construction and elaboration. *Neuropsychologica* 2007;45:1363–1377.

18. Land MF. Do we have an internal model of the outside world? *Philos Trans R Soc B* 2014;369:20130045.

19. Carey N. *The Epigenetics Revolution.* Columbia University Press, New York, 2012.

20. Testa-Silva G, Verhoog MB, Linaro D, et al. High bandwidth synaptic communication and frequency tracking in human neocortex. *PLoS Biol* 2014;12(11): e1002007. doi: 10.1371/journal. pbio.1002007.

21. Squires L. Gliotransmission. In: Brady ST, Siegel GJ, Albers RW, Price DL (eds.), *Basic Neurochemistry*, 8th edn. Elsevier Academic Press, New York 2012.

22. Coolidge FL, Wynn T. Cognitive prerequisites for a language of diplomacy. In: Tallerman M, Gibson KR (eds.), *The Oxford Companion to Language Evolution.* Oxford University Press, Oxford, 2012.

23. Fuster JM. *The Prefrontal Cortex: Anatomy, Physiology, and Neuropsychology of the Frontal Lobe.* Lippincott-Raven, Philadelphia, PA, 1997.

24. Bruner E. Morphological differences in the parietal lobes within the human genus: a neurofunctional perspective. *Curr Anthropol* 2010;51:S77–S88.

25. DeSmet HJ, Paquir P, Verhoeven J, Mariën P. The cerebellum: its role in language and related cognitive and affective functions. *Brain Lang* 2013;127:334–342.

26. Renfrew C, Frith C, Malafouris L. *The Sapient Mind: Archeology Meets Neuroscience.* Oxford University Press, New York, 2009.

27. Marean C. When the sea saved humanity. *Scientific American* August 2010.

28. Wadley L. Announcing a still bay industry at Sibudu Cave, South Africa. *J Hum Evol* 2007;52:681–689.

29. Marean CW. Pinnacle Point Cave 13B (Western Cape Province, South Africa) in context: the Cape Floral kingdom, shellfish, and modern human origins. *J Hum Evol.* 2010;59(3–4):425–443.

30. Opperman S. *Out of Eden: The Peopling of the World.* Robinson, London, 2004.

31. McBrearty, S. Palaeoanthropology: sharpening the mind. *Nature.* 2012;491(7425):531–532.

32. Watson E, Forster P, Richards M, Bandelt HJ. Mitochondrial footprints of human expansions in Africa. *Am J Human Genet* 1997;61:691–704.

33. Gibbons A. Y chromosome shows that Adam was African. *Science* 1997;278(5339):804–805.

34. Schlebusch CM, Lombard M, Soodyall H. MtDNA control region variation affirms diversity and deep sub-structure in populations from southern Africa. *BMC Evol Biol* 2013;13:1–20.

35. Rito T, Richards MB, Fernandes V, et al. The first modern human dispersals across Africa. *PLoS One* 2013;8:e80031.

36. Tishkoff SA, Gonder MK, Henn BM, et al. History of click speaking populations of Africa inferred from mtDNA and Y chromosome genetic variation. *Mol Biol Evol* 2007;24:2180–2195.

37. Pickrell JK, Patterson N, Barbieri C, et al. The genetic prehistory of southern Africa. *Nat Commun* 2012. doi: 10.1038/ncomms2140.

38. Henn BM, Cavalli-Sforza LL, Feldman MW. The great human expansion. *PNAS* 2012;109:17758–17764.

39. Knight A, Underhill PA, Mortensen HM, et al. African Y chromosome and mtDNA divergence provides insight into the history of click languages. *Curr Biol* 2003;13:464–473.

40. Crawford MA, Broadhurst CL, Guest M, et al. A quantum theory for the irreplaceable role of docosahexanoic acid in neural signaling throughout evolution. *Prostaglandins Leukot Essent Fatty Acids* 2013;88:5–13.

41. Crawford MA. Docosahexaenoic acid in neural signaling systems. *Nutr Health* 2006;18(3):263–276.

42. Bazinet RP, Laye S. Polyunsaturated fatty acids and their metabolites in brain function and disease. *Nat Rev Neurosci* 2014;15:771–785.

43. Ramsden CE, Faurot KR, Zamora D, et al. Targeted alteration of dietary n-3 and n-6 fatty acids for the treatment of chronic headaches: a randomized trial. *Pain* 2013;154(11). doi: 10.1016/j.pain.2013.07.028.

44. Elston GN. Pyramidal cells of the frontal lobe: all the more spinous to think with. *J Neurosci* 2000;20:RC95.

45. Elston GN. Cortex, cognition and the cell: new insights into the pyramidal neuron and prefrontal function. *Cerebral Cortex* 2003;13:1124–1138.

46. Bruner E. Geometric morphometrics and paleoneurology: brain shape evolution in the genus Homo. *J Hum Evol* 2004;47:279–303.

47. Bruner E, Manzi G, Arsuaga JL. Encephalization and allometric trajectories in the genus *Homo*: evidence from the Neanderthal and modern lineages. *PNAS* 2003;100:15335–15340.

48. Bruner E, De La Cuétara JM, Holloway R. A bivariate approach to the variation of the parietal curvature in the genus *Homo*. *Anat Rec* 2011;294:1548–1556.

49. Orban GA, Caruana F. The neural basis of human tool use. *Front Psychol* 2014;5:310.

50. Bruner E. The evolution of the parietal cortical areas in the human genus: between structure and cognition. In: Broadfield D, Yuan M, Schick K, Toth N (eds.), *The Human Brain Evolving*. Stone Age Institute Press, Gosport, IN, 2010.

51. Overmann KA. Finger counting in the upper Paleolithic. *Rock Art Res* 2014;31:63–80.

52. Coolidge FN, Overmann KA. Numerosity, abstraction and the emergence of symbolic thinking. *Curr Anthropol* 2012;53:204–225.

53. Cavanna, AE, Trimble MR. The precuneus: a review of its functional anatomy and behavioural correlates. *Brain* 2006;129:564–583.

54. Weaver AH. Reciprocal evolution of the cerebellum and neocortex in fossil humans. *PNAS* 2005;102:3576–3580.

55. Vandervert LR, Schimpf PH, Liu H. How working memory and the cerebellum collaborate to produce creativity and innovation. *Creat Res J* 2007;19:1–18.

56. Dunbar RIM. Neocortex size as a constraint on group size in primates. *J Hum Evol* 1992;20:469–493.

57. Barrett L, Henzi SP, Dunbar RIM. Primate cognition: from "what now" to "what if?" *Trends Cogn Sci* 2003;7:494–497.

58. Schultz S, Nelson E, Dunbar RIM. Hominin cognitive evolution: identifying patterns and processes in the fossil and archaeological record. *Phil Trans R Soc B* 2012;367:2130–2140.

59. Richards MP, Pettit RB, Stiner MC, Trinkaus E. Stable isotope evidence for increasing dietary breadth in the European Mid-Upper Palaeolithic. *PNAS* 2001;98:6528–6532.

60. Pearce E, Shuttleworth A, Grove M, Layton RH. The costs of being a high-latitude hominin. In: Dunbar RIM, Gamble C, Gowlett JAJ (eds.), *Lucy to Language*. Oxford University Press, Oxford, 2014.

61. Grove M. Amplitudes of orbitally induced climate cycles and patterns of hominin speciation. *J Archaeol Sci* 2012;39:3085–3094.

62. Pearce E, Bridge H. Is orbital volume associated with eyeball and visual cortical volume in humans? *Ann Hum Biol* 2013;40(6):531–540.

63. Balzeau A, Holloway RL, Grimaud-Herve D. Variations and asymmetries in regional brain surface in the genus Homo. *J Hum Evol* 2012;62:696–706.

64. Pearce E, Stringer C, Dunbar RIM. New insights into differences in brain organization between Neanderthals and anatomically modern humans. *Proc R Soc London B* 2013;280B. doi: 10.1098/rspb.2013.0168.

65. McNabb J. The importance of conveying visual information in Archeulean society: the background to the visual display hypothesis. *Hum Evol* 2011;1:1–23.

66. Dunbar RIM, Gamble C, Gowlett JAJ. *Lucy to Language*. Oxford University Press, Oxford, 2014.

67. Mithen S. The music instinct: the evolutionary basis of musicality. *Ann NY Acad Sci* 2009;1169:3–12.

68. Higham T, Basell L, Jacobi R, et al. Testing models for the beginnings of the Aurignacian and the advent of figurative art and music: the radiocarbon chronology of Geißenklösterle. *J Hum Evol* 2012;62(6):664–676.

69. Conard NJ, Bolus M. Radiocarbon dating the appearance of modern humans and timing of cultural innovations in Europe: new results and new challenges. *J Hum Evol* 2003;44(3):331–371.

70. Higham T, Douka K, Wood R, et al. The timing and spatiotemporal patterning of Neanderthal disappearance. *Nature* 2014;512:306–309.

71. Gilpin W, Feldman MW, Aoki K. An ecocultural model predicts Neanderthal extinction through competition with modern humans. *PNAS* 2016;113(8):2134–2139.

Unraveling of Brain Networks in Neurological Conditions
Nature's Reductionism

Contemporary neurology, neuroscience, and mathematical network analyses have tackled our most pressing brain disorders with a "network approach." These include extensive brain networks such as the default mode network (DMN) that is impaired in Alzheimer's disease and the salience network that unravels in frontotemporal dementias and traumatic brain injury – hence the concept of networktopathies. At a molecular level, some unravel at the junctions or synapses – synaptopathies – such as many psychiatric disorders and Gulf War Illness.

Among anatomically modern humans (AMH), the protracted time between birth and development of the body – and more specifically brain maturity – allowed sufficient time for vast connectivity to take place for the change from discrete intelligences to a cognitively fluid intelligence. In Mithen's model of "Cathedrals of Intelligences," the change was from the "isolated" intelligences within the brain of natural history, technical, social, linguistic, and general intelligence with little interaction (also referred to as a Swiss Army knife configuration), to a cognitive fluid mentality with extensive interaction. It simply provides time for connections between specialized intelligences to be formed within the mind. The consequences of this cognitive fluidity were the development of art, spirituality, complex tools, and language. Viewed in another way, consciousness can be seen to have developed as an integrating system for the various knowledge centers that were entrapped within domains of separate intelligences. An approximate timeline was that of *Purgatorius* and *Northarctus* between 65 and 50 mya, an evolutionary switch from hardwired-type behavioral responses to a generalized type of intelligence that allowed learning from experience. Although general intelligence required an increase in brain size, the cost–benefit ratio appeared biologically worth it. *Proconsul*, at about 35 mya, had developed a further increase in general intelligence as well as social intelligence. Subsequently, technical and natural history intelligences evolved, and so did linguistic intelligence. The latter was integral to social intelligence and presumably developed ~2 mya. Enhanced language capacity followed and enabled information processing about a conspecific's mind, or one's own mind. The new cognitive fluidity was assumed to have developed due to new connections and was not associated with increase in brain size or due to speed of information processing, although the latter also occurred in stages.

Provisioning for food may have prompted the development of natural history intelligence followed by technical intelligence. Hence, the different specialized intelligences no longer functioned in isolation, and by becoming interconnected the stage was set for more complex human abilities. Our closest cousins, the Neanderthals, may have represented a "missing cognitive link." By studying evidence of Neanderthal communication systems, Mithen developed his *Hmmmm* model; a holistic, manipulative, multimodal, musical, and mimetic system that designated them as the "singing Neanderthals" surviving about 250 000 years. Mithen envisaged them as very emotional people, expressing their emotions through body language, gestures, and utterances, while lacking cognitive circuitry inherent among AMH for more advanced sociality and tool-making, in coping with their environmental challenges. One possibility is that the missing cognitive link might have been related to enhanced working memory. Connectivity between all of Mithen's five intelligences was later interpreted by Ramachandran and others as the factor that likely sparked the big bang of human intelligences [1,2]. Further brain networking occurred in the approximated sequences presented in Table 7.1.

Contemporary Brain Networking Hypotheses

Our brain's network architecture has been conceived of as a "small-world organization" that combines a plentiful level of restricted neighborhood-type clustering that enables efficient local information handling. At the same time, the network organization features a number of long-distance links rendering good global communication that serves to integrate information between geographically different brain regions. This network architecture is viewed as representing an optimum balance between local short-range and global long-range cerebral connectivity. The human brain network is therefore a compromise between the two extremes of a lattice (minimizes cost but not global integration) and random (large number of long-distance fibers with elevated wiring cost). Such topology (from Greek *topos* and the way in which constituent parts of a system are interrelated) is also a characteristic of other familiar complex systems including social and scientific networks, as well as human-created systems such as airline hubs and the stock market [15].

The Rise of New "Neuro" Disciplines

Unsurprisingly, advances in the understanding of the complex human connectome are only possible and best achieved by similarly networking between disparate disciplines in science and the humanities. This has spawned new disciplines altogether within the last two decades, such as network mathematics. This has benefited functional neurosurgical approaches and the treatment of neuro-oncological conditions and traumatic brain injury (TBI) [16–18]. Other emerging neuro-related disciplines include neuro-ergonomics [19], neuro-economics [20], and neuro-art history [21], all of which have had significant input into our understanding of the workings of the human mind. Neuro-archeology, in particular, owes its emergence to distinguished investigators such as Renfrew, Wynn and Coolidge, and Bruner, to name a few who have championed its inception [9,22,23].

The likely reason for the increasing number of disciplines involved in human connectomal analyses and elucidation is that such a complex entity benefits from these diversified approaches. For example, archeologists delve into material remains that allow them to infer past human behaviors, while cognitive archeologists venture into the possible

Table 7.1 A summary of the approximate time course of the principal networking evolution of the human mind

Stage	Archeological evidence	Presumptive time of development	Reference
1. Frontoparietal circuitry, dorsal and ventral visual streams development	Oldowan stone tools, flakes, australopithecines	~2.6 mya	[3]
2. Technical intelligence, procedural memory, and conceptual thought	Archeulean hand axes, blades, *Homo erectus*	~1.9 mya	[4]
3. Symbolic thought		~500–300 kya	[5]
4. Mirror neuron circuit to stage 7 and theory of mind	AMH	~50 kya?	[6]
5. Autonoesis, mental time travel	AMH	~50 kya?	[7]
6. Executive function	Hohlenstein–Stadel Lionman, AMH	40–30 kya	[8]
7. Enhanced working memory to stage 7		~30 kya	[9]
8. Spirituality, shamanism, cave art, imagistic communication		~30 kya	[10]
9. Emotional intelligence and social emotion		?	[11]
10. Recursive language		~50 kya	[12,13]
11. Metacognition (introspection)		?	[14]

cognitive capacities and thought processes that may be gleaned from these recreated behaviors. Cognitive neuroscientists concern themselves with the neurobiological processes responsible for observed behaviors, and neuroscientists study the genetic, epigenetic, and molecular structure of the neural systems in organisms to help elucidate the processes at work [24]. As already noted, the profound escalation in white matter is a defining feature of modern humans. Modern neurology is now concerned with processes that unravel the human connectome, as increasingly connectivity-based neuroradiological imaging is refining neurological diseases and allowing earlier diagnoses. Examples of connectomic abnormalities amenable to resting-state functional MRI scanning include Alzheimer's disease and other dementias, TBI, multiple sclerosis, minimally conscious states, epilepsy, autism, and schizophrenia. There are important clinical implications of the functional network disruption diagnosis detected by fMRI, as distinct patterns of network disruption in the major neurodegenerative diseases can be detected much earlier and these may represent what Pievani et al. have termed "intermediate clinical phenotypes between pathology and clinical syndromes" [25].

Several intrinsic connectivity networks have been reported. These include the default mode network (DMN) that is of relevance in Alzheimer's disease, the salience network for frontotemporal lobe dementia, the basal ganglia–thalamocortical circuitry which is disrupted in Parkinson's disease and dementia with Lewy bodies, and the attentional network [26]. In Alzheimer's disease there is a close link between global energy metabolism and the disease pathology that follows both temporally and spatially the DMN. Network dysfunction appears to occur in parallel with metabolic dysfunction, in both cognitive aging and Alzheimer's disease. Sensitivity and specificity for DMN imaging in Alzheimer's disease and healthy normal controls have been reported at 85 percent and 77 percent respectively [27]. Brain connectivity studies have revealed that with Alzheimer's disease, the A-beta and tau deposition takes places in the highly interconnected hub regions, with subsequent spread to the much larger network. Similar findings have been reported for alpha synuclein in Lewy body disease and the spread of tau protein, TDP 43, and FUS in frontotemporal lobe dementia. It has been proposed that the misfolded proteins initially spread intraneuronally and, similar to prions, might induce misfolding of adjacent normal proteins. Thereafter presynaptic cellular and then postsynaptic cellular involvement occurs, with one proposal being a possible network-centered dysregulation of the excitation–disinhibition imbalance in local microcircuits. Hence the network theory of neurodegenerative disease pathophysiology is seen to proceed from a primary neuronopathy, spreading to the local microcircuitry then affecting the long-range disease fiber networks and presenting as a networkopathy [28,29]. This affords an identification of the five most common dementia subtypes and presymptomatic network disruption with the identification of subgroups, most likely to benefit from disease-modifying therapies. Potential therapies with positive results in phase 1 Alzheimer's disease trials in this regard include the recalibration of networks by transcranial magnetic stimulation or deep brain stimulation, for example, that have shown improvement in network metabolism-related functions and cognitive performance [30,31].

Frontotemporal Lobe Disorders

Frontotemporal lobe disorders (FTDs) are probably among the most common brain disorders. The inferior frontal lobes, anterior temporal lobes, and the uncinate fasciculus and processes affecting these circuits may be viewed as a kind of "ground zero" for the study of modern mind evolution. These syndromes are particularly intriguing conditions from a neurobehavioral point of view, and of course at the same time often devastating for the individuals and the families so afflicted. The manifold frontotemporal lobe syndromes are, however, yielding invaluable insights into human mind evolution and at the same time pointers to potential therapies. Their relatively covert, frequently subtle presentations and diverse etiologies pose major challenges in diagnosis and treatments. Yet these are the most plastic areas of the brain, providing opportunities for successful interventions.

FTDs and their neurobiological substrates and principal fiber tracts, most notably the uncinate fasciculus, represent unique human illnesses. These encompass widely differing pathophysiologies, including frontotemporal lobe dementias, chronic traumatic encephalopathy, TBIs, vascular dementias, neurotoxicological syndromes, and mild

FTD phenocopy subtypes [32]. Some, such as the last of these, may stabilize for decades and even improve, in contradistinction to the traditional dementias such as Alzheimer's disease [33]. Networktopathies and synaptopathies represented by TBI, post-traumatic stress disorder (PTSD), as well as molecular derangements such as Gulf War Illness (GWI), have been associated with FTD presentations. GWI, primarily a synaptopathy associated with acute-phase lipids, may present as an FTD syndrome together with other polysyndromic presentations, making diagnosis inordinately difficult. Furthermore, neuroimmunological disorders with inflammation and autoimmune disorders have also been implicated in FTD [34,35]. Metabolic syndromes tend to target the more posterior association areas resulting in the Alzheimer's spectrum of cognitive dysfunction, whereas the more anterior association cortices of the frontal and anterior temporal lobes may be more prone to trauma, toxins, and stressors of various kinds [36]. These in turn target the default mode network and salience networks, respectively, that can be imaged by functional MRI scans [26].

Recent wars have highlighted two signature syndromes that afflict a significant number of deployed personnel. Both affect brain regions with syndromes that are difficult to diagnose and treat. Mild and moderate traumatic brain injury (mTBI) and GWI fall within the domain of FTD [37]. These constitute a panoply of disorders in which the presentation is predominantly behavioral, more so than with cognitive impairments. They are characterized by marked heterogeneity of clinical presentations with respect to behavior, cognition, neurological syndromes, and pathology. Deciphering these syndromes and their causes is pivotal for potentially effective treatments, which elude us at the present time.

Behavioral and cognitive disorders are especially likely to occur in the scenario of constant stimulation and complicated nature that is part of the information age. This requires sustained attention, effective executive function, and insightful reasoning for optimal decision-making, appropriate impulse control, and inhibition of responses. The extensive networks and highly evolved cells – such as pyramidal, spindle, and fork cells – that are characteristic of the association cortices, in particular, are targeted. No effective treatments currently exist and the pharmaceutical industry has recently de-emphasized research in these areas.

Making Sense of the Numerous Presentations

FTDs are infamous for defying diagnosis, sometimes for years, with misdiagnoses and incorrect treatments common. This is largely due to the relatively subtle behavioral presentations, which are frequently missed by standard neuropsychological tests, let alone cognitive screening tests. The latter include the Mini-Mental State Examination (MMSE) that has no frontal lobe tests and the Montreal Cognitive Assessment (MOCA) that has some cognitive frontal tests but provides no behavioral information. Even specific frontal lobe batteries such as the Frontal Assessment Battery (FAB) have no behavioral components. FTD have extremely varied and protean presentations, with up to 19 different syndromes delineated, for example [38]. A global FTD database (https://ftdregistry.org), designated as a contact and research registry, is currently gathering prospective data on people with FTD and their cognitive and behavioral impairments. The memory-centric approach to dementias in general may divert attention from many other early presentations, such as dysociality, abulia/apathy, and change in personality [39]. A relatively rapid, comprehensive, screening, bedside-type testing approach has been proposed by the author to help delineate the disparate presentations to allow more precise subgroups to be recognized so that potential therapies might stand a better chance of success [40].

Modern Neuroimaging Approaches

Brain network science (small world, rich club hubs), the hodological effects of lesions and clinically apparent diaschisis syndromes (at rest, functional, connectional), demand that the entire brain be evaluated no matter where the lesion location. With more uniform subgroup identification, targeted treatments are more likely to be successful. These can be accomplished by using diffusion tensor imaging, metabolic positron emission tomography (PET) and resting-state brain network imaging [41].

Paving the Way for Therapeutics

Neuropharmacological options are scarce and efficacy in these disorders is dismal. FTD syndromes are predominantly a serotonergic rather than the acetylcholine deficiency syndrome that characterizes Alzheimer's disease. Trazodone is the only pharmotherapeutic success to date in this group of illnesses, in particular for frontotemporal lobe dementia. Such neurotransmitter therapies, however, have limited effects. The longstanding acetylcholine-enhancing medications such as donepezil have recently been trounced by a European meta-analysis that concluded the benefits were below the minimally relevant thresholds and it was not cost-effective [42]. The earliest neurobiological defect of cognitive disorders may well be at the neurovascular level, with both clinical and neuroimaging studies supporting impaired cerebrovascular reactivity impairment as the first sign of compromise. This underscores the essential role of physical exercise that induces both generalized cardiovascular and cerebrovascular health, as well as neurotrophic factors that lead to neurogenesis and angiogenesis, and augment brain circuitry.

Much greater promise appears to be in the realm of lifestyle/behavioral interventions in people with mild cognitive impairment in general. These include the administration of a high-seafood diet with docosahexapentanoic acid (DHA) and eicosapentanoic acid (EPA), together with monitored physical exercise and structured cognitive exercise applications. These have shown profound cognitive, behavioral, and neuroimaging improvements in dementia patients [43]. Physical exercise has particularly potent brain protective effects and has been shown to reduce the incidence of dementia by up to 50 percent [44]. Healthy diet adherence, such as a Mediterranean-type diet has consistently shown reduction in cardiovascular disease, dementia, and cancer. A principal mechanism in this regard may be the effects on working memory, which may be regarded as the core frontal lobe function central to all other processes, including attention, memory, executive function, and inhibition. Specific working memory cognitive exercises have been developed, such as Brain HQ (www.brainhq.com) and Cogmed (www.cogmed.com/program), that may be particularly relevant for those presenting within the mild cognitive impairment spectrum.

Traumatic Brain Injury and Gulf War Illness

TBI is often regarded as a signature injury of recent wars such as Operation Enduring Freedom (OEF), Operation Iraq Freedom (OIF), and Operation New Dawn (OND). A major part of the reason for this is that, in contemporary military combat, the ratio of survivors who died from their combat wounds has increased from 2:1 in World War II, to 2.6:1 in the Vietnam War, 2.8:1 in the Korean War to 7.4:1 in OIF [45]. The increased survival rate in general allows a relatively greater survival of those with head injuries. However, a significant increase in suicide has been realized in those who survive. For example, the US Department of Defense Suicide Event Report (DoDSER) program documented 2553 suicide attempts and 812 suicides among active service members in a three-year surveillance period [46]. TBI research has revealed a complex pathophysiological process that includes microvascular injury and neurometabolic uncoupling that are superimposed on the primary injury processes such as subdural, contusion, and diffuse axonal injury [47]. In addition, the microvasculopathy, perivascular edema, and microthrombosis that also lead to selective neuronal loss as well as tissue hypoxia all conspire to make this a widely dispersed networktopathy [48]. These assertions have since been demonstrated by the latest neuroimaging techniques, specifically diffusion tensor imaging and resting-state network imaging, which show that TBI impairs "small-world topology" similarly to what has been demonstrated in Alzheimer's disease, schizophrenia, and aging. The small-world neural architecture is in turn dependent on the unimpaired long-distance connections as well as the local interactive circuitry. Brain networks are composed of small-world networks with strong local connectivity as well as having proficient and efficient long-distance connections. The impaired long-distance axonal connections translate into impaired network function and consequently cognitive dysfunction [49]. The "hub failure hypothesis" posits that most, if not all, brain diseases are in essence system disorders. Damage occurs to hubs with a consequent redistribution of hub nodes, which has been documented so far in TBI, Alzheimer's disease, multiple sclerosis, Parkinson's disease, and epilepsy. The primary clinical deficit or impairment seen with hub failure, no matter the disease process, manifests with cognitive deficits in three principal domains: attention, working memory, and executive function [50].

Newly Appreciated Subtypes of TBI

The advent of non-conventional warfare, such as the use of improvised explosive devices (IEDs) ushered in a different kind of injury: blast injuries. Cernak reviewed the potential mechanisms responsible and delineated a number of different phases. The primary blast has components of an overpressure wave of ~100–250 psi, followed by an underpressure wave. Secondary injury may occur due to debris as well as blunt and penetrating injury. A tertiary injury may be consequent to acceleration and deceleration forces on the body and brain. Quaternary effects may occur due to burns from heat or flashes and quinary effects may occur and be attributed to effects of radiation or bacterial infection [51]. Blast traumatic brain injury (bTBI) may be regarded as a synaptopathy, with neuronal synapses undergoing stretching and shearing with a temporary disconnection of neural circuitry transpiring. Clinically this manifests with the bTBI symptoms of immediate loss of consciousness and dizziness that is attributed to a "synaptic disconnection" injury. The synaptic cleft (gap) is altered and "dislocated," with the scaffolding proteins and cellular adhesion molecules disrupted by the shear forces. Neurotransmitter transmission and clearance are altered, and glutamate- and calcium-mediated neurotoxicity may occur with oxidative stress (Figure 7.1) [52]. This has support from neurobiological research into bTBI, both from clinical and rodent animal data. In an important study by Zuckerman et al., exposure to experimental blastwave effects in rodents caused significant spatial

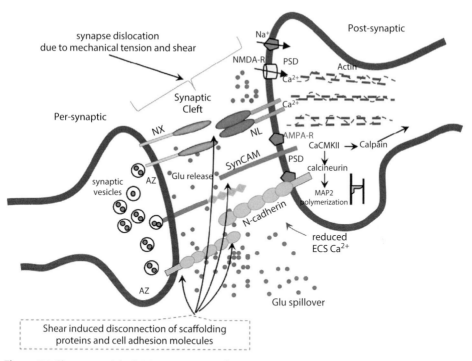

Figure 7.1 Blast traumatic brain injury: a synaptopathy.

Source: Przekwas A, Somayaji MR, Gupta RK. Synaptic mechanisms of blast-induced brain injury. *Front Neurol* 2016 doi: 10.3389/fneur.2016.00002. Reproduced under the CC BY 4.0 license https://creativecommons.org/licenses/by/4.0/

learning impairment in 23.6 percent and elicited well-defined behavioral responses very similar to mTBI-like and PTSD-like responses. In 10.9 percent there was also a comorbid PTSD and mTBI. MRI brain scanning did not reveal abnormalities in any of these groups [53]. Contrary to teaching that concussion and mild TBI resolves rapidly within weeks to months, new clinical and rodent studies show the opposite. Not only may the symptoms persist for years, but they might even worsen. This is more common in repetitive TBI than after a single TBI [54,55].

A different kind of temporally related network damage occurs with chronic traumatic encephalopathy (CTE). Known for decades under previous names such as dementia pugilistica, it was first recognized in boxers. This condition is now acknowledged in a number of sports, foremost in American football but also in other contact sports such as ice hockey and soccer, as well as in military-related blast injuries. Both subconcussive and repetitive concussions are etiologically related. CTE differs from other neurodegenerative diseases both clinically and pathologically. Clinically, behavioral deficits are more pronounced than cognitive deficits such as dysmemory and executive dysfunction. Similar to FTD, there may be profound sociopathies, lack of empathy, aggression, explosivity, depression, and suicidality. Gross pathological findings include frontal and temporal atrophy; microscopically, tau and TAR DNA-binding protein 43 pathology and axonal degeneration are evident. In a brain bank analysis of 202 demised football players (termed a convenience sample), of those who played in the National Football league, 110 of 111 had a neuropathological diagnosis of CTE [56]. CTE stages I–IV occur with gradual progression from the front of the brain to the back. Initially the abnormalities involve the frontal and temporal lobes, then the brainstem and later involve the parietal and occipital lobes, which is very different from an Alzheimer's disease-type progression. These stages may be readily delineated by tau PET scanning and by tau pathological diagnosis [57]. Other differences include pathology subtypes. An isolated severe TBI episode is associated with amyloid beta pathology very similar to Alzheimer's disease. Repetitive brain injury, on the other hand, is associated with a predominant tauopathy typical of CTE and dementia pugilistica of boxer's brains [58].

Gulf War Illness

Toxic Wounds and Synaptopathies

GWI has been referred to as a "toxic wound" related to the Gulf War (1991), Desert Shield, and Desert Storm. For the 25 years following those wars, up to one-third of combatants have been frequenting multiple different medical specialties with polysymptomatic presentations typical of multisystem illness. Of those exposed, 25–32 percent have several or all of the listed symptoms, including fatigue, headaches, cognitive dysfunction, musculoskeletal pain, respiratory, gastrointestinal, and dermatologic problems. In addition, brain cancer occurs at increased rates, as do neuropsychological and brain imaging abnormalities. These have since been encompassed in specific criteria such as the Kansas, Haley, and Institute of Medicine criteria that help make the diagnosis. A review by ten centers concluded that psychiatric causes have been ruled out and that exposure to pyridostigmine bromide and permethrin (insecticide) pesticides are causally associated with GWI and the neurological dysfunction in Gulf War veterans. Many other potential causes examined, including exposure to sarin and cyclosarin and to oil-well fire emissions, are also associated with neurologically based health effects, though their contribution to development of the disorder known as GWI is less clear [35].

Unraveling at the Molecular Level

Acute-phase lipid abnormalities, mitochondrial toxicity, and synaptic abnormalities have been identified in GWI, which is regarded primarily as a neurological and not a psychiatric condition. Endocrine and autonomic nervous systems disturbances feature prominently, in addition to the other syndromes mentioned. Neuroscientific progress with GWI first documented the elevation of acute-phase lipids, including phospholipids, that was reported by Hokama et al. in 2008 [59]. Lipid metabolism pathways can influence inflammation and endocrine functions are deranged in GWI. As phosphocholine and sphingomyelin levels increase (these lipids primarily contain omega-6 and omega-9 fatty acids) this results in lower free phosphocholine. Phosphocholine is a metabolite of phosphotidylcholine and sphingomyelin, which is used endogenously for synthesis of Ach. As a consequence, lysosomal and perioxisomal dysfunctions occur, as well as increased astroglial activation. In addition, axonal transport impairment occurs, with microtubule structure, transport, and tubulin – a neuronal transport protein – affected. The dysfunctional lipid metabolism in GWI was supported by animal studies of pyridostigmine bromide, as well as stress-exposed rats in which it was shown that pyridostigmine bromide lowers brain levels of phosphocholine as opposed to rats exposed to stress only [34]. The high-bandwidth synapses in the human brain are also affected, with at least one mechanism so far demonstrated. The study by Zakirova et al. implicated impairment of the multiprotein signaling complexes or signalosomes, with one of the proteins affected being synaptophysin in cortex and hippocampus, associated with astrogliosis [60,61].

Clinical studies support these basic neuroscience discoveries. For example, neuropsychological studies revealed significant differences in the prefrontal cortex activity engaged in a working memory task between GWI and control groups. The implication was that the GWI group needed to allocate more resources to the working memory demands in relation to controls. Neuroimaging studies in those diagnosed with GWI revealed loss of white matter integrity in corticocortical and corticospinal areas. Diffusion tensor imaging studies revealed significant changes in axial diffusivity, particularly in the inferior frontooccipital fasciculus (IFOF) [35]. As meditation has been shown to "brain build" prefrontal cortex white matter tracts, these findings have implications for meditation as a potential therapy for GWI, as will be discussed in Chapter 12.

Implications of GWI Pathophysiology for Other Neurotoxicological Conditions

The similarity of the health problems of GWI veterans and those of other occupational groups with organophosphate exposures include farmers, sheep dippers, insecticide applicators, agricultural nursery workers, and chemical plant workers. Identification of future treatments for the GWI veteran population will have far-reaching implications for treating other groups of ill patients for whom there are currently no effective treatments.

References

1. Mithen S. *The Prehistory of the Mind.* Phoenix, London, 1998.

2. Ramachandran VS. *The Tell-Tale Brain.* W.W. Norton, New York, 2011.

3. Stout D, Toth N, Schick K, Chaminade T. Neural correlates of Early Stone Age toolmaking: technology, language and cognition in human evolution. *Phil Trans R Soc B* 2008;363:1939–1949.

4. Johnson-Frey SH. The neural bases of complex tool use in humans. *Trends Cogn Sci* 2004;8:71–78.

5. Barham LS. Systematic pigment use in the Middle Pleistocene of South-Central Africa. *Curr Anthropol* 2002;43:181–190.

6. Arbib MA. From mirror neurons to complex imitation in the evolution of language and tool use. *Ann Rev Anthropol* 2011;40:257–273.

7. Corballis MC. Mental time travel: a case for evolutionary continuity. *Trends Cogn Sci* 2013;17:5–6.

8. Suddendorf, T. Foresight and evolution of the human mind. *Science* 2006;312:1006–1007.

9. Renfrew C, Frith C, Malafouris L. *The Sapient Mind: Archeology Meets Neuroscience.* Oxford University Press, New York, 2009.

10. Lewis Williams D. *The Mind in the Cave.* Thames and Hudson, London, 2002.

11. Jablonka E, Ginsberg, S, Dor D. The co-evolution of language and emotions. *Phil Trans R Soc B* 2012;367:2152–2159.

12. Lieberman P. The evolution of human speech. *Anthropology* 2007;48:39–66.

13. Fitch TW. *The Evolution of Language.* Cambridge University Press, Cambridge, 2010.

14. Fleming SM, Dolan RJ. The neural basis of metacognitive ability. *Phil Trans R Soc B* 2012;367:1338–1349.

15. Bullmore E, Sporns O. The economy of brain network organization. *Nat Rev Neurosci* 2012;13:336–349.

16. Hart MG, Ypma RJ, Romero-Garcia R, et al. Graph theory analysis of complex brain networks: new concepts in brain mapping applied to neurosurgery. *J Neurosurg* 2016;124(6):1665–1678.

17. Gkigkitzis I, Haranas K, Kotsireas I. Biological relevance of network architecture. *Adv Exp Med Biol* 2017;988:1–29.

18. Al-Anzi B, Gerges S, Olsman N, et al. Modeling and analysis of modular structure in diverse biological networks. *J Theor Biol* 2017;422:18–30.

19. Parasuraman R, Rizzo M. *Neuroergonomics: The Brain at Work.* Oxford University Press, Oxford, 2006.

20. Camerer C, Loewenstein C. Neuroeconomics: how neuroscience can inform economics. *J Econ Lit* 2005;43:9–64.

21. Onians J. *Neuroarthistory: From Aristotle to Pliny to Baxandall and Zeki.* Yale University Press, New Haven, CT, 2007.

22. Coolidge FL, Wynn T. *The Rise of Homo Sapiens: The Evolution of Modern Thinking.* Wiley-Blackwell, London, 2009.

23. Reyes LD, Sherwood CC. Neuroscience and human brain evolution. In Bruner E (ed.), *Human Paleoneurology.* Springer, New York, 2015.

24. Stout D, Hecht E. Neuroarcheology. In: Bruner E (ed.),. *Human Paleoneurology.* Springer, New York, 2015.

25. Pievani M, De Haan W, Wu T, Seeley WW, Frisoni GB. Functional network disruption in the degenerative dementias. *Lancet Neurol* 2011;10:829–843.

26. Seeley WW, Menon V, Schatzberg AF, et al. Dissociable intrinsic connectivity networks for salience processing and executive control. *J Neurosci* 2007;27(9):2349–2356.

27. Kapogiannis D, Mattson MP. Disrupted energy metabolism and neuronal circuit dysfunction in cognitive impairment and Alzheimer's disease. *Lancet Neurol* 2011;10:187–198.

28. Zhou J, Greicius MD, Gennatas ED, et al. Divergent network connectivity changes in behavioural variant frontotemporal dementia and Alzheimer's disease. *Brain* 2010;133:1352–1367.

29. Zhang HY, Wang SJ, Liu B, et al. Resting brain connectivity: changes during the progress of Alzheimer disease. *Radiology* 2010;256:598–606.

30. Laxton AW, Tang Wai DF, McAndrews MP, et al. A phase 1 trial of deep brain stimulation of memory circuits in Alzheimer's disease. *Ann Neurol* 2010;68:521–534.

31. Cotelli M, Calabria M, Manenti R, et al. Improved language performance in Alzheimer disease following brain stimulation. *JNNP* 2011;82:794–797.

32. Bang J, Spina S, Miller BL. Frontotemporal dementia. *Lancet* 2015;386:1672–1682.

33. Kipps CM, Hodges JR, Hornberger M. Nonprogressive behavioural frontotemporal dementia: recent developments and clinical implications of the "bvFTD phenocopy syndrome." *Curr Opin Neurol* 2010;23(6):628–632.

34. Abdullah L, Evans JE, Montague H, et al. Chronic elevations of phosphocholine containing lipids in mice exposed to Gulf War agents pyridostigmine bromide and permethrin. *Neurotoxicol Teratol* 2013;40:74–84.

35. White RF, Steele L, O'Callaghan JP, et al. Recent research on Gulf War Illness and other health problems in veterans of the 1991 Gulf War: effects of toxicant exposures during deployment. *Cortex* 2016;74:449–475.

36. Arnsten AFT, Wang M. Targeting prefrontal cortical systems for drug development: potential therapies for cognitive disorders. *Annu Rev Pharmacol Toxicol* 2016;56:339–360.

37. Jawaid A, Rademakers R, Kass JS, Kalkonde Y, Schulz PE. Traumatic brain injury may increase the risk for frontotemporal dementia through reduced progranulin. *Neurodegener Dis* 2009;6(5–6):219–220.

38. Kertesz A. *The Banana Lady and Other Stories of Curious Behavior and Speech.* Trafford Publishing, Bloomington, IN, 2006.

39. Terracciano A, An Y, Sutin AR, Thambisetty M, Resnick SM. Personality change in the preclinical phase of

Alzheimer disease. *JAMA Psychiatry* 2017;74(12):1259–1265.

40. Hoffmann M, Schmitt F, Bromley E. Comprehensive cognitive neurological assessment in stroke. *Acta Neurol Scand* 2009;119:162–171.

41. Carrera E, Tononi G. Diaschisis: past, present and future. *Brain* 2014;137: 2408–2422.

42. Courtney C, Farrell D, Gray R, et al. Long-term donepezil treatment in 565 patients with Alzheimer's disease (AD2000): randomized double-blind trial. *Lancet* 2004;363:2105–2115.

43. Köbe T, Witte AV, Schnelle A, et al. Combined omega-3 fatty acids, aerobic exercise and cognitive stimulation prevents decline in gray matter volume of the frontal, parietal and cingulate cortex in patients with mild cognitive impairment. *Neuroimage* 2016;131:226–238.

44. Podewils LJ, Guallar E, Kuller LH, et al. Physical activity, APOE genotype, and dementia risk: findings from the Cardiovascular Health Cognition Study. *Am J Epidemiol* 2005;161:639–651.

45. Armonda RA, Bell RS, Vo AH, et al. Wartime traumatic cerebral vasospasm: recent review of combat casualties. *Neurosurgery* 2006;59:1215–1224.

46. Corr WP. Suicides and suicide attempts among active component members of the U.S. Armed Forces, 2010–2012: methods of self-harm vary by major geographic region of assignment. *MSMR* 2014;21:1–24.

47. Maas AIR, Stocchetti N, Bullock R. Moderate and severe traumatic brain injury. *Lancet Neurol* 2008;7:728–741.

48. Veenith TV, Carter EL, Geeraerts T, et al. Pathophysiologic mechanisms of cerebral ischemia and diffusion hypoxia in traumatic brain injury. *JAMA Neurol* 2016;73:542–550.

49. Pandit AS, Expert P, Lambiotte R, et al. Traumatic brain injury impairs small world topology. *Neurology* 2013;80:1826–1833.

50. Stam CJ. Modern network science of neurological disorders. *Nat Rev Neurosci* 2014;15:683–695.

51. Cernak I. Blast injuries and blast-induced neurotrauma: overview of pathophysiology and experimental knowledge models and findings. In: Kobeissy FH (ed.), *Brain Neurotrauma: Molecular, Neuropsychological, and Rehabilitation Aspects.* CRC Press, Boca Raton, FL, 2015.

52. Przekwas A, Somayaji MR, Gupta RK. Synaptic mechanisms of blast induced brain injury. *Front Neurol* 2016. doi: 10.3389/fneur.2016.00002.

53. Zuckerman A, Ram O, Infergane G, et al. Controlled low-pressure blast-wave exposure causes distinct behavioral and morphological responses modelling mild traumatic brain injury, post-traumatic stress disorder, and comorbid mild traumatic brain injury-post-traumatic stress disorder. *J Neurotrauma.* 2016. doi: 10.1089/neu.2015.4310.

54. Dams-O'Connor K, Tsao JW. Functional decline 5 years after blast traumatic brain injury. *JAMA Neurology* 2017;74:763–764.

55. MacDonald CL, Barber J, Joran M, et al. Early clinical predictors of 5-year outcome after concussive blast traumatic brain injury. *JAMA Neurology* 2017;74:821–829.

56. Metz J, Daneshvar DH, Kiernan PT, et al. Clinicopathological evaluation of chronic traumatic encephalopathy in players of American football. *JAMA* 2017;318(4):360–370.

57. Stein TD, Alvarez VE, McKee AC. Chronic traumatic encephalopathy: a spectrum of neuropathological changes following repetitive brain trauma in athletes and military personnel. *Alzheimers Res Ther* 2014;6:4.

58. DeKosky ST, Blennow K, Ikonomovic MD, Gandy S. Acute and chronic traumatic encephalopathies: pathogenesis and biomarkers. *Nat Rev Neurosci* 2013;9: 192–200.

59. Hokama Y, Empey-Campora C, Hara C, et al. Acute phase phospholipids related to the cardiolipin of mitochondria in the sera

of patients with chronic fatigue syndrome (CFS), chronic *Ciguatera* fish poisoning (CCFP), and other diseases attributed to chemicals, Gulf War, and marine toxins. *J Clin Lab Anal* 2008;22(2):99–105.

60. Zakirova Z, Tweed M, Crynen G, et al. Gulf War agent exposure causes impairment of long term memory formation and neuropathological changes in a mouse model of Gulf War Illness. *PLoS One* 2015;10(3):0119579.

61. Testa-Silva G, Verhoog MB, Linaro D, et al. High bandwidth synaptic communication and frequency tracking in human neocortex. *PLoS Biology* 2014;12(11):e1002007.

Neurological Diseases as Networktopathies with Disconnection Phenomena

New insights from cerebral neuroimaging research have shown that the brain is composed of multiple interdigitated large-scale networks – numbered at 17 based on our current ability to analyze this. This explains why not only lesions may cause symptoms, but also areas in the brain remote from the lesion. Furthermore, all neurological diseases present, with a greater or lesser degree, impairments in working memory and attentional and executive dysfunction. These provide both an understanding of the nature of the deficit as well as treatment opportunities, notably the neuroplastic potential.

Clinical Neurological Lesions as Clues to the Connectome

Clues to the connectomal nature of the brain come from clinical neurological lesions that frequently present with syndromes best explained by a diaschisis phenomenon. A definition of cerebral diaschisis is the recognition by examination or neuroradiological means of distant neurophysiological alterations as a direct consequence of a focal lesion such as a stroke or tumor. After a brain lesion, intact brain areas can assume the role or function of the areas that have been damaged – a kind of surrogate activity, termed vicariation. This process may take the form of excitatory or inhibitory effects and, as we will see later, this can be modulated by electrical or magnetic stimulation.

Diaschisis subtypes may be focal (diaschisis at rest and functional) or connectional. These subtypes are important to distinguish to enable differentiation from vicariation and neuroplastic processes. Focal diaschisis at rest refers to a decrease or hypometabolism in the absence of any stimulation or through activation procedures. Functional diaschisis, on the other hand, refers to altered responsivity of another distant cortical region in the context of normal physiological-type activation procedures of a neural system remote from a lesion when challenged by physiological activation. With functional diaschisis, for example, a left subcortical lesion with right cerebellar hypometabolism may only occur with motor activity of the right limb but no cerebellar hypometabolism is noted when there is no activity – that is, during rest.

Pathophysiologically, there may be distant excitability that is attributed to a loss of inhibition due to the hemisphere with the lesion. With circumscribed strokes, a frequent finding is an enduring impairment of inhibitory gamma-aminobutyric acid (GABA) transmission to the normal hemisphere or contra-lesional cortex, with the over-activation usually appearing soon after stroke and decreasing as time passes or recovery takes place. Relevant neuroimaging or neurophysiological tests can be employed to monitor this process and potential treatments. These include resting-state fMRI, MRI–DTI, diffusion spectrum imaging, a variant for fiber-crossing detection, magnetoencephalography (MEG), high-density electroencephalography (HdEEG), and electrocorticography (EcoG). The principal advantages of the electrophysiological modalities such as MEG and EEG is in their much higher temporal resolution but lower spatial resolution. For example, upsurge in beta activity (16–26 Hz) can be detected by EEG or MEG and transcranial magnetic stimulation can dampen this overactivity, as will be discussed later. Diaschisis is viewed as a target for neuromodulation by procedures such as transcranial magnetic stimulation and direct current stimulation, which will be discussed further in Chapter 12.

Connectional diaschisis refers to the effects of focal brain lesions that have extensive remote alterations that are apparent in both hemispheres in terms of connectivity. Connectional diaschisis may take two forms – context-specific or not – and is independent of focal diaschisis. Connectional diaschisis may be seen within motor, sensory, or attentional domains. At the present time the differentiation of diaschisis, neuroplasticity (positive or maladaptive), or vicariation cannot be made with certainty. Neuroplasticity itself can be positive, trending to recovery, or maladaptive [1].

Mapping Brain Connectivity with Newer Neuroradiological Tools

The approximately 50 Brodmann areas depicting histologically based different areas were reported over 100 years ago by the anatomist Korbinian Brodmann in 1909, and these are still used extensively today. More recently, newer functional neuroimaging capabilities by DTI and functional MRI intrinsic connectivity network analysis has allowed the delineation of four principal intrinsic connectivity networks by independent component analysis. These included the default mode network, salience network, dorsal attention network, and motor network [2]. In an ambitious study of 1000 healthy young adults, Yeo et al. assessed the human cortical networks by intrinsic functional connectivity MRI (fcMRI) for the purposes of providing contemporary reference maps. Spatial measurement applications may be performed by using DTI which measures diffusion of water with noninvasive mapping of white matter tracts, and fcMRI, which measures intrinsic functional correlations among the various brain regions. A seven-network system was derived from these measurements, which included sensory visual and somatomotor cortices. The associated cortical networks included the dorsal attention, ventral attention, frontoparietal, limbic, and default mode networks. A 17-network classification was also reported that was derived by separating the basic seven networks into smaller subnetworks. These measurements have revealed that secondary and tertiary association cortices comprise the vast majority of the human cerebral cortex of multiple functionally coupled networks [3]. An even more ambitious project has redefined the brain map from 52 Brodmann areas to 360 areas [4].

The ground zero of human functional connectivity expansion appears to be in the midline. The most impactful lesions on brain connectivity have been recorded when medially placed cerebral lesions occur that affect the temporoparietal junction (BA 5 and 7) and the prefrontal cortex and frontal eye field areas (BA 46 and 8). Using diffusion imaging noninvasive mapping of highly connected networks, a densely connected structural core of the human brain emerged, with critical components being the posterior medial cortex

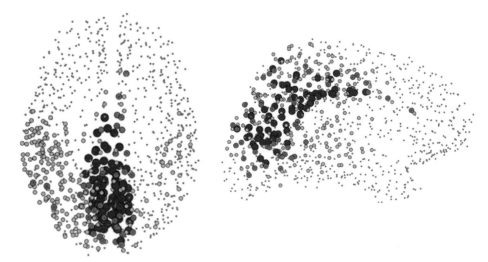

Figure 8.1 A densely connected structural core of highly connected networks in the human brain. The highest "network score" was recorded for the posterior cingulate, precuneus, cingulate isthmus, and paracentral lobules in both hemispheres. Left, anterior posterior; right, sagittal depiction.
Source: Hagmann P, Cammoun L, Gigandet X, et al. Mapping the structural core of human cerebral cortex. *PLoS Biol* 2008;6(7):e159. https://doi.org//10.1371/journal.pbio.0060159 Reproduced under the CC BY 4.0 license https://creativecommons.org/licenses/by/4.0/

and parietal cortical regions. There are links from there through a multitude of connector hubs that are linked with frontal and temporal cortices, which are regarded as playing a crucial role in integrating cerebral information processes. Using six different network measures, Hagmann et al. were able to identify eight different anatomical subregions that composed the structural core network. These were the cuneus, precuneus, the paracentral lobe, superior temporal sulci, cingulate isthmus, superior parietal cortex, and inferior parietal cortex in both hemispheres [5]. This correlates with evidence of the precuneus, in particular, having the highest energy consumption of any part of the cortex [6]. This core region probably represents the substrate for influencing other large-scale cerebral networks and integrating these with many other networks [7,8] (Figure 8.1).

Network Imaging by Intrinsic Functional Connectivity

Network imaging by intrinsic functional connectivity is able to decipher objective abnormality in most neurological diseases. In many neurological diseases, normal structural MRI brain imaging frequently confounds the diagnostic process. Newer MRI-based network imaging has had a number of significant impacts. So far evidence for improved diagnosis, early diagnosis, and more sensitive diagnoses have been reported for traumatic brain injury (TBI), multiple sclerosis, depression, Alzheimer's disease, Parkinson's disease, frontotemporal lobe dementia, and migraine. Management may also be improved and be more accurate in understanding network analyses, which has been helpful in providing critical information for epilepsy surgery, for example [9]. The importance of detecting these network changes lies in the supposition that these may be the most sensitive and earliest surrogate markers for recovery. A new understanding of the connectome is that the network dysfunction also affects the intact, non-lesioned hemisphere. Already, rodent data have demonstrated an increase in the "small worldness" of a sensory network within three days post-stroke, becoming normal at about two months [1]. These observations have prompted the concept of an additional subtype of diaschisis, connectomal diaschisis. The small-world impairment has also been seen clinically in TBI patients [10]. In Parkinson's disease two different dynamic functional connectivity patterns were identified that correlated with disease severity [11].

Interactions between Complex Networks and the Brain

Many other very complex networks interact with the brain networks. The various "omics," including genomics, proteinomics, lipidomics, epileptomics, as well as matrisomes and microbiomes, are immensely complex systems that interact with the human connectome [12].

Following the era of genomics, then proteomics, more recently the era of lipidomics has yielded many critical insights for the study of the lipidome, lipid messengers such as prostaglandins and in the understanding of signaling between neurons, astrocytes, oligodendrocytes, and microglia. The retina and brain have the highest concentrations of DHA of any tissue, and it is especially abundant in photoreceptors and synapses. DHA is a key component in mechanisms providing neuroprotection, anti-inflammatory effects, vision, and memory processing. These critical processes have given rise to the concept of DHA signalolipidomics, which relates synaptic functions and neuroprotection (via NPD1) and neurotrophin agonists [13–15].

For example, cerebral small-vessel disease (SVD) is the most proximate, responsible mechanism in 25–30 percent of people with stroke and the number one cause of decline and disability among the adult population. Cerebral SVD is due to a complex interaction of environmental and genetic factors. Matrisome refers to the aggregate of proteins that constitute the extracellular matrix (ECM). This comprises a complexity of cross-linked proteins whose functions include binding to cell surfaces via adhesion receptors by proteins such as integrins and the regulation of various growth and cellular secretory factors. The matrisome of the cerebral blood vessels includes the basement membrane, a critical interface structure between the brain and the microvasculature. Derangements of this part of the matrisome are now considered a major cause of SVD, both acquired and familial. The latter includes inherited conditions such as CADASIL, CARASIL, HANAC, COL4A1, and COL4A2. As the major proportion of matrisome protein is expressed in the endothelial basement membrane, which also interacts with pericytes and astrocytes, it occupies a strategic position as part of the neuro-gliovascular unit [16]. It comes as no surprise, therefore, that vascular dysregulation precedes that of A-beta deposition in dementias such as Alzheimer's disease, ascribed to impaired clearance as opposed to an A-Beta overproduction. Vascular dysregulation has been touted as the causal role for Alzheimer's disease since 1900, in contradistinction to the amyloid hypothesis. Also, an age-dependent BBB (blood–brain barrier) breakdown with misfolded protein deposition and related toxicity with increased permeability correlates with clinical cognitive dysfunction [17].

Microbiome Insights

Our bodies and our resident microbes work together, both in sickness and in health. The extensive host microbiome interaction within our bodies occurs at the genomic, intracellular, intercellular, and cerebral network levels. Our gut–brain axis has an epigenetic component that serves as a mediator between the genetic and environmental interface [18]. Hence, we are superorganisms (humans and their microbes) termed holobiont. The term hologenome refers to the combination of our genetic and the microbe genetic material. Furthermore, our psychobiome refers to the effect our gut organisms (bacteria, viruses) have on our mind, conferring states of well-being, altered mood, depression, or anxiety.

The Effect of Microbe Symbiosis on Pace of Evolution

Our symbiosis with microbes allowed a much more rapid pace of evolution. The very much more rapidly evolving microbes adapted to new or different food sources, which may have led to the formation of new species due to environmental stressors, such as climate. The microbiota adapts much more rapidly than the host. The ability to change a biological response in our bodies within our own lifetime may be explained by this theory, termed the "hologenome theory of evolution," first conceived by Richard Jefferson [19]. This has led to a more personalized food-intake approach, bearing in mind the physiological response of what we eat and how it impacts our health in general, as well as longevity. Nutritional factors directly influence our cellular genetic machinery, from which emerging fields such as nutrigenomics have surfaced with a more precise evaluation of food constituents and their effects on gene expression and health [18,20,21].

The Rise of Network Medicine

The initial hype surrounding the Human Genome Project was one of the factors that spawned the relatively recent emergence of personalized medicine and precision. The realization since, that only a miniscule number of diseases are the result of mono- or oligogenic inherited disorders and the promise of these being amenable to correctional therapy, has dwindled. The increasing complexity of superadded environmental factors and more complex genetic factors, most notably epigenetic mechanisms, has dawned on researchers who must now integrate these into the recognizable clinical phenotype. A vast amount of bioinformatics data have also emerged from the various "omic" databases (omic – collective quantification and characterization of biological molecules that confer function and structure of the organism) that have to be integrated with the genetic and environmental information that together have given rise to the relatively new concept of network medicine.

Earlier in medical history, the reduction of disease states into progressively more cellular or molecular pathology realms was associated with so-called "magical bullets." This was exemplified by treatments for infectious disease, such as penicillin for syphilis and streptomycin for tuberculosis. As Malina pointed out in her review, this was also the basis of the renowned Massachusetts General Hospital weekly Clinicopathological Conference (CPC) tradition. As noted by McKeown, mortality and morbidity with tuberculosis, for example, correlated with nutritional and economic improvement and not vaccines, sanatoriums, or antimicrobial therapies [22]. At the present time, the dismal output of about 20–30 new pharmaceutical agents per year also illustrates the relative myth of molecular targets to combat a phenotypic disease state. Drug targets are only one of many factors that make up a vast network of biological systems that interact. Drug side-effects are also an important consideration as having adverse effects on these complex systems. A good example has been the recent abandonment of vitamin therapies, by health-minded people without specific vitamin deficiencies, as actually causing more adverse effects than benefits. Reviews of many studies have not found overall benefit, and some have documented potential harm with routine supplementation of vitamins or micronutrients. This was encapsulated in a recent prominent editorial entitled "Enough is enough: stop wasting money on vitamin and mineral supplements" [23]. Pathophysiology in human disease states need to be considered as complex interacting networks of many biological systems that include genomics, proteinomics, lipidomics, metabolomics, and various environmental factors [24].

References

1. Carrera E, Tononi G. Diaschisis: past, present and future. *Brain* 2014;137:2408–2422.

2. Ibrahim GM, Cassel D, Morgan BR, et al. Resilience of developing brain networks to interictal epileptiform discharges is associated with cognitive outcome. *Brain* 2014;137:2690–2702.

3. Yeo BTT, Krienen FM, Sepulcre J, et al. The organization of the human cerebral cortex estimated by intrinsic functional connectivity. *J Neurophysiology* 2011;106:1125–1165.

4. Thomas Yeo BT, Eickhoff SB. A modern map of the human cerebral cortex. *Nature* 2016;536:152–154.

5. Hagmann P, Cammoun L, Gigandet X, et al. Mapping the structural core of human cerebral cortex. *PLoS Biology* 2008;6(7):e159.

6. Raichle ME, MacLeod AM, Snyder AZ, et al. A default mode of brain function. *PNAS* 2001;98:676–682.

7. Greicius MD, Krasnow B, Reiss AL, Menon V. Functional connectivity in the resting brain: a network analysis of the default mode hypothesis. *PNAS* 2003;100:253–258.

8. Fox MD, Snyder AZ, Vincent JL, et al. The human brain is intrinsically organized into dynamic, anti-correlated functional networks. *PNAS* 2005;102:9673–9678.

9. Besson P, Brandt SK, Proxi T, et al. Anatomic consistencies across epilepsies: a stereotactic-EEG informed high resolution structural connectivity study. *Brain* 2017;140:2639–2652.

10. Pandit AS, Expert P, Lambiotte R, et al. Traumatic brain injury impairs small world topology. *Neurology* 2013;80:1826–1833.

11. Kim J, Criaud M, Soo Cho S, et al. Abnormal intrinsic brain functional network dynamics in Parkinson's disease. *Brain* 2017;140:2955–2967.

12. Bernasconi A. Connectome based models of the epileptogenic network: a step towards epileptomics? *Brain* 2017;140:2525–2527.

13. Marcheselli VL, Hong S, Lukiw WJ, et al. Novel docosanoids inhibit brain ischemia reperfusion mediated leukocyte infiltration and pro inflammatory gene expression. *J Biol Chem* 2003;278:43807–43817.

14. Mukherjee PK, Marcheselli VL, Barreiro S, et al. Neurotrophins enhance retinal pigment epithelial cell survival through neuroprotectin D1 signaling. *PNAS* 2007;104:13152–13157.

15. Brady ST, Siegel GJ, Albers RW, Price DL. *Basic Neurochemistry*, 8th edn. Elsevier Academic Press, New York, 2012.

16. Joutel A, Haddad I, Ratelade J, Nelson MT. Perturbations of the cerebrovascular matrisome: a convergent mechanism in small vessel disease of the brain? *J Cereb Blood Flow Metab* 2016;36:143–157.

17. Iturria-Medina Y, Sotero RC, Toussaint PJ, et al. Early role of vascular dysregulation on late onset Alzheimer's disease based on multifactorial data driven analysis. *Nat Commun* 2016. doi: 10.1038/ncomms11934.

18. Stilling RM, Dinan TG, Cryan JF. Microbial genes, brain & behaviour: epigenetic regulation of the gut–brain axis. *Genes Brain Behav* 2014;13:69–86.

19. Zilber-Rosenberg I, Rosenberg E. Role of microorganisms in the evolution of animals and plants: the hologenome theory of evolution. *FEMS Microbiol Rev* 2008;32:723–735.

20. Müller M, Kersten S. Nutrigenomics: goals and perspectives. *Nat Rev Genet* 2003;4:315–322.

21. Arnold C. The other you. *New Scientist,* January 12, 2012:31–34.

22. McKeown T. *The Role of Medicine: Dream, Mirage or Nemesis?* Nuffield Provincial Hospitals Trust, London, 1976.

23. Guallar E, Stranges S, Mulrow C, Appel LJ. Enough is enough: stop wasting money on vitamin and mineral supplements. *Ann Intern Med* 2013;159:850–851.

24. Malina D. Putting the patient back together: social medicine, network medicine and the limits of reductionism. *N Engl J Med* 2017;377:2493–2499.

The Sensitivity and Vulnerability of the Prefrontal Cortex to Changes in Daily Rhythms

The primate prefrontal cortex (PFC) is most developed in humans and enables integration of recalled past experiences to implement the most appropriate motor response. These molecular processes are based on pyramidal cell activity and their networks that may occur in the absence of external stimuli. Dopamine is the principal neurotransmitter involved, but is part of a fragile process susceptible to error. Even minor changes in the brain's neurochemical milieu can lead to network failure. The inverted U-shaped curve of too much or too little dopamine leads to failure. These prefrontal cortical functions are particularly prone to physiological processes such as arousal, fatigue, or stress, as well as external or environmental influences. Hence PFC function is inherently capricious and is considered an Achilles heel in our cognitive abilities. However, these brain areas are particularly plastic and network connections can be strengthened or inhibited rapidly and so provide great flexibility in the behavioral repertoire. These relatively volatile prefrontal functions and vulnerabilities also confer unique human mental disorders. Understanding these mechanisms supports interventions such as meditation and cognitive behavioral therapies that "brain build," in addition to pharmacological options.

The Human Connectome: Macroscopic Hardwired Tracts and Neurochemical Tracts

The core PFC functions include working memory, inhibition, attention, set shifting, and error monitoring. These primary processes allow our most advanced human cognitive activities to process our actions, emotions, thoughts, and language. However, there is considerable vulnerability within these systems as even relatively minor stressors (emotional upset, fatigue, disturbed sleep, alcohol, medication, hormonal imbalance, and other environmental factors) can impair tasks that are complex and require flexible cogitation. In contradistinction, minor stress may improve more elementary tasks or those that have been well mastered and been ingrained in the basal ganglia circuitry through extensive practice, for example [1,2].

PFC Regulation, Amygdala-Based Regulation, and Stress

PFC and amygdala-based regulation are related to the amount of stress. The PFC connects to all parts of the brain through four principal routes (Figure 9.1). The dorsolateral route connects to the motor and sensory cortices and mediates thought and action. The dorsomedial PFC is concerned with the process of error monitoring. The ventromedial

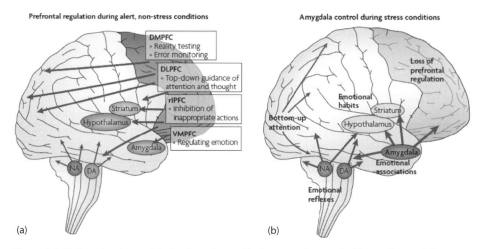

Figure 9.1 Prefrontal and amygdala circuits and stress. The brain may be switched from reflective (left) to reflexive behavior (right) in response to stress.

Reproduced by permission from Springer Nature from Arnsten AFT. Stress signaling pathways that impair prefrontal cortex structure and function. *Nat Rev Neurosci 2009;10*:410–422.

route connects to the subcortical components, the amygdala, hypothalamus, and nucleus accumbens, which mediate emotional responses. The right inferior PFC effectuates inhibitory responses [3]. Together these major circuits guide high-level decision-making, behavior, and emotional responses in a relatively stress-free environment augmented by the ascending monoaminergic fiber tracts. The latter have optimal levels of effect in an inverted U-shaped fashion [4,5]. The amygdala also connects to the brainstem and hypothalamus. With elevated stress, a surge in noradrenaline and dopamine release occurs which has the effect of hindering PFC function and "top-down control," resulting in impaired working memory, attention, and appropriate inhibitory responses. A bottom-up, amygdala-controlled process takes over, together with the sensory cortices, whereby stimuli that are visual, auditory, or somatosensory-related predominate. This becomes a more emotive and reflexive response as opposed to a slower, more calculated response [6,7].

In addition to the major cerebral networks discussed in Chapters 3 and 4, the principal cerebral neurochemical tracts include the fast-acting excitatory (glutaminergic) and inhibitory (GABA)-ergic amino acid-type neurotransmitters. There are also eight (dopamine, serotonin, norepinephrine, acetylcholine, histamine, oxytocin, vasopressin, and orexin) slower-acting modulatory neurochemical tracts that are "wired" differently. They arise from the brainstem, hypothalamus, and basal forebrain, and have widely projecting ramifications delivering more diffuse, slower-acting, and longer-lasting actions promulgated by the G-protein cascade that transduces the signal from these neurotransmitters. This chemical architecture allows the coordination of many neurons, as well as many neuronal circuits in response to a particular threat.

DLPFC network activity is due to pyramidal cell firing that is modulated by GABA, termed lateral inhibition. Goldman Rakic's research has shown that these interneurons (chandelier and basket cell types) will induce a neuron to fire during the delay period that follows a particular stimulus. However, due to what has been termed "spatial tuning," the pyramidal cell neuron firing has a preference in one direction as opposed to another direction (for example, 90-degree versus 270-degree orientation). This constitutes the neural basis of spatial working memory or representational information. The pyramidal cell networks are found predominantly in layer three, are connected with each other by NMDA dendritic synapses, and have the ability to fire in the delay period [8]. This circuitry, with its spatial tuning capacity, can be amplified by dopamine. Another neurochemical process that can augment pyramidal cell firing and connectivity to bolster working memory is calcium.

There is a differential PFC neurochemical innervation by the monoamines, serotonin, dopamine, noradrenaline, and acetylcholine. For example, decreased prefrontal serotonin impairs reversal learning, which is a measure of cognitive flexibility requiring adjustment of behavior in the context of previous reward-related occurrences established that now need to be reversed. Dopamine depletion, on the other hand, impairs set formation. Set formation refers to a tendency to exhibit certain behavioral approaches because past experiences have been favorable. Noradrenaline depletion affects set shifting (switching tasks in a non-conscious manner), whereas acetylcholine affects serial reversal learning (SRL). SRL refers to the ability to discriminate between two differently rewarded stimuli in which the reward contingency is then altered by multiple reversals. When testing animals display fewer errors after repeated reversals with a task, it implies they have behavioral flexibility. These neurotransmitter systems are also involved in so-called state-dependent systems such as attention (dopamine, acetylcholine), arousal (noradrenaline, dopamine), stress (noradrenaline), and affect (serotonin or 5HT), which in turn may amplify/augment these differing executive functions [9]. Executive function as a generic label encompasses the core components of working memory, response inhibition, attention, and set shifting or cognitive flexibility. These core components may be altered in various ways to yield the clinical phenotypes of obsessive compulsive disorder (OCD), depression, attention deficit hyperactivity disorder (ADHD), bipolar disorder schizophrenia, and neurodegenerative diseases such as frontotemporal lobe dementias, Alzheimer's disease, and Parkinson's disease.

Dopamine

Dopamine is regarded as the principal neurotransmitter within the extensive frontal subcortical circuits, discussed in Chapter 5, with dopamine and acetylcholine predominating in the left hemisphere and norepinephrine and 5HT in the right hemisphere. Previc proposed his hypothesis of the dominance of dopamine in the frontal subcortical circuits as a key neurotransmitter critical in heat management as it promoted cooling of our brain and bodies in the thermally stressed condition of the arid East African Rift Valley during the last 2–3 million years [10]. This allowed superior toleration of hyperthermia and heat stroke and additionally may have enabled early hominoids to use chase hunting to their advantage as the less heat-tolerant herbivores succumbed to overheated muscles or chase myopathy [11,12]. Dopamine presumably became exapted for executive function and regarded as a key neurochemical factor in the human intelligence, becoming the most important neurotransmitter in our brain's evolution, and fundamental to the core frontal attributes of cognitive flexibility, working memory, abstraction, temporal sequencing, and motor planning [13]. It has also been postulated that further dopamine expansion occurred, on account of upregulated calcium metabolism related to increased aerobic activity and an overall increase in tyrosine (dopamine precursor) consequent to increased meat intake [14]. Of clinical relevance today is the pharmacological advisory of dopamine-blocking medications (risperidone, quetiapine, haloperidol) and neuroleptic malignant syndromes or malignant hyperthermia syndrome that may be precipitated.

At a neuronal level, dopamine action affects the signal-to-noise ratio specifically on the PFC pyramidal, glutaminergic cell G-protein linked receptors that are located on the dendritic shafts and spines of glutaminergic pyramidal neurons, as well as acting on the GABA-ergic neuronal dendrites. In this manner, dopamine regulates the critical and core processes of working memory, as well as reasoning and language. All the great apes and humans have the hallmark of dopamine input to all cerebral regions, in contrast to the scarce rodent dopaminergic innervation. There are also regional differences with dopaminergic distribution, most concentrated in the association cortices within layers 1, 5 and 6 [15]. Humans differ further in that they have a more extensive prefrontal dopaminergic input compared to great apes. These factors together give credence to the dopaminergic evolutionary hypotheses that dopamine, in particular, was a major factor in human culture, tool-making, exploration, and manifold scientific advances [13]. The same capabilities, however, have also predisposed humans to the many hyperdopaminergic syndromes that include bipolar disease, autism, schizophrenia, ADHD, and neurodegenerative disease [16].

Acetylcholine

The acetylcholine axons of great apes and humans have varicosities that have been linked to a role in cortical plasticity, mediating self-awareness, social learning, advanced tool-making, and higher-level learning capacity [17]. The five muscarinic G-protein linked receptors (M1–M5) mediate these modulatory effects, whereas the ligand-gated ion channel nicotinic receptors transmit both excitatory and inhibitory effects upon pyramidal cells and GABA interneurons. The phenotypic cognitive output translates into working memory and cognitive flexibility [18].

Serotonin

Similarly with serotonin innervation, an overall increase of cortical efferent fibers has been noted among the great apes in comparison to other mammals. To date, 14 serotonergic G-protein coupled receptors, as well as a single ion channel receptor (5-HT 3) have been described. These modulate a number of different processes that include inhibition, learning, and memory. The serotonin receptors located on pyramidal cells, their dendritic shafts, and interneurons, enable signal modulation of localized circuits in relation to extrinsic stimuli [19]. An important clinical perspective is that of the serotonergic innervation within the orbitofrontal cortex, which modulates inhibition regulation, emotional processing, and self-control [20].

Noradrenaline

Both noradrenaline and dopamine exert critical excitatory innervation for wakefulness, which allows neurons to engage in information processing [21,22]. They also have modulatory effects that augment PFC connections while engaging in working memory operations. Both noradrenaline and dopamine display "inverted U-shaped" effects on working memory, with either too much or too little of either neurotransmitter impairing PFC performance. Noradrenaline stimulates different receptors depending on how much has been released, displaying the highest affinity for α2-adrenergic receptors with lower affinity for beta-adrenergic and α1 receptors [23]. Optimal levels of noradrenaline for alertness without undue stress occur with α2A-receptor stimulation [24,25].

With significant stressors, elevated noradrenaline levels stimulate more of the α1-receptors and β1-receptors, with consequent impairment of PFC activity [26,27]. Both dopamine and noradrenaline release occurs during acute stress, whereas mild stress increases only dopamine release [28]. Depletion of noradrenaline or blocking of PFC α2A-receptors leads to working memory dysfunction, whereas stimulation of α2A-receptors augments working memory function [29]. Alternatively, high levels of PFC α1-receptor stimulation decreases spatial working memory function [30,31]. In the setting of cognitive impairment attributed to stress, these can be ameliorated by issuing α1-receptor antagonists. Important clinical consequences include the success demonstrated with using α1-receptor antagonists such as prazosin benefiting those with PTSD [32,33]. Similarly, β-receptor antagonist treatment has also been shown to improve cognitive flexibility in association with stress. Dopamine effects on working memory occur through the D1 receptor group (D1 and D5), also with an inverted U-shaped effect with both excessive stimulation or blocking of the D1 receptor family leading to working memory function deterioration [34,35]. D1 blockade by D1 antagonists ameliorates working memory impairment during stress. These findings support complementary roles for noradrenaline and dopamine, with α2A-receptor stimulation enhancing PFC network firing with overall signal increase, and D1 receptor stimulation decreasing firing to non-preferred inputs and so shaping neuronal firing with decreased "noise" [36].

The Mosaic Cognitive Evolution

Primate and hominoid imitation ability and behavior were pivotal to the cultural evolution, leading Subiaul to refer to this ability as an "all-purpose learning mechanism." Evolution of the imitation circuitry components included anatomical and chemical aspects, as well as reorganization of circuits, the latter termed mosaic circuits. The mosaicism refers to prefrontal cortical, temporal parietal, and cerebellar components. The major cognitive domains of attention, memory, language, and tool use are all based on mosaic patterns. The mosaic pattern itself was modeled on the imitation behavior circuitry, which has auditory, tactile, and visual dimensions [37]. Both serotonergic and dopaminergic chemical networks and their receptors feature in the OFC inhibitory control mechanisms. However, serotonin depletion and not dopamine have been correlated with impairment of OFC inhibitory control. Studies by Walker et al. in marmosets and monkeys demonstrated the more in-depth differential contributions of these two neurotransmitters in inhibitory control. Those animals with OFC serotonin depletion were shown to have stimulus-bound responses to discrimination extinction and conditioned reinforcement tests, indicating that OFC serotonin function may be to prevent potentially competing and task-irrelevant inputs from guiding their responses. Dopamine depletion did not display such behavioral responses [38].

The Idiosyncratic PFC Network Vulnerabilities and the Concept of Dynamic Network Connectivity

Normal daily physiological variations precipitated by arousal, stress, fatigue, and impaired sleep can significantly alter PFC working memory functions. In disease states such as stroke, dementias, neuropsychiatric diseases as well as the aging process, PFC function is invariably affected [39,40]. Some of the molecular mechanisms concerned with the exquisitely controlled PFC network connectivity include intracellular signaling operations that influence the relative strength of a particular network from one moment to the next, called dynamic network connectivity [41]. For example, network connections can be diminished by the opening of potassium channels found on dendritic spines or upgraded by closing these channels or by opening other depolarizing channels via nicotinic receptors.

The Microcircuitry and Intracellular Signaling Pathways that Mediate PFC Working Memory

A variety of circuit modulation and intracellular mechanisms can strengthen or weaken PFC network connections. Such mechanisms act relatively rapidly and bestow flexibility but also confer vulnerabilities on cognitive function. However, improved insights into molecular processes pave the way for potential therapeutic targets. The intricacies of these processes are beyond the scope of this book, but the avid reader requiring more information is referred to the excellent treatise by Amy Arnsten [42].

Reducing excitability: Ca^{++} entry through NMDA channels opens small conductance Ca^{++} activated K^+ (SK) channels that decrease NMDA actions with an overall reduction in excitability. Glutamate spillover affects metabotropic glutamate receptors (perisynaptic mGluR1/5). When stimulated, these reduce PFC network firing and improve working memory [43,44].

Increasing excitability: calcium may activate Ca^{++}/calmodulin-dependent kinase II (CaMKII) as well as protein kinase C (PKC) that can be released in the context of stress exposure. Both can impair PFC function [45]. Increases in cyclic AMP weaken PFC network firing through the opening of cyclic AMP-regulated potassium channels. Cyclic AMP may also open HCN and KCNQ channels through the mechanism of protein kinase A (PKA) signaling. These markedly reduce network activity and working memory function [46].

Effects of Chronic Stress on the PFC

More extensive network changes have been documented, such as loss of dendritic spines in layer two and three pyramidal neurons [47,48], and the PFC and hippocampal connections that are important for memory consolidation are disrupted. In rodents these changes are slowly reversible when the stress subsides [49,50].

Dopamine D1 Receptors and "Noise"

Dopamine D1 receptors may shape networks by weakening "noise." D1 receptors are found on PFC spines and release c-AMP when stimulated. The output takes the form of an inverted U response, whereby either too little or too much stimulation of D1 receptors decreases PFC working memory capacity. Insufficient D1 stimulation causes "noisy" cell firing during the delay period after a stimulus. Moderate D1 stimulation leads to suppression of the neuron's non-preferred direction firing. This enhances what is termed spatial tuning. A high-level D1 stimulation in response to severe stress causes complete cessation of firing [36].

Specific Adrenergic Stimulation

Strengthening PFC network activity with improvement in working memory capacity can be augmented by α2A-adrenergic receptor stimulation, which inhibits production of c-AMP [46].

PFC Vulnerability to External, Environmental or Internal Genetic Insults

Prefrontal cortical functions are uniquely labile, with impairments ensuing after a single event or within hours to days. This fragility of the apical component of our cognitive abilities is presumably due to the molecular signaling complexity of the PFC microcircuits. An important evolutionary insight may be why the PFC has mechanisms that weaken network activity or firing. An increase in Ca^{++} and c-AMP through negative feedback mechanisms may translate into survival value by curbing excessive excitotoxicity and electrical activity that may cause brain damage and seizures, respectively [41]. Chronic stress exposure leads to PFC structural changes as occurs with PTSD. Through the improved understanding of the stress-signaling mechanisms due to a variety of metabolic, environmental, and genetic assaults, insights into therapies become more likely.

The Benefits Mechanistic of Insights into Microcircuitry for Treating PTSD

Post-traumatic stress disorder is a debilitating psychiatric disorder with a lifetime prevalence of ~8 percent, which develops in ~15 percent of individuals exposed to trauma. There may be a role for non-coding RNAs (ncRNAs), including microRNAs (miRNAs), in ameliorating the impact of severe stress or trauma syndromes [51,52]. PTSD has a close association with the uncinate fasciculus syndrome and so may present with overlap syndromes with frontotemporal syndromes [53]. Prazosin and meditation are both notable breakthrough therapies in the treatment of PTSD that will be further discussed in Chapter 10. Neurotoxicological syndromes such as heavy metal poisoning, lead in particular, as well as solvents, may present with the primary syndromes of working memory impairment, disinhibition, and cognitive flexibility syndrome disorders.

The COMT genotype regulates dopamine availability and influences where a person is situated on the D1 inverted U curve. DAG kinase inhibits PKC signaling, which if altered genetically may lead to bipolar disorder [54]. Translocation genes, DISC1 regulated phosphodiesterase, which causes catabolism of the c-AMP signaling system, leads to neuropsychiatric disorders such as schizophrenia [55].

References

1. Broadbent, D. *Decision and Stress.* Academic, London, 1971.

2. Hockey, GRJ. Effect of loud noise on attentional selectivity. *Q J Exp Psychol* 1970;22:28–36.

3. Goldman-Rakic, PS. Circuitry of primate prefrontal cortex and regulation of behavior by representational memory. In: Plum F (ed.), *Handbook of Physiology, The Nervous System, Higher Functions of the Brain* vol. V. American Physiological Society, Bethesda, MD, 1987.

4. Price JL, Amaral DG. An autoradiographic study of the projections of the central nucleus of the monkey amygdala. *J Neurosci* 1981;1:1242–1259.

5. Price JL, Carmichael ST, Drevets WC. Networks related to the orbital and medial prefrontal cortex: a substrate for emotional behavior? *Brain Res* 1996;107:523–536.

6. Ghashghaei HT, Barbas H. Pathways for emotion: interactions of prefrontal and anterior temporal pathways in

the amygdala of the rhesus monkey. *Neuroscience* 2002;115:1261–1279.

7. Debiec J, LeDoux JE. Noradrenergic signaling in the amygdala contributes to the reconsolidation of fear memory: treatment implications for PTSD. *Ann NY Acad Sci* 2006;1071:521–524.

8. Kojima S, Goldman-Rakic PS. Delay-related activity of prefrontal neurons in rhesus monkeys performing delayed response. *Brain Res* 1982;248(1):43–49.

9. Robbins TW, Roberts AC. Differential regulation of fronto-executive function by the monoamines and acetylcholine. *Cerebral Cortex* 2007;17(suppl. 1): i151–i161.

10. Previc FH. Dopamine and the origin of human intelligence. *Brain Cogn* 1999;41:299–350.

11. Bortz WM II. Physical exercise as an evolutionary force. *J Hum Evol* 1985;14:145–155.

12. Carrier DR. The energetic paradox of human running and hominid evolution. *Curr Anthropol* 1984;25:483–495.

13. Passinghim RE, Stephan KE, Kotter R. The anatomical basis of functional localization in the cortex. *Nat Rev Neurosci* 2002;3:606–616.

14. Leonard WR, Robertson MS. Comparative primate energetics and hominid evolution. *Am J Phys Anthropol* 1997;102:265–281.

15. Lewis DA, Melchitzky DS, Sesack SR, et al. Dopamine transporter immunoreactivity in monkey cerebral cortex: regional, laminar and ultrastructural organization. *J Comp Neurol* 2001;432:119–136.

16. Willamson PC, Allman JM. *The Human Illnesses: Neuropsychiatric Disorders and the Nature of the Human Brain.* Oxford University Press, Oxford, 2011.

17. Sarter M, Parikh V. Choline transporters, cholinergic transmission and cognition. *Nat Rev Neurosci* 2005;6:48–56.

18. Levin ED, Simon BB. Nicotinic acetylcholine involvement in cognitive function in animals. *Psychopharmacology* 1998;138:217–230.

19. Jakab RL, Goldman-Rakic PS. Segregation of serotonin 5HT 2A and 5HT 3 receptors in inhibitory circuits in the primate cerebral cortex. *J Comp Neurol* 2000;417:337–348.

20. Soubrie P. Reconciling the role of central serotonin neurons in human and animal behavior. *Behav Brain Sci* 1986;9:319–364.

21. McCormick DA, Pape HC, Williamson A. Actions of norepinephrine in the cerebral cortex and thalamus: implications for function of the central noradrenergic system. *Prog Brain Res* 1991;88:293–305.

22. Seamans JK, Durstewitz D, Christie BR, Stevens CF, Sejnowski TJ. Dopamine D1/ D5 receptor modulation of excitatory synaptic inputs to layer V prefrontal cortex neurons. *PNAS* 2001;98:301–306.

23. Arnsten AFT. Through the looking glass: differential noradrenergic modulation of prefrontal cortical function. *Neural Plast* 2000;7:133–146.

24. Arnsten AFT, Goldman-Rakic PS. Alpha-2 adrenergic mechanisms in prefrontal cortex associated with cognitive decline in aged nonhuman primates. *Science* 1985;230:1273–1276.

25. Li B-M, Mei Z-T. Delayed response deficit induced by local injection of the alpha-2 adrenergic antagonist yohimbine into the dorsolateral prefrontal cortex in young adult monkeys. *Behav Neural Biol* 1994;62:134–139.

26. Birnbaum SG, Gobeske KT, Auerbach J, Taylor JR, Arnsten AFT. A role for norepinephrine in stress-induced cognitive deficits: α-1-adrenoceptor mediation in prefrontal cortex. *Biol Psychiatry* 1999;46:1266–1274.

27. Ramos BP, Colgan L, Nou E, et al. The beta-1 adrenergic antagonist, betaxolol, improves working memory performance in rats and monkeys. *Biol Psychiatry* 2005;58:894–900.

28. Deutch AY, Roth RH. The determinants of stress-induced activation of the prefrontal cortical dopamine system. *Prog Brain Res* 1990;85:367–403.

29. Ramos B, Stark D, Verduzco L, van Dyck CH, Arnsten AFT. Alpha-2A-adrenoceptor stimulation improves prefrontal cortical regulation of behavior through inhibition of cAMP signaling in aging animals. *Learn Mem* 2006;13:770–776.

30. Birnbaum SG, Yuan PX, Wang M, et al. Protein kinase C overactivity impairs prefrontal cortical regulation of working memory. *Science* 2004;306:882–884.

31. Arnsten AFT, Mathew R, Ubriani R, Taylor JR, Li B-M. α-1 noradrenergic receptor stimulation impairs prefrontal cortical cognitive function. *Biol Psychiatry* 1999;45:26–31.

32. Taylor F, Raskind MA. The α1-adrenergic antagonist prazosin improves sleep and nightmares in civilian trauma posttraumatic stress disorder. *J Clin Psychopharmacol* 2002;22:82–85.

33. Raskind MA, Thompson C, Petrie EC, et al. Prazosin reduces nightmares and other PTSD symptoms in combat veterans: a placebo-controlled study. *Am J Psychiatry* 2003;160:371–373.

34. Sawaguchi T, Goldman-Rakic PS. D1 dopamine receptors in prefrontal cortex: involvement in working memory. *Science* 1991;251:947–950.

35. Zahrt J, Taylor JR, Mathew RG, Arnsten AFT. Supranormal stimulation of dopamine D1 receptors in the rodent prefrontal cortex impairs spatial working memory performance. *J Neurosci* 1997;17:8528–8535.

36. Vijayraghavan S, Wang M, Birnbaum SG, et al. Inverted-U dopamine D1 receptor actions on prefrontal neurons engaged in working memory. *Nature Neurosci* 2007;10:376–384.

37. Subiaul F. Mosaic cognitive evolution: the case of imitation behavior. In Broadfield D, Yuan M, Schick K, Toth N (eds.), *The Human Brain Evolving*. Stone Age Institute Press, Gosport, IN, 2010.

38. Walker SC, Robbins TW, Roberts AC. Differential contributions of dopamine and serotonin to orbitofrontal cortex function in the marmoset. *Cerebral Cortex* 2009;19:889–898.

39. Arnsten AFT, Vijayraghavan S, Wang M, et al. Dopamine's influence on prefrontal cortical cognition: actions and circuits in behaving primates. In: Bjorklund A, Dunnet S, Iversen L, Iversen S (eds.), *Dopamine Handbook*. Oxford University Press, Oxford, 2009.

40. Arnsten AFT. Stress signaling pathways that impair prefrontal cortex structure and function. *Nat Rev Neurosci* 2009;32:267–287.

41. Arnsten AFT, Paspalas CD, Gamo NJ, et al. Dynamic network connectivity: a new form of neuroplasticity. *Trends Cogn Sci* 2010;14:365–375.

42. Arnsten AFT. Fleeting thoughts. In: Stuss DT, Knight RT (eds.), *Principles of Frontal Lobe Function*. Oxford University Press, Oxford, 2013.

43. Hagenston AM, Fitzpatrick JS, Yeckel MF. mGluR-mediated calcium waves that invade the soma regulate firing in layer V medial prefrontal cortical pyramidal neurons. *Cereb Cortex* 2008;18:407–423.

44. Runyan JD, Dash PK. Distinct prefrontal molecular mechanisms for information storage lasting seconds versus minutes. *Learn Mem* 2005;12:232–238.

45. Partridge LD, Swandulla D, Muller TH. Modulation of calcium-activated non-specific cation currents by cyclic AMP-dependent phosphorylation in neurons of Helix. *J Physiol* 1990;429:131–145.

46. Wang M, Ramos BP, Paspalas CD, et al. α2A-adrenoceptor stimulation strengthens working memory networks by inhibiting cAMP-HCN channel signaling in prefrontal cortex. *Cell* 2007;129:397–410.

47. Holmes A, Wellman CL. Stress-induced prefrontal reorganization and executive dysfunction in rodents. *Neurosci Biobehav Rev* 2008. doi:10.1016/j.neubiorev.2008.11.005.

48. Radley JJ, Rocher AB, Miller M, et al. Repeated stress induces dendritic spine

loss in the rat medial prefrontal cortex. *Cereb Cortex* 2006;16:313–320.

49. Cerqueira JJ, Mailliet F, Almeida OF, Jay TM, Sousa N. The prefrontal cortex as a key target of the maladaptive response to stress. *J Neurosci* 2007;27:2781–2787.

50. Radley JJ, Rocher AB, Janssen WG, et al. Reversibility of apical dendritic retraction in the rat medial prefrontal cortex following repeated stress. *Exp Neurol* 2005;196:199–203.

51. Snijders C, de Nijs L, Baker DG, et al. MicroRNAs in post-traumatic stress disorder. *Curr Top Behav Neurosci* 2017. doi: 10.1007/7854_2017_32.

52. Girgenti MJ, Duman RS. Transcriptome alterations in posttraumatic stress disorder. *Biol Psychiatry* 2017. doi: 10.1016/j.biopsych.2017.09.023.

53. Constanzo ME, Jovanovic T, Pham D, et al. White matter microstructure of the uncinate fasciculus is associated with subthreshold posttraumatic stress disorder symptoms and fear potentiated startle during early extinction in recently deployed Service Members. *Neurosci Lett* 2016;618:66–71.

54. Papaleo F, Crawley JN, Song J, et al. Genetic dissection of the role of catechol-O-methyltransferase in cognition and stress reactivity in mice. *J Neurosci* 2008;28:8709–8723.

55. Millar JK, Pickard BS, Mackie S, et al. DISC1 and PDE4B are interacting genetic factors in schizophrenia that regulate cAMP signaling. *Science* 2005;310:1187–1191.

10 Implications for Treatment and Management
A Network-Based Approach

Neuropharmacological therapies such as those forming the mainstay of psychiatry are limited in that they largely target the ascending neurotransmitter modulatory systems. These conform to only part of the brain's networks and are intrinsically limited and non-specific, with limited benefits for those affected. More robust and enduring therapies involve the manipulation of the brain's inherent capacity for neuroplasticity. Such brain training is even more appealing because of the concept of generalization and transfer. A brain-training program may enhance a particular skill, but the effects may be more widespread within the brain circuitry. Preliminary data point to a possible "transfer effect" to a more general cognitive performance improvement that may translate to other cognitive functions. The molecular substrate of these plastic changes in the motor and sensory networks, for example, is in the form of rapid dendritic spine formation and slower spine elimination during sleep.

Physical exercise and dietary factors have already been shown to improve general cognitive processing capacities. Meditation may facilitate specific prefrontal region brain building that is important in focusing and social abilities. More specific interventions include mirror feedback therapy, transcranial magnetic stimulation, and transcranial direct current stimulation. The latter modalities enable advantageous stimulation or inhibition of different parts of the brain networks that are altered by injury or disease.

Working with the brain's own neuroplasticity has been relatively less emphasized in the current era, with a more predominant focus on pharmacological pill-centric approaches. A gene-centric approach had also been initially promising in lieu of the recently completed Human Genome Project. Lastly, memory-centric diagnoses may have obscured other important symptoms and dementias other than Alzheimer's disease. A triadic focus is advocated, with an intensification of disease mechanism elucidation (connectomics), an emphasis on neuroplastic mechanisms for most conditions, and pill therapy for some. However, most important are the primary and secondary prevention opportunities through brain fitness rules adherence. This has never been more urgent with the advent of the tsunamis of Alzheimer's disease and vascular dementias imminent. From the reviews earlier, the fundamental architecture of the brain is one of a massive evolutionary surge in white matter growth, brain networks, and connectivity that are supported by clinical observations such as diaschisis. The daily formation and dismantling of neuronal assemblies is a normal part of the brain's activity. Electrophysiological studies have long recorded the orchestrated neuronal networks and their specific patterns in various neurological states from seizures to encephalopathy and cognitive exercises, by amplifying electrical signals [1].

Even though vision evolved as the primary sense organ among mammals and even more so specifically among primates, processing of visual percepts from the environment occurs by retinal cone and rod cells, but these are not the only functions of the eyes. Light duration, frequency, and intensity are also processed, but by another type of retinal cell, termed the intrinsically photosensitive retinal ganglion cells (ipRGCs), comprising 1–3 percent of retinal cells. These ipRGCs process a photopigment, melanopsin, that activates the suprachiasmatic nucleus (SCN), which diminishes melatonin output. Melatonin is a sleep-inducing hormone secreted by the pineal gland. The pineal gland is also called "the third eye," taking on a more plausible role as an "eye" in fish, reptiles, and amphibians, in whom light stimulates the pineal gland through their much thinner skulls. This fact underscores our evolutionary brain–light linkages and dependencies. The ipRGCs also activate hypothalamic orexin-secreting neurons, which lead to arousal. Orexin is deficient in narcolepsy, for example [2]. The pineal gland also secretes pinoline, a neuroprotective antioxidant agent [3].

The function of the central SCN pacemaker is in keeping both 24-hour time and seasonal time. Multiple peripheral body clocks are tied to the SCN, which all express clock genes that influence metabolism and stimulate the immune system. Given these crucial functions, inadequate natural light exposure is a risk factor for a number of conditions, including cardiovascular disease, metabolic disease, and depression. The connection from the SCN to the peripheral body clocks located in the amygdala and habenula explains the depression from inadequate or irregular light exposure or even being out of synchronization with the solar day [4]. The central SCN transmits information to peripheral tissue body clocks. Approximately 20 000 cells in the SCN control peripheral tissue body clocks through a network of transcriptional factors that act as epigenetic modifiers, influencing cognition, memory, and metabolism [5].

Heliotherapy

Not surprisingly, sleep experts recommend 30–60 minutes of direct sunlight daily, with the best exposure time around midday to capitalize on the UV light output which is then at its maximum.

Modern-day shift work and staggered work schedules have caused a disconnection of the central clock, peripheral body clocks, and internal rhythms in such workers. Such circadian dysynchrony causes impaired cognition based on core processes being disrupted, such as attention and working memory, as well as promoting cardiovascular disease and metabolic dysfunction. Using artificial lighting at night will cause persistent SCN stimulation and block melatonin release, a sleep onset trigger. The intrinsic photosensitive retinal ganglion cells (ipRGCs) are also especially sensitive to blue wavelengths (460–480 nm) generated by light emitting diodes (LEDs) that are ubiquitous among screens of many devices such as iPads, smartphones, and computers. It follows that planned rest from such continued light stimulation or using programs to adapt to longer wavelength orange lighting of screens would be of benefit. Blue LED technology surfaced during the late 1990s and has lower energy requirements as well as superior lighting in comparison to incandescent lights. The SCN is most sensitive to short-wavelength blue light, with blue LEDs having a twofold deleterious impact on nocturnal melatonin suppression compared to yellower incandescent lighting.

Sleep Hygiene

The brainstem ascending neurotransmitter system interplay induces an intricate, orderly sequence of sleep stages. EEG analysis of sleep staging N1, N2, N3, and REM sleep is determined by various rhythms and frequency analyses. For example, the awake EEG features alpha (8–13 Hz) and beta (14–25 Hz) rhythms. During sleep, theta (5–7 Hz) and delta (0.5–4 Hz) predominate, although sigma (12–16 Hz) and gamma (30–80 Hz) may also be identified. The average night sleep of eight hours contains six cycles of ~90 minutes duration each, with the cycles usually following in an orderly sequence, but with a progressive lengthening of REM in the latter part of the sleep period. Sleep stages are primarily classified by the EEG, but also take into account the recordings of eye movements by electro-oculography and limb movements by electromyography. During NREM sleep, slow waves (theta and delta waves) originate in the frontal lobes and propagate posteriorly. In REM sleep, gamma waves (30–80 and 80–150 Hz) arise which are similar to the waking frequencies involved with attention and working memory processing. The gamma waves connect different brain regions and are the likely mechanism whereby linking to many different sensory domains during REM sleep occurs, as well as activation of the medial prefrontal regions and the amygdala. The amygdala and related fear circuitry are involved in anxious dreams [6]. During REM sleep, atonia prevents skeletal muscle activity, preventing dream enaction.

This complex sleep staging and its benefits were forged in our evolutionary past. Although mammalian sleep has profound variations among species, there are some spectacular examples that shed light on human sleep; perhaps the most significant event in our history was the tree-to-ground transition. This occurred around the time of *Homo erectus* ~1.8 mya, and had decisive cognitive sequelae and is viewed as a major attainment in human evolution. This event necessarily coincided with the use of fire and tool production [7]. A most notable cognitive enhancement was that of episodic memory, which is a critical function of sleep, especially with respect to consolidation of memory with the newly formed, labile memories transferred into existing memory networks [8]. The improved sleep and accompanying stages also augmented REM sleep and dreaming, providing a neural podium that in turn fostered innovation and creativity [7]. Together the sleep electrophysiological events sculpt the brain during a 24-hour cycle, with the slow NREM phases pruning new neural connections and the subsequent dreaming REM forming new connections relevant to the recent daily experiences. The pervasive slow-wave activity during NREM sleep can be viewed as communication channels between distant brain regions that process new informational items for storage into long-term memory. Certain parts of the brain are up to 30 percent more active during REM sleep. These are processes during which information relating to autobiographical memories, emotions, and socially related experiences are updated rather than processing external information that occurs during the waking hours. The sometimes bizarre visual auditory and somatosensory aspects of dreams woven together in an intriguing metaphorical nature, specific to the person, are a glimpse into the workings of this information processing, which is geared toward integrating new concepts and making sense of interpersonal and social intricacies. The concept of emotional intelligence, which encompasses the regulation of our own emotions and the recognition in others and how we interact with them, is regarded as a key feature and function of REM dreaming. Improving our ability to recognize emotions in others, their signals from certain eye movements, facial expressions, and body gestures, all combine for more rational and more appropriate decision-making, improving collaboration and fostering alliances, the essence of emotional intelligence.

REM sleep also facilitates the updating of information by integrating new experiences with the repository of the person's long-term storage of individualized memories. This process stimulates creativity; the newly formed memories and the entire cache of one's autobiography are amalgamated by wide-ranging neuronal ensembles that link disparate brain regions. Novel solutions to obdurate problems, with sometimes revolutionary approaches and solutions, emerge after REM sleep and dreaming. Many examples in history of creative solutions after a good night's sleep have been reported by engineers, artists, musicians, and scientists, with their creative solutions emerging after a specific dream. August Kekule's snake, biting its tail, and his revelation of the circular chemical ring structure of the benzene molecule is a good example [9].

Both the augmentation of emotional advancement or intelligence and creativity, engendered by REM sleep, are regarded as major factors in the remarkable human cognitive evolution. Matthew Walker's groundbreaking research and insights into sleep prompted him to describe dreaming as a "creative incubator in which the brain will cogitate vast swaths of acquired knowledge and extract overarching rules and commonalities – the gist. We awake with a revised Mind Wide Web that is capable of divining solutions to previously impenetrable problems. In this way REM dreaming is informational alchemy." He uses a very apt term, "ideasthesia," seen as a pivotal factor in human cognitive and behavioral evolution [10].

The waking brain neurochemical and electrical processing comes at a price, with the high-level metabolism requiring disposal mechanisms, which is accomplished through the glymphatic system. This system mediates a marked increase in metabolic refuse elimination, up to 20-fold. This is accompanied by an approximate 60 percent dilated interstitial space and contraction of the neuroglial cells, aiding the exchange of cerebrospinal fluid (CSF) within the interstitial fluid perfusion for clearance of many products, notably amyloid and tau proteins.

Amyloid-β production, increased by awake-state neural activity, is flushed out during sleep [11]. The deposition of amyloid, for example, begins in the medial frontal lobes, the origin of NREM electrical waves. People with sleep-related problems are more likely to develop neurodegenerative disease such as Parkinson's and Alzheimer's disease within a four-year period, as reported in the SHARE trial [12]. In general, sleep disturbances are one of the earliest symptoms associated with Alzheimer's disease. Sleep deprivation studied in mice was associated with a marked rise in amyloid-β deposition concentration [13]. Sleep deprivation interferes at a molecular level, causing amyloid-β deposition. Healthy middle-aged men with cerebrospinal fluid of amyloid-$\beta 42$ measurements and polysomnographic evaluation revealed a 6 percent decrease in levels after one night of good-quality sleep, not seen in those with sleep deprivation. Notably, with the default mode network being the most active region in the awake state, it happens to be the location of maximum amyloid-β accumulation. Chronic sleep disturbance escalates brain amyloid-$\beta 42$ and overall risk of Alzheimer's disease and other dementias [14,15].

People with PTSD present with daytime flashbacks, night-time nightmares, disturbed REM sleep, and obtrusive memories, for example, and are at increased risk for dementia. Their experiences have left them with elevated noradrenaline levels that counter the development of normal and sustained REM sleep and dreaming. Their nightly emotional experiences and traumatic memories cannot be reconciled by dreaming on account of their disturbed neurochemical milieu. So far, the only interventions with some success include the noradrenaline blocker prazosin, and meditation.

Our current approaches, with widespread use of hypnotics, are therefore problematic in that they cause an impairment of the sleep architecture with an approximate 50 percent compromise in brain cell connections formed in learning processes. In addition, meta-analyses reveal an excess of mortality due to stroke, cardiac infarcts, and obesity, as well as an overall increase in mortality of up to 5.3 OR when using more than 132 pills annually [16]. The objective benefit has also been determined to be no better than placebo. In Walker's phraseology, "Ambien laced sleep became a memory eraser rather than engraver" [10].

The Concept of Criticality and Sleep

Physics insights into the neuroscience of sleep come from the concept of criticality and sleep. Criticality relates to a physics principal often observed in the natural world, featuring the interaction of very large numbers of components. Some examples include water transformation from liquid to steam, grains in collapsing sand piles, and flocks of migrating birds. All of these examples have points of criticality at which an "avalanche" of activity is suddenly precipitated. Cerebral networks are yet another example and are hypothesized to operate close to a critical point, the function being the enhancement of its information-processing ability. Such mechanisms confer flexibility to tackle unpredictability, often encountered in the natural environment, and so enabling these biological systems to reorient and adapt more rapidly [17]. Large, interconnected neuronal systems are presumed to operate near such a critical transition zone, known as resting-state networks, and these complex systems operate near a critical point, finely balanced between volatility and stability [18,19]. There is also a criticality role of sleep and dreaming function, whereby these serve as a protective mechanism to counter "super-critical behavior" that would be injurious to brain function. The molecular processes involved, as already noted, are the synaptic pruning and plasticity rendered during sleep and dreaming for optimization of the brain's future responses [20,21].

Recommendations for Improved Sleep and Sleep Hygiene

1. Respect the 24-hour solar light cycle with set, regular hours for retiring and waking.
2. Abide by your chronotype and juxtapose as far as possible with work schedules.
3. Prioritize night-time sleep hygiene with limitation of pre-bedtime electronic, bright light, and excessive noise exposure. Ensure low ambient temperature and minimize noise. Use low-intensity, background "white noise" apps if needed.
4. Avoid activities that impair sleep, such as high-level cognitive activity (endogenous). Avoid the extension of the work schedule by correspondence such as emails (may increase cortisol release).
5. Avoid caffeine-containing stimulants such as coffee, energy drinks, soft drinks, or chocolate for several hours prior to retiring. Avoid substance abuse.

6. Limit substances that interfere with sleep architecture such as alcohol. Alcohol increases initial slow-wave sleep, but there may follow a disruption of subsequent REM sleep often with early morning waking, associated with impaired memory formation and dreaming.

7. Become cognizant that anxiety, stress, depression, and post-traumatic stress disorder all release cortisol and adrenaline, which interfere with sleep; attend to these treatments separately.

8. Chronic illness (chronic pulmonary disease, cardiac failure, arthritis, acid reflux, cancer, hyperthyroidism) and effects of commonly associated medications (steroids, antidepressants, anti-hypertensives, decongestants, stimulant weight loss medications) require review and medication pruning as far as possible.

9. Micronutrient deficiency correction, most commonly vitamins B and C, calcium, and magnesium deficiencies.

10. Polyuria management, which is common with prostate abnormalities and diuretic therapies.

11. Hormonal imbalance correction – for example, estrogen level fluctuations may affect melatonin release.

12. Treat sleep apnea with physical fitness, CPAP, or mandibular advancement devices.

13. Become cognitively fit to enhance cognitive reserve.

14. Monitor sleep with simple, unobtrusive, actigraphic devices to gain insights into personal sleep characteristics such as duration and changes in response to activities.

15. Keep a dream log to assist in the understanding of dreams and their potential analysis.

16. Augment the 24-hour sleep–wake cycle with brief daytime sleep ("power naps") to improve cognitive performance and reduce mortality [22,23].

Recommended Key Performance Indicators

Measuring and monitoring by you: Use a sleep health scale, such as the SATED scale, with scores ranging from zero to ten, with ten being the optimal score [24]; and the widely used sleepiness scale, the Epworth scale (normal is <10). Record total sleep duration; the optimum is 7–8 hours per night. Sleep quality can be recorded using electronic aids (Withings, Apple, Garmin devices).

Measuring and monitoring by medical professionals: WatchPAT for REM/NREM, sleep architecture, apnea index, oxygen desaturation or employ a formal sleep study (polysomnography).

Physical Exercise

The benefits of physical exercise (PE) to brain and body health are potent. Engaging in PE leads to improvements in overall body health, brain function, and increased cognitive reserve. PE induces new brain cell growth in at least two brain areas, as well as both gray and white matter growth. These new neurons that connect with others lead to increased neuronal circuits and brain padding or cognitive reserve. Cognitive reserve is a buffer against future brain insults such as stroke, dementia, and age-related deterioration. Recent cardiovascular and neurovascular clinical reviews and editorials have strongly advocated that physical exercise be regarded as a vital sign. There is also a complex and

Table 10.1 Physical exercise perspectives of specific job fitness requirements

Federal Bureau of Investigation (FBI) fitness test for men 20–29 (less for women and less for older age categories)	
Push-ups, minimum in 1 min	29
Sit-ups ≤1 minute	38
Sprint, 300 m	≤59 s
Run 1.5 miles	≤12.5 min
Navy Seals entry level requirements (competitive level differs)	
Push-ups, minimum in 2 min	42
Sit-ups, minimum in 2 min	50
Swim 500 yards	≤12.5 min
Pull-ups minimum no time limit	6
Run 1.5 miles (boots, long pants)	≤11.5 min

direct interaction between the health of the body overall and brain health. The two are tightly intertwined. The critical energy supply to the brain is provided by the microvasculature, the small brain blood vessels and the neurovascular unit, which are the first to suffer impairment in the context of poor physical form. Small-vessel disease is now regarded as the underlying neuropathological process and earliest pathophysiological process of many dementias and hence it becomes critical to investigate vascular factors and pathology before the disease escalates and becomes irreversible [25]. Much clinical and basic sciences research supports physical exercise as a major factor in the prevention of dementia and cardiovascular disease. An impressive study that was scientifically rigorous, the Caerphilly study, included, in addition to PE, other factors as well, such as smoking cessation, weight control, and healthy eating. However, of these, physical exercise was the most powerful, with specific example exercises being two miles of walking or ten miles of cycling per day. This study reported a 60 percent reduction in mild cognitive impairment (MCI) and dementia, a 50 percent reduction in both vascular disease and diabetes, and a 60 percent reduction in the all-cause mortality category [26].

Some occupations demand a certain entry level of fitness capabilities (Table 10.1). However, basic brain and body fitness is a prerequisite for all who make decisions for themselves and who are entrusted with others, whether a parent, spouse, company CEO, or national figurehead.

Scientific research has revealed that the following effects of PE may be realized:

Hardware
1. brain chemicals are released (BDNF) that stimulate brain growth;
2. neurogenesis or new brain cell formation;
3. synaptogenesis or new connections are formed;
4. angiogenesis or new brain blood vessel formation [27].

Software
1. improved working memory (the brain's operating system);
2. improved episodic memory;

3. improved attention;
4. improved executive function.

Feel-good neurotransmitters released
1. brain "marijuana" (endocannabinoids);
2. brain "morphine" (opioids).

Feel-good effects
1. alleviation of depression;
2. alleviation of anxiety;
3. improved sleep (adenosine production).

Reduction in the top four major diseases
1. dementia (~50 percent reduction);
2. cardiovascular disease;
3. strokes;
4. cancers [28,29].

What Happens When You Don't Exercise?

1. Brain atrophy (shrinkage) that correlates directly with obesity.
2. Speed of information processing decreases (word finding and memory problems).
3. Executive function decreases (the PFC is more sensitive to effects of aging compared to other brain areas and has the most rapid age-related loss in volume; it is also the region most sensitive to more physically active lifestyles).
4. Weight gain and increased BMI lead to vascular (heart attack, stroke, kidney, retinal disease) and/or metabolic conditions (diabetes), which in turn affect all organs.
5. Depression [30,31].

Side-Effects of Exercise

In addition to the beneficial effects, as with any intervention, adverse effects may occur. Endocannabinoid and opioid production lead to your own natural high that is safe and with minimal side-effects [32,33]. Side-effects may result as a consequence of the natural high experienced after moderate to intense exercise, sometimes called the "runner's high," leading to unrestrained exercise. This results in overuse injuries and withdrawal states when injury renders one unable to exercise.

Type of Exercise: Physical Activity (PA) and Physical Exercise (PE)

1. PA refers to the monitoring of non-exercise activity only, measured by tri-axial accelerometers, referred to as actigraphy.
2. PE refers to specific exercises to improve overall fitness, and is monitored by fitness devices that include time, speed, and distance parameters.
3. PE may be monitored by more advanced measurements such as VO_2 max (the maximum rate of oxygen consumption during intense exercise, where V = volume, O_2 = oxygen, max = maximum), measured in milliliters of O_2 per minute per

kilogram of weight; lactate threshold is useful for competitive athletes and those who are able to participate in high-intensity aerobic exercises.

How to Exercise

Screening

Screening is important before you start and should include the following:

1. Cardiovascular assessment encompassing:
   a. ECG rhythm strip
   b. cardiac stress testing;
2. physiotherapy consultation for:
   a. balance
   b. coordination
   c. musculoskeletal status.

Basic PE Components

1. aerobic (becoming cardiovascular fit – running, cycling, swimming, kayaking);
2. anaerobic (improving fitness – interval training sessions);
3. strength training (this has many benefits, including hypertension and weight reduction);
4. yoga (improves flexibility, stretching, correcting muscle imbalance due to specific sports);
5. balance.

Electronic Monitoring Devices

1. actigraphy devices: Nike Fitbit, Withings Pulse Monitor
2. GPS-based devices: Garmin, Apple Watch, chest heart rate monitoring.

Exercise Intensity

Exercise intensity is guided by maximum heart rate (MHR) percentage, subjective exertion and benefits. Calculation of MHR for a particular age and gender is by the following formula:

$$MHR = 217 - (0.85 \times age)$$

A simplified version of MHR by the CDC target heart rate formula can be used (220 – age). For moderate-intensity physical activity one should aim for 50–70 percent of MHR. For example, the MHR of a 50-year-old person would be $220 - 50 = 170$; therefore, the moderate-intensity levels for a person aged 50 would be:

- 50 percent: $170 \times 0.50 = 85$
- 60 percent: $170 \times 0.60 = 102$
- 70 percent: $170 \times 0.70 = 119$.

Thereafter the intensity of exercise, using running as an example, is evaluated according to the individual heart rate parameters (mild, moderate, intense):

- Mild: MHR 50–60 percent. Relatively easy pace of activity with regular breathing and early, aerobic/cardiovascular training effects.

- Moderate: MHR 60–70 percent. The pace remains comfortable, conversation possible, breathing deeper and more frequent, increased aerobic training effects.
- Moderate: MHR 70–80 percent. Moderate pace, more difficult to hold conversation, optimal aerobic/cardiovascular training.
- Intense: MHR 80–90 percent. Further increase in pace, with more labored breathing, leading to improved anaerobic capacity and improvements of speed of individual activity.
- Intense: MHR 90–100 percent. Sprinting pace, cannot sustain for long periods, labored breathing, with anaerobic benefits, increased muscular power and endurance.

Measurements of PA

PA, or basic movement, can be measured by number of steps taken per day using an actigraphy device:

- sedentary: <5000
- low activity: 5000–7499
- somewhat active: 7500–9999
- active: 10 000–12 499
- highly active: ≥12 500.

Metabolic Equivalent Approach to Exercise

By way of brief overview, quiet sitting is considered 1 MET (metabolic equivalent); sleeping is rated at 0.9; and walking at a slow pace is rated at 2. An approximate range of MET values vary from 0.9 (sleeping) to 23 (running at 22.5 km/h or a 4:17 minutes per mile pace). From a scientific point of view, 1 MET is defined as the amount of oxygen consumed while sitting at rest and is equal to 3.5 ml O_2 per kilogram of body weight × time (minutes) (3.5 ml $O_2 \cdot kg^{-1} \cdot min^{-1}$) or one MET is 58.2 W/m^2. A convenient grading scale is:

- light: <3.0
- moderate: 3–6
- vigorous: ≥6.

We can compute weekly METs/per hour × hours per week (aim for 9–15 hours per week) or minutes per week (aim for 500–1000 minutes per week). Table 10.2 offers some examples of activities and their METs.

Advanced Measurements Used by Athletes

- VO_2 max estimation
- vVO_2 max estimation
- lactate threshold
- beat to beat
- stress monitoring.

VO_2 max is an accurate and objective measure of fitness as it calculates aerobic endurance and cardiovascular fitness. It may be conceived as a kind of "horse power" of your cardiovascular system. Various formulas exist for this measurement:

- VO_2 max estimation by the Uth–Sorensen–Overgaard–Pedersen test: VO_2 max = 15 × HR max/HR rest;

Table 10.2 Example METs

Activity	MET/hour of activity
Walking (km/h)	
slowly	2.0
6.4	5.0
7.2	7.0
Running (km/h)	
10	10.0
13	12.9
15	14.6
Cycling (km/h)	
15	5.9
20	7.4
25	8.4
30	9.8
Swimming (km/h)	
2	4.3
2.5	6.8
3.0	8.9
3.5	11.5
4.0	13.6
Kayaking/rowing (km/h)	
8	10.3
12	13.5
16	16.4
20	19.1
Selected sports/activities	
Weight training	10.9
Yoga	3.2
Fishing from bank	2–3
Fishing from stream	3–4
Gardening	4.4
Shoveling snow	5.1
Housework	5–7
Alpine skiing	5–9
Aerobic dancing	6
Volleyball	6
Tennis	6–8
Fencing	6–10
Equestrian	7
Curling	7.4

Table 10.3 Some notable values of VO$_2$ max in ml/kg^2/min

Example	VO$_2$ max
Low-fitness human	11
Average untrained man	35–40
Average untrained woman	27–31
High-fitness human	50
Best human Olympic athlete	96
Cheetah	130
Siberian Iditarod dog	240
Pronghorn antelope	300

- Cooper test: VO$_2$ max = d12 – 505/45 (d12 is distance in meters covered in 12 minutes) [34].
  Table 10.3 offers some average VO$_2$ max values.
- VO$_2$ max and cognitive function: In addition to athletic fitness, exercise has both general and specific effects on cognitive function:
  - general: several different cognitive domains improve after months of aerobic exercise;
  - specific: executive function is improved more than other cognitive domains.

Functional neuroimaging research has shown that white matter connectivity improves with better VO$_2$ max, and that lower microstructural integrity of brain white matter is related to higher mortality [35]. The volume of white matter hyperintensities has also been correlated with decreased cognitive functioning [36].

vVO$_2$ max estimation is a measure of efficiency of your body. Although your VO$_2$ max or the "horse power" of your cardiovascular system is important, how efficiently your body transfers this power to overall speed via the legs or arms is what counts – hence velocity at VO$_2$ max is reported in units of speed, typically meters per second. The velocity at maximal oxygen uptake (vVO$_2$ max) is the peak running pace that can be maintained for an average of about six minutes running at maximal oxygen uptake. For a trained athlete, this may be a four-minute-mile pace or running at about 24 km/h or more. The vVO$_2$ max measurement is therefore dependent on VO$_2$ max as well as running economy.

Heart rate variability (HRV) can be easily measured using a number of wearable electronic devices. It reflects autonomic control of the cardiovascular system, with an increase in variability when parasympathetic activity dominates and a decrease with increased sympathetic activity. HRV can be used as an indicator of daily stress in a person's life, allowing an early and appropriate adjustment. HRV can also be used as a prognostic indicator in cardiac syndromes such as heart failure and acute myocardial infarction [37].

Fitness age is a very convenient and effective method of rapidly computing a person's biological – as opposed to chronological – age. Using a formula with inputs from resting and maximal heart rates, waist circumference at the level of the navel, age, gender, and amount and intensity of physical activity, a fitness age number is generated which may be older or younger than the chronological age. Typically, fit elderly people may be one or more decades younger by fitness age! The website for this calculation can be found at www.ntnu.edu/cerg/vo2max. These formulas are based on the estimated cardiorespiratory fitness researched by the Norwegian University of Science and Technology group [38].

Recommended Key Performance Indicators

Measuring and monitoring by you:

1. Overall activity measured in metabolic equivalents (MET). Some examples of a MET per hour: sitting, 1; slow walk, 2; Yoga, 3.2; brisk walk, 3.5; cycling, 7.5; swimming, 9; weight training, 10; running, 10; kayaking, 10; sprinting, 23. Aim for 9–15 MET hours per week.
2. You can record the number of steps per day (for example, 10 000 is good) with smartphones or electronic fitness devices.
3. Keep a log of timed distance and speed data from activities you do, such as walking, running, swimming, cycling, or kayaking with the aid of electronic monitoring devices (e.g., Garmin, Fitbit).

Measuring and monitoring by medical professionals:

1. Garmin devices measure VO_2 max.
2. VO_2 max may also be computed using the formula VO_2 max $= 15 \times$ HR max/HR rest (Uth–Sorensen–Overgaard–Pedersen test).
3. VO_2 max can be computed using VO_2 max $=$ d12 $-$ 505/45 where d12 is distance in meters covered in 12 minutes (Cooper test).
4. vVO_2 max estimation is used for competitive athletes. The vVO_2 max is computed by measuring the distance run in meters at maximum heart rate for a time of 6 min, and is recorded in meters per second.
5. Measure heart rate variability (HRV), which allows estimation of stress monitoring by specific Garmin devices (Vivoactive 3).
6. Record fitness age as a comparison to your biological age (Garmin devices) or from the website www.ntnu.edu/cerg/vo2 max.

Brain Foods

The Lyon Heart Study, published almost 20 years ago, reported a dramatic reduction of 50–70 percent in recurrent coronary artery disease, myocardial infarct, angina, and stroke among those in the Mediterranean diet arm [39]. Since then, similarly impressive data have been accruing in studies with the Mediterranean (M) diet, with reductions of dementia by up to 50 percent, myocardial infarction (MI) reduction by 37 percent, and stroke by ~35 percent. Adherence to an M diet after MI was almost threefold better as opposed to taking a statin drug. The M diet also showed a ~30 percent improvement over a low-fat diet in terms of cardiovascular events compared to statin use, with a 24 percent reduction. In addition, significant reductions in depression and cancer were also reported. Primary prevention of cardiovascular diseases in high-risk patients using the M diet also reduced cardiovascular death, infarction, and stroke by ~30 percent [40–43]. Global disorders of metabolism such as diabetes mellitus and obesity are associated with cognitive aging and Alzheimer's disease, and extensive data from animal and human studies have shown that lifestyle alterations improve global energy metabolism (caloric restriction and exercise). These measures are effective in preventing and even reversing cognitive impairment and attenuating brain atrophy associated with aging and Alzheimer's disease [44,45]. A higher intake of a prudent diet was associated with 30 percent reduction in myocardial infarction, as well as stroke on a global basis [46,47].

Cerebral white matter lesions or leukoaraiosis and white matter hyperintensity volume (WMHV) reduction, which is associated with cognitive decline, was also lessened by following the M diet [48]. An amelioration in mild cognitive impairment and conversion to Alzheimer's disease has also been reported [49]. Although the M diet is the most extensively studied to date, other diets with similar core compositions and relatively void of processed ingredients have also been shown to be effective. Examples include the Nordic, Okinawan, modified Atkins, Paleo, and Rosedale diets [50–54].

However, there is increasing awareness of what is thought to be our "original diet" or a high-fat, low-carbohydrate diet also known as the Banting diet, described in 1864 by William Banting of London, England [55]. This consists of seven foodstuffs: fish, meat, eggs, nuts, dairy produce, leafy vegetables, and low-carbohydrate fruits, predominantly berries. Carbohydrates were not an essential part of the Neolithic human diet, and now adays insulin resistance manifests in people who consistently consume >50 g per day of carbohydrates. Insulin resistance results in weight gain, elevated blood pressure, fat deposition in the abdominal organs – especially the liver – elevated uric acid, elevated glucose levels, impaired arterial dilatation, endothelial dysfunction, whole-body inflammation, mitochondrial dysfunction, and impaired physical exercise capability. High carbohydrate intake and insulin resistance in turn manifest with six principle widespread conditions today: obesity; myocardial infarction; stroke; type 2 diabetes mellitus; type 3 diabetes (Alzheimer's disease); non-alcoholic fatty liver disease (NAFLD); and cancer. Rather than a random collection of diseases, these are different expressions of the same disease or insulin resistance, and should be labeled as such to allow effective prevention and treatment. A key requirement in those with insulin resistance is to limit carbohydrates to no more than 25–50 g per day [56]. Noakes has compiled evidence that pursuing the correct diet is more effective than pharmacotherapy for our major global diseases of diabetes mellitus type 2, hypertension, and obesity [57].

What has worked, therefore, are those diets that all include composite food items in combinations that very likely contribute to success. However, what has not worked is the studying of food items or substances in isolation, nor vitamin supplementation studies that have seen some spectacular failures [58]. Nutritional factors are potent determinants of our brain health. For whatever reason, serotonin production has been outsourced to our gut, the bacterial microbiome being responsible for about 90 percent of its production. Microbiome health is key to our physical and mental well-being and is surprisingly capricious. For example, only two weeks of a suboptimal fast-food diet can alter the bacterial gut populations (microbiome) in a deleterious manner, with increased gastrointestinal inflammation that depletes serotonin. The by-products of inflammation convert serotonin into tryptophan, which in turn generates neurotoxic metabolites that are linked to depression, Alzheimer's disease, and schizophrenia [59]. The extensive and rapid communication between the gut and the brain is composed of neural networks, the vagus nerve, and neurotransmitters such as serotonin. The gut has an extensive nervous system, also called the enteric nervous system, and the resident bacteria and viruses, the gut microbiome, number ~200 trillion cells, elaborating neurochemicals and conferring immune functions integral to our health. Hence, diet is vitally important, as what you eat influences genes and alters them by epigenetic mechanisms even for future generations.

Because of the brain's large energy consumption, energy transfer from nutrients to neurons is integral to optimal brain function. The close link between brain-derived neurotrophic factor (BDNF), mediated synaptic plasticity, and energy metabolism is an example. BDNF is prolific in cognitive (hippocampus) and metabolic regulatory (hypothalamus) areas [60,61]. IGF-1 is also involved in hippocampal regions, influencing nerve growth, neurotransmitter synthesis processing, and synaptic plasticity [62]. Food-derived signals or energy metabolism are translated into synaptic plasticity via the mTOR (mammalian target of rapamycin) and Akt activation pathways. Omega-3 fatty acids also influence synaptic plasticity and cognition [63,64].

The concept of intermittent metabolic switching (IMS), or various methods of fasting, has been gaining popularity in improving brain health. Although most of the data to date stem from rodent models, some impressive results have been reported. The physiological basis is best understood in evolutionary terms. Those individuals whose bodies and brains performed well while undergoing a variety of fasting states were clearly in an advantageous position with respect to obtaining nutrients, ongoing reproduction, and overall survival. The change or switch in metabolism in supplying cellular fuel source is attended by molecular and cellular modifications with respect to cerebral neural networks in the brain, with an overall enhancement of function as well as improved ability to ward off disease, injury, and stress. Differing IMS protocols of intermittent fasting in animals have been employed, including alternate day fasting (ADF), by fasting for 24 hours at a time, and daily time restricted feeding (TRF) by fasting for 16 hours at a time. These induce depletion of liver energy glycogen stores and consequently adipose cells release fatty acids, which in turn are converted into ketone bodies (beta hydroxybutyrate and acetoacetate), also termed the glucose to ketone switch. An overall enhancement of physical performance, cognition, and motor function has been reported by such IMS protocols. Physiologically, an upregulation of neurotrophic factors and antioxidants occurs, as well as various DNA repair systems, including protein deacetylase and autophagy, being engaged. Both neuroprotection and mitochondrial biogenesis ensue. Human trials are now underway, but there is already a large body of evidence of benefit, including the ketogenic diet, that is both neuroprotective and successful in reducing drug-resistant epilepsy syndromes [65].

Six taste senses guide our intake of foods, with the first four being beneficial indicators and the latter two heralding potential "poisons":

1. salt: critical electrolyte for all animals;
2. sweet: complex sugars, high-density energy food;
3. umami: protein, savory detection, high-density energy food;
4. fat detection receptor: high-density energy food;
5. sour: acid, H^+ detection, food decomposition;
6. bitter: toxin detection.

These assist in supplying what the body needs. There are no strict rules with respect to proportions or calorie counting, but only general guidelines. Both quality of food and portion sizes are important in optimal nutrition. In addition, the closer one can follow what has been termed an ancestral type of diet as the overall general guiding principle, the better. A synopsis of these guidelines follows.

What the Body Needs

- Fish should be preferably wild in origin and shellfish should be evaluated for potential heavy metals such as mercury and arsenic.

- Fruit and vegetable consumption should be fibrous; oranges instead of orange juice.
- Some saturated fats are healthy and the obsession with low-fat diets has paradoxically increased cardiovascular disease.
- Large type A LDL particles are healthy and are reduced by a low-fat diet, whereas the small, dense type B LDL particles, driven by high sugar intake, are predominantly responsible for atherogenic dyslipidemia (clogging of blood vessels in the heart, brain, kidneys).
- Meat, whether red or white, should be from free-range animals.
- Dairy products should be full-fat and not reduced or fat-free; healthy saturated fats contain vitamins A and D.
- Maintain an anti-nutrient awareness with respect to grains, which should probably not be consumed in excess and when consumed should be whole grains.

Overview

The cornerstone to healthy eating involves eating moderate- to high-fat foods as opposed to the frequently promoted low-fat foods, minimizing grain consumption, drastically reducing sugar intake that causes heart attacks, strokes, diabetes, obesity, fatty liver, and dementia. Food quality, quantity, and timing of intake are all important. High-quality foods are outlined below; portion size in general involves one plate and one serving. Meal timing involves eating the majority in the first half of the waking day. Practice intermittent fasting for 12–16 h once per week and monthly 24 h fasts.

The key wholefoods include (1) seafood; (2) eggs; (3) red/white meat (free range); (4) fruit (berries); (5) regular-fat dairy; (6) tubers (potatoes, sweet potatoes, carrots); (7) cruciferous vegetables (broccoli, cabbage); (8) legumes (peas, beans, lentils); (9) probiotics (fermented dairy, yogurt, pickles, olives, sauerkraut); (10) prebiotics (garlic, onions, leeks); (11) nuts, seeds, and spices (curcumin, cinnamon, oregano, chili peppers, thyme, basil). In general, this may be achieved by following the original diet of Banting, or others such as the Mediterranean, Nordic, Pegan, or Okinawan diets.

Avoiding What the Body Does Not Need

- refined sugars: cane sugar, corn syrup, sodas, diet sodas;
- processed fats and oils: trans-fats, vegetable oils;
- processed dairy products: low-fat or fat-free dairy;
- processed meats;
- avoidance of meats contaminated with antibiotic use;
- cigarettes and substance abuse;
- avoidance of insecticides and toxins;
- avoidance of unnecessary vitamins and supplements;
- water purification – be aware of potential heavy metals (arsenic, mercury).

The Relation of Nutrition to Sleep and Exercise

- In the diurnal cycle, ghrelin increases with lack of sleep, which initiates hunger and feeding. Hence the best diet adherence can be derailed if sleep is impaired.
- Physical activity and nutrition are synergistic and both stimulate brain growth factors such as BDNF.

Microbiome Awareness and Monitoring

- Avoid unnecessary antibiotic use.
- Consider use of probiotics in yogurts, for example.
- There is a "Godzilla" within us of 200 trillion cells – respect it.

A Proposed Evolution-Based Diet: The Legacy Diet and the Macronutrient Index

- Beneficial foods category – small portion sizes! For example, portion sizes for fruit typically refer to one average-sized apple, one banana, or about a dozen blueberries.
- Appropriate portion sizes for other foods can be reviewed at the website (www.nhlbi .nih.gov/health/educational/wecan/eat-right/distortion.htm).
- From the lists below:
  - score one point for each category only in the right frequency intake;
  - minus one point for any component in the deleterious nutrition category taken at any time, daily or weekly;
  - maximum macronutrient index score: 20.

Intake 5–7 times per week

1. Fruits deciduous – apples, pears, plums, grapes, berries
2. Fruits tropical – mango, papaya, pineapple
3. Fruits citrus – oranges, grapefruit, mandarin
4. Vegetables – broccoli, cabbage, cauliflower, tomatoes, peas
5. Nuts, seeds
6. Eggs – preferably from free-range hens
7. Yogurt with probiotics, milk, cheese
8. Grains (whole, not refined) – oats, barley, rye, wheat, bran, muesli
9. Coffee (ground beans), black or green tea, dark chocolate
10. Alcohol ≤30 g/d for men (2 units), ≤20 g/d for women (1.5 units)

Intake 3–4 times per week

1. Fish – pelagic (preferably wild)
2. Shellfish – oysters, clams, mussels, scallops
3. Crustaceans – shrimp, lobster
4. Meat (white) – chicken, turkey, preferably free-range
5. Tubers – potatoes, sweet potatoes, yams, carrots, cassava
6. Leafy vegetables – lettuce, spinach
7. Complex starches – maize, rice
8. Legumes – beans, lentils, peas, peanuts
9. Spices – curcumin, oleander, cinnamon

Intake 1–2 times per week

1. Meat (red) preferably free-range or bison

Intake 0 times per week: deleterious nutrition category – subtract points

1. Added refined sugar, sucrose, high-fructose corn syrup (HFCS)
2. Sodas, soft drinks – diet or regular

3. Trans-fatty acid containing foods (e.g., margarine)
4. Processed meats due to nitrate content
5. Fat-free dairy products (yogurt, milk)

Recommended Key Performance Indicators

Measuring and monitoring by you: body mass index (BMI), aim for 19–25; blood pressure ≤130/90. BMI estimation at www.nhlbi.nih.gov/health/educational/lose_wt/BMI/bmicalc.htm

Measuring and monitoring by medical professionals (do 1–4 in all and if indicated include 5–8):

1. Evaluate for metabolic syndrome – blood glucose, HbA1C, fasting insulin, HDL, triglycerides, homocysteine, GGT (NAFLD), albumin/globulin ratio, uric acid, omega 3/6 ratio.
2. Inflammation – C-reactive protein, IL-6, TNF alpha.
3. Vitamin D, B12, folate.
4. Hormone levels – thyroid (TSH, T4).
5. Micronutrients – magnesium, selenium, iodine, zinc, copper, iron.
6. Other vitamins – E, B1, B2, B3, B6, B9.
7. Toxins and deleterious heavy metals – lead, mercury, manganese, cadmium, arsenic.
8. Consider discontinuing drugs that may alter memory and cognition, including anticholinergics, antianxiety, antipsychotic, hypnotics (sleeping tablets), and statins.

Cognitive Exercises

Studies from different parts of the world have supported the role of building cognitive reserve and slowing dementia when engaging in differing cognitive activities. A French study examining the value of travel, knitting, and performing "odd jobs" correlated with a decreased risk of subsequent dementia [66]. A Chinese community study that involved gardening activities also correlated with a relative decrease in incident dementia [67]. A New York-based study of non-demented elderly people who participated in 13 different leisure-based activities showed that those with high activity involvement (>6 activities), when compared to those with low activity involvement (≤6 activities), showed a marked decrease (38 percent) in their risk of subsequent dementia [68]. Activities such as reading, music, board/card/puzzle games, computer gaming, learning new languages, meditation, and Tai Chi (meditation in motion) are all activities that have shown positive results in this regard.

Biophilia and Nature Therapy

Biophilia refers to our close affiliation with nature and its attendant health effects [69]. Dating to 1987, recreation within natural environments has decreased by ~25 percent in the USA, attributed to the surge in indoor electronic entertainment [70]. Yet other evidence points to our unique affinity for aquatic environments – lacustrine (lake), marine, and riverine – presumably linked to our aquatic evolutionary past [71,72].

The attentional brain network, of which the PFC is a major hub, is engaged when external focus and attention are required. It is metabolically expensive. Multimedia electronic devices engage this attentional network and disengage the DMN, our "idling brain circuit," which is involved in fostering creativity [73,74]. Biophilia exposure promotes revitalizing processes to the PFC attentional circuitry cortex that are taxed during multitasking activities (attention fatigue). This has been termed the attention restoration theory [75]. A biophilic exercise test used a specially designed Remote Associates Test (RAT) involving hiking in various western US wilderness regions. The test group recorded a 50 percent improvement in performance compared to a control group after the fourth day. The proposed mechanisms of influence pertaining to the natural environment and brain health were the engagement of the DMN with introspection and positive emotions [76].

Another aspect of biophilic cognitive enhancement (improved cognitive scores, less anxiety and depression), as well as cardiovascular and immune benefits, was shown in people walking in Japanese forests. Immune effects included a ~40 percent increase of natural killer cell activity attributed to inhaling phytoncides (aromatic volatile substances released by trees) [77]; there was also decreased prefrontal cortical flow, as shown by near-infrared spectroscopy in the forest bathing group [78]. Japanese forest bathing or Shinrin-Yoku has accordingly been promoted within Japan since 1982 [79]. Other biophila studies, such as the one by MacKerron, used a GPS-based, mobile application called "Mappiness" that tracked the location of people in natural surroundings. At specific intervals they recorded their status in questionnaires, graded from 1–100 for extent of happiness. Increased contentment occurred when outdoors [80]. Other proposed mechanisms of biophilic engagement include epigenetic-related DNA methylation and altered gene expression [81].

Animal-Assisted Therapy and Animal-Assisted Intervention

Interacting or being associated with animals pays dividends in both health and illness. Pet interaction can lead to a decrease in anxiety, depression, and post-traumatic stress disorder (PTSD), as well as facilitating sociality and emotional health of the owners [82–84]. In addition to the animal-assisted studies, a dementia study was conducted with robotic animals. A robotic seal was used in an Australian PARO study that was constructed to display emotion and be responsive to both touch and voice, with the benefit of practically no maintenance and improved safety [85]. Therapy trials using horses (equine therapy or hippotherapy) have been beneficial in those with PTSD and autism spectrum conditions and for people with musculoskeletal abnormalities such as paraplegia or hemiparesis. In the Saratoga War Horse project, veterans with PTSD tested with the Beck Depression Inventory-II and PTSD checklist showed a significant 58 percent improvement. The neurobiological basis is attributed to oxytocin release as well as PFC activity modulation. Oxytocin release occurs when petting a dog in both the humans and the petted dog, similar to studies in primates and rodents [86].

Meditation

People engage in stimulus-independent thought for a considerable part of their waking day, termed mind wandering, that includes contemplation of the future that is associated with DMN activity of the brain. The evolutionary perspective correlates this activity with capabilities of mental time travel, planning, reasoning, and various roleplay scenarios. An excess of such activity is presumed to be the cause of various neuropsychiatric conditions,

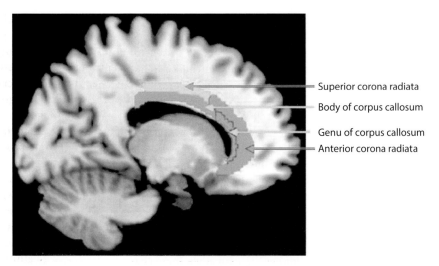

Superior corona radiata
Body of corpus callosum
Genu of corpus callosum
Anterior corona radiata

Figure 10.1 Meditation and brain building shown by MRI fractional anisotropic values for white matter connectivity in the anterior cingulate gyrus. The superior corona radiata (purple), body of the corpus callosum (red), genu of the corpus callosum (blue), and left anterior corona radiata (green) increased in efficiency and integrity.
Source: Tang Y-Y, Lu Q, Gen X, et al. Short-term meditation induces white matter changes in the anterior cingulate. *PNAS* 2010;107:15649–15652. Reproduced with permission.

including depression and anxiety; meditation is promoted as a possible attenuation of mind wandering, to help people "live in the moment." This was supported by the study of Killingsworth and Gilbert that people with wandering minds were relatively less happy: "A wandering mind is an unhappy mind" [87]. Several medical and neurological conditions reported benefits through mindfulness training, including anxiety, depression, PTSD, and chronic pain conditions [88–91]. Of specific interest is that mindfulness meditation was associated with an increased mononuclear cell telomerase activity, viewed as a measure of life expectancy and aging [92].

Meditation induces "brain building," with experienced meditators showing neuro-imaging evidence for both increased gray and white matter within the medial fronto-polar cortex [93,94]. In addition, several other brain regions revealed volume increases, including the hippocampus, inferior parietal lobe, and posterior cingulate cortex [95]. Experienced meditators also have larger hippocampal volumes. Mindfulness training induces neuroplasticity within these brain regions and has been correlated with objective improvements in metacognition (Figure 10.1) [96,97].

Closely related to meditation is eudaimonia, a human characteristic that incorporates intellectual activities, personal fulfillment, and virtuosity, in contradistinction to the concept of hedonic well-being. Eudaimonia has been correlated with lower risk of cardiovascular disease and depression [98]. A positive association was also been reported with eudaimonia, well-being, and right insular cortical gray matter volume [99]. On the contrary, a negative association has been noted with depression and insula volume [100].

Musicality

Rhythm is a key element of music but is also a feature in more fundamental human activities such as walking, running, and in tasks requiring complex coordination. The origins of rhythmicity in the human brain may well be related to bipedalism in the Late Miocene period. Rhythm relies on motor and sensory frontoparietal circuitry that underlies efficient bipedalism. The augmentation of sensorimotor control for bipedalism requirements may have been an initial contributor to brain enlargement, with added prospects for involvement in other tasks such as foraging, language development, and social interaction.

In Mithen's view, music and language evolved from the demands for vocal grooming that took over from tactile grooming of hominids, with their changes in social life and foraging and need for improved communication 6–7 mya. He postulated that gestures and music-like vocalizations would have increased and evolved into what he termed *Hmmmm* [101]. Extant primates today exhibit these fundamental aspects, with both geladas and gibbons referred to as "musical apes" as they synchronize their vocalizations with others, using a variety of melodies and rhythms. Geladas have a lip-smacking activity (rapidly opening and closing their mouth). The facial movements involved in lip-smacking appear speech-like, suggesting that this may have been an early step toward eventual human speech evolution [102]. Together, these characteristics may be regarded as early precursors for language-like activity. Both apes use their musical communication for social interaction. Making music together may be viewed as a low-cost form of cooperation that promotes social bonding and fosters group cooperation [103]. A common ancestral musical protolanguage evolved into the *Hmmmm* of Neanderthals, and in more separate circuitry for musicality and eventual language for more efficient communication of information and concepts among AMH ~200 kya [104]. Today, clinical studies reveal that the neural networks for language and music are relatively independent of each other and exhibit a degree of double dissociation. Musical ability or attributes can be "eroded" to an extent by the demands of language acquisition [105]. Other clinical studies support rhythmic auditory stimulation therapy for people with stroke, Parkinson's disease and TBI [106–108]. With aphasia, melodic intonation therapy (singing rather than speaking phrases and sentences) may work by decreasing the hyperactive right homologous Broca's area, which could be causing inhibitory effects in the impaired left Broca's region.

Insightful views by Tomlinson in his treatise of "A million years of music" reflected that the music neurobiological circuitry is relatively ancient, one of our newer cultural endowments, termed the "original human mental machinery," long preceding language and evolving by technological and social forces. His sagacious premise was that technosociality formed the basis of musicality and was bound to early hominin experiences of both motion and emotion that enabled musical information to transmit emotive communicative acts. This is turn led to more cognitive flexibility, increasing theory of mind, the capacity to think about others, and "thinking at a distance," all of which evolved in a prelinguistic phase [109]. There is ample neurophysiological support for such observations. Auditory processing emanates from a core superior temporal lobe area radiating posteriorly to the parietal lobes and anteriorly to the temporal lobes. From there, bidirectional circuitry impinges on every prefrontal cortical area. This extensive circuitry allows auditory information to be integrated into memory systems and motor programs. Particularly robust connections in the PFC are to the medial PFC (anterior cingulate cortex) and frontopolar cortex. Connections to the anterior cingulate cortex enable a synchronization of motor expression, attention and arousal, motivation, autonomic functions, memory circuits, emotion, and social engagement [110,111]. The anterior cingulate cortex (ACC) has particularly robust affiliation with hippocampal, memory-related circuits, the amygdala, and the frontopolar cortex. Barbas et al. inferred that the FPC, auditory association cortical, and ACC connections may be the neurophysiological basis of using symbolic representations of internalized organized thought [112].

The basic emotions, whether considered in terms of four categories (anger, fear, sadness, joy), or six, seven, or eight do not always present as dramatic, intense, fully developed responses. Much more frequent day-to-day emotional experiences are variations in degree of these basic emotions along intensity dimensions. This was encapsulated by Plutchik's cone model of emotion, with the apex of the cone accommodating the lower-intensity emotions, indicating more subtle differences or less divergence, whereas the other end of the cone depicts the basic emotions at their highest intensities. The idea behind the cone was that music mostly elicits or augments the "partial" emotions rather than the extreme emotion subtypes [113,114].

Brain pathology and musical abilities may lead to a large variety of syndromes, from impaired musical emotion to newly acquired musicophilia, musical hallucinations, loss of musical abilities, or newfound expertise in music. Music therapy is based on the premise that the modulation of attention, cognition, emotion, and behavior can improve both psychological and physiological well-being of people, whether afflicted by brain illness or not [115]. In Parkinson's disease, for example, improvements may be induced due to music-evoked priming and arousal of the brain's motor systems, mediated by auditory stimulation. This may be a function of entrainment of the motor circuitry by the music's beat. Music therapy has also benefited people with Alzheimer's disease, Tourette's syndrome, post-stroke visual neglect, memory, inattention, and working memory [115–117]. The postulated mechanisms include possible enhanced cerebral connectivity and activation of motor cortical areas by processes such as entrainment, whereby one rhythmic frequency impacts another neuronal ensemble to a point of synchronization, or they influence each other [118]. It has been demonstrated that neurons fire in unison with musical input, and in that manner music modulates cerebral rhythms. Different types of music have been investigated from a therapeutic point of view, and the music of Mozart, in particular, has received much attention. Light and sound can entrain neurons, something that can readily be seen on EEG recording with flashing lights, photic stimulation and entrainment, and in a pathological sense when one has photosensitive epilepsy [119].

Music can be regarded as a type of nutrient for the nervous system – the neurostimulation resetting the nervous system. The pioneering French doctor Alfred Tomatis, known for the sound stimulation program called the Tomatis method, referred to the importance of sound and music by saying "The ear is a battery to the brain." Music can be uplifting by stimulating the dopaminergic reward system, and hypothetically music resynchronizes the brain through entrainment. Music is a high-value commodity across all human cultures due to the basic underlying reward system being stimulated with dopamine released by the striatal components, the caudate, and accumbens nuclei. Music as an abstract stimulus can initiate euphoria, shown by a PET brain study (using ^{11}C-raclopride) of striatal dopamine release at peak emotional arousal [120]. In this regard, the so-called Mozart effect is sometimes referred to as a universal type of music that has not been influenced by individual linguistic and cultural rhythms. One of the reasons postulated is that Mozart started composing at the age of five, before his native German language was able to influence his compositions to a significant degree. Many benefits of musical instrument playing have been claimed, many with scientific foundations, including the enhancement of working memory, mathematics, and verbal skills [121]. Importantly the transfer of the music effect may be more generalized and apply to the domains of general attention, working attention, and executive function, all of which are impoverished after stroke, causing amusia, for example [122].

A Proposed Regimen For Cognitive Exercises and "Brain Building"

A long list of activities has been shown to be of benefit, and many others not mentioned may qualify:

1. computerized exercises such as BrainHQ, Cogmed, Posit, Lumosity, Brain Age. These yield a number of different scores that can track improvement or worsening over time;
2. board games, such as chess and Stratego. These two in particular have inherent attributes that involve working memory by contemplating many moves ahead and their consequences. This specific ability may be one of the earliest indicators of incipient cognitive failure in people as they age;
3. card games;
4. sudoku;
5. book clubs and discussion groups;
6. learning a second language;
7. pursuing a qualification, diploma, or degree;
8. engagement in educational courses, such as the Great Courses program;
9. literary arts – reading, writing, poetry;
10. culinary arts – cooking or baking classes;
11. visual arts – viewing museum paintings or engaging in art production or therapy;
12. music – singing, instrument playing, performing, or passive listening;
13. biophilia, outdoor exercise, interaction with nature (Japanese forest therapy);
14. animal companionship and interaction;
15. meditation, spirituality. Meditation does not require monitoring. However, smart phone-based devices can be used to access services such as Headspace.com, and the Muse device (www.choosemuse.com), which can guide and monitor meditation.

Recommended Key Performance Indicators

Measuring and monitoring by you: brain activity quotient (AQ) with BrainHQ (www .BrainHQ.com) recommended for 0.5 hours, three times per week. You can also use computerized games and exercises that can track brain scores.

Measuring and monitoring by medical professionals: (1) computerized testing (CNS-VS) for working memory, speed of information processing, attention, executive function, perceptions of emotions (POET subtest), and inhibition; (2) King Devick test; (3) cerebrovascular reserve (transcranial Doppler); (4) cognitive reserve (PET brain scan).

Socialization

Sociality was a major factor in initial human brain enlargement, attributed to coping with group dynamics and polyadic relationships as being cognitively very demanding. Sociality improves brain network integrity and promotes cardiovascular and immune health. Sociality induces oxytocin, endorphin, and vasopressin secretion in the brain, which have neuroprotective, anti-inflammatory, anti-anxiety, and antidepressant effects. Group membership makes us healthier and more resilient, and develops stronger immune systems. A study of prospective stroke studies (NOMASS) revealed that socially isolated people were twice as likely to have another stroke within five years compared to those in significant personal relationships [123]. Social isolation has also been reported in association with cardiovascular disease, rheumatoid arthritis, renal disease, cancer, and overall mortality [124–128]. The social brain circuitry includes lateral temporal, hippocampal, inferior parietal and prefrontal regions, with a critical hub in the CA2 region of the hippocampus [129,130]. Clinically, decreased inhibitory neuronal counts in the CA2 in people with bipolar disease and schizophrenia are findings supported by mouse data that are relevant to possible future treatment prospects for neuropsychiatric disease [131]. Oxytocin has been identified as a mediator of social neuroprotection after cerebrovascular ischemia, demonstrating both anti-inflammatory and antioxidant properties in rodent studies. At a molecular level, decreased neutrophil infiltration, decreased pro-inflammatory cytokines (interleukin 6), and lipopolysaccharide (LPS) and superoxide production by microglial cells have been documented [132]. Humans have been deemed super-cooperators by Nowak. The mechanisms responsible for the relatively advanced level of cooperation among humans stem from sociality, and several mechanisms have been identified as leading to the high level of cooperativity within our species. Assisting one another is referred to as direct and indirect reciprocity, as one favor may beget a reciprocal one; network reciprocity relates to advantages of groups, such as contiguously dwelling neighbors; kin selection relates to a preferred cooperativity with blood relatives, relative to strangers. Together these have made humans super-cooperators, which led Nowak to research future possibilities, such as curbing overexploitation of our current environmental resources. His intergenerational goods game suggested that decisions made by democratic group voting as opposed to individual decision-making tended to counter overexploitation of resources [133,134]. Further support for cooperating within a team structure comes from engineering, arts, science, humanities, patents, and manuscript publishing. Over a 50-year period, 2.1 million patents and 19.9 million manuscripts were reviewed by Wuchty et al., who found that team cooperativity dominated over single authorship and production [135].

Super-connectivity is also important with respect to optimal diversification of contacts. Networks or social organizations with a relative excess of strangers may impede exchange of new concepts or ideas, on the one hand, while networks dominated by a preponderance of personal friends may similarly stunt innovation. An optimal ratio was envisaged by Uzzin and Dunlap which explained success stories of cooperativity, such as their example of the famous musical *West Side Story* [136,137]. Social information is critical to survival and optimal interaction in groups. The inferential brain hypothesis, proposed by Koscik and Tranel, posits that human brains have progressed from primarily perceptual processing to inferential processing [138].

Looking further into the future, the trend of human evolution has been a progressive escalation in the networking domains. Initially our own brain sensorimotor networks and intracortical connectivity expanded and then evolved outside the brain to interaction with other minds, or intercortical connectivity, facilitated by the mirror neuron system. Nowadays the brain–machine interface extends connectivity even further. Direct brain-to-brain communication, or the transmission of information between two humans not utilizing our sensory or motor networks, has been accomplished by the combination of brain-to-computer interfaces using EEG encoding of binary (0,1) information bits. The remote subject was stimulated by computer-to-brain communication (transcranial magnetic stimulation) that generated phosphenes which were also encoded in binary information bits [139].

The electronic age has certain social impediments. Many social media platforms exist, such as Twitter, Instagram, Snapchat, and Facebook, and these are manifestations of extended human sociality. However, there are limits to electronic communication. Despite hundreds of millions of users, Facebook users, for example, have not developed group sizes any larger than our ancestral hunter-gatherer traditional group size of 100–250 individuals. Pollet et al. noted that engaging in social network sites does not translate into greater "offline social network size" nor to emotionally closer friendships among offline network members [140].

Our social brain circuitry evolved to engage a polysensory input and multimodal output, fashioned over millions of years, that include components of communication such as:

1. numerous facial expression that impart subtle, covert, and other vital nuances to communication (Ekman claims over 10 000);
2. nonverbal communication relayed through body language such as stances and postures;
3. speech intonation or prosody that relays different, and at times even the opposite, message compared to spoken content [141,142].

Socialization and Brain Health Proposals

1. Socialize for brain development that has particular importance for children, teenagers, and young adults. The major fiber network for social and emotional competency, the uncinate fasciculus, continues to mature into the fourth decade.
2. Socialize for brain health as the process releases oxytocin, vasopressin, and endorphins, which have anti-inflammatory and neuroprotective properties.
3. Participation in group meetings, sport clubs, group discussion, dancing, group dinners, and performing arts.
4. Emphasize interpersonal face-to-face opportunities to benefit from communication mediated in the nonverbal domains, not captured by electronic communication devices.
5. Electronic communication nevertheless remains invaluable, but ancillary, facilitative, not a substitute for face-to-face interactions. It complements but should not replace face-to-face encounters.

Recommended Key Performance Indicators

Performance measures by you: Modified Social Network Index – participation once every two weeks with up to 12 different social groups (spouse, parents, child, neighbors, relatives, volunteers, work colleague, student, sport groups, social clubs, religious group, charity groups). Score out of 12 (maximum).

Measuring and monitoring by a medical team: CRP, interleukin-6, brain network integrity by MRI brain scan fractional anisotropy [143,144].

Summary of Lifestyle Interventions

The earliest neurobiological defect of cognitive disorders may well be at the neurovascular level, with both clinical and neuroimaging studies supporting impaired cerebrovascular reactivity impairment as the first sign of compromise. This underscores the essential role of physical exercise which induces both generalized cardiovascular and cerebrovascular health as well as neurotrophic factors that lead to neurogenesis and augment brain circuitry. Great promise appears to be held in the realm of lifestyle/behavioral interventions in people with mild cognitive impairment. These include the administration of a high-seafood diet with docosahexapentanoic acid (DHA) and eicosapentanoic acid (EPA) administration, together with monitored physical exercise and structured cognitive exercise applications. These have shown profound cognitive, behavioral, and neuroimaging improvements in dementia patients [145]. Physical exercise has particularly potent brain-protective effects and has been shown to reduce the incidence of dementia by up to 50 percent [146]. Healthy diet adherence, such as a Mediterranean-type diet, has consistently shown reductions in cardiovascular disease, cancer, and dementia, in excess of statins, for example. Working memory may be regarded as the core frontal lobe function central to all other processes, including attention, memory, executive function, and inhibition. Specific working memory cognitive exercises have been developed, such as Cogmed [147].

Once biochemical toxins, infections, and inflammatory abnormalities have been corrected, the lifestyle/behavioral interventions can be initiated. Once optimization of lifestyle/behavioral factors has been attained, augmentation of the brain's plasticity with neurostimulatory devices such as the PoNS device can be pursued.

Medical Treatment

Neurostimulation Devices

There are local effects with neurological deficit and other deficits, and also effects triggered more remotely due to network effects. Otherwise-intact neuronal assemblies may manifest with impaired function (clinical deficits) due to these network influences. The brain can enter a kind of dysrhythmia that may have the electrophysiological correlate of EEG-observed slow-wave activity in a variety of illness states such as TBI and dementia. With targeted and specific stimulation, both of these processes can be ameliorated, as will be seen later. Even the damaged area may benefit from stimulation, as has been noted in stroke patients where so-called learned non-use occurs and constraint-induced therapy (CIT) is shown to be clinically effective. CIT has since demonstrated success in a number of brain cognitions, including multiple sclerosis, TBI, cerebral palsy, focal dystonia, aphasia, and spinal cord injury. The mechanism of action is presumably on the basis of a reorganization of cerebral networks by persistent sensory modulation [148].

Neurostimulation has been tried with physiological interventions such as physical exercises, and also cognitive (hypnosis, neurofeedback) and various other modalities such as magnetic (TMS, d-TCS), electrical (PoNS, Cefaly, vagal nerve stimulation), sound, and light stimulation.

Neuropharmacological stimulation or neuromodulation capitalizes on the state-dependent ascending neurotransmitter systems that ramify throughout the cerebral cortex. Sometimes referred to generically as the RAS, modulation may be effective by resetting the brain's integral balance of excitation inhibition, although this is a purely hypothetical premise. Autonomic nervous system activity may also be in a state of imbalance, as occurs with PTSD, for example, where a deleterious signal-to-noise ratio is present. The balance between the sympathetic and parasympathetic nervous system may be achieved by a number of exercises that include meditation, yoga, hypnosis, and biofeedback, for example. None of these processes are likely to be successful unless optimal neuronal conditions for recovery are provided. These include the powerful restorative effect of the right quantity and quality of sleep, nutrients, and cognitive and physical stimulation.

Laser Therapy

Lasers can produce light of very pure frequencies that can be aimed in a very focused and specific direction. Hence the acronym LASER – light amplification through stimulated emission radiation. The exact frequency is important as one wavelength may portend healing and another be able to sever tissue. For example, low-intensity lasers (cold lasers) stimulate healing at the cellular level, whereas high-intensity lasers (hot lasers) are used in surgery to cut away diseased tissue. The healing frequency is 660 nm (red light), with frequencies up to 840 nm of potential benefit.

Brain stimulation applied transcranially with low-level light laser therapy (LLLT) is the application of directional low-level laser power in the red and near-infrared wavelength parameters in the hopes of neurobiological modulation and therapeutic effects. The underlying LLLT mechanism of action is the absorption of photon energy by the mitochondrial enzyme cytochrome oxidase, the final enzyme of mitochondrial respiratory chain reactions.

LLLT is noninvasive and is being intensively investigated as a modality for cognitive impairment, neurodegeneration, and cerebrovascular disorders, with evidence for cognitive enhancement and neuroprotection through mitochondrial respiration augmentation [149].

Brain Electrographic Devices

There is evidence that after brain injuries of various kinds, some of the interacting neural networks and their associated interneurons are involved, with an "imbalance" between excitation and inhibition function. This has been termed a "noisy" brain and leads to an impairment of regulating sensory input. The common symptoms after various brain lesions – such as photophonophobia, working memory problems, inattention fatigue, and tinnitus – may be explained by such neuronal assembly dysfunction. Improvement after various stimulation strategies may help reset these, with one of the possible mechanisms being through activating the interneuron assemblies. Although speculative, internal sources of stimulation that may be achieved by meditation, yoga, and hypnosis may similarly function in ameliorating the "noisy" brain networks. External stimulation devices, whether through using magnetism or electrical means, may activate the interneuronal networks by way of stimulation via the tongue or other branches of the trigeminal nerve, the connection to the reticular activating system (RAS) (used here as a generic term for the eight different neurotransmitter systems), that ramifies widely throughout the brain [150]. Similarly, the autonomic nervous system can be in a state of imbalance, with relative excess of sympathetic versus parasympathetic activity, as is the case with PTSD, anxiety, and hyperactivity disorders, for example. This, too, can be modulated and balance restored by augmenting the parasympathetic nervous system, the signal-to-noise ratio, and social engagement [151].

The PoNS (portable neuromodulation stimulator) has long been touted for cerebral rehabilitation. It has been estimated that the electrical stimulation of the 15 000–50 000 lingual (tongue) nerve fibers that traverse the fifth cranial nerve (lingual division) and seventh cranial nerve (facial nerve) transmit neural signals to the brain stem and cerebellum. A recently completed clinical trial of TBI and imbalance had positive results, and on this basis the company is now seeking FDA approval for this indication. Support for one of the presumed mechanisms of action has recently been reported by studying high- and low-frequency PoNS stimulation with 64-channel EEG. Brain activation was recorded that included increased alpha and theta activity, which were associated with reflection and relaxation (http://heliusmedical.com).

Further evidence for the modulation of brain networks by stimulation comes from studies using noninvasive transcutaneous vagal nerve stimulation applied to the ear. Resting-state network connectivity was measured specifically in the amygdala–lateral prefrontal network in people with mild-to-moderate depression. Clinical improvement in depression and anxiety was associated with increases in this intrinsic connectivity network [152]. Vagal nerve stimulation has also emerged as a modality for treatment-resistant depression [153]. An extensive literature exists for the more invasive form, first developed for medication-refractory epilepsy, which has also shown improvement in the core frontal function of working memory [154].

Transcranial direct current stimulation: Maintaining working memory underlies the processing of most cognitive tasks. Working memory training together with frontoparietal transcranial direct current stimulation (tDCS) has shown behavioral improvement as well as the suggestion of transfer of improved performance gains in tasks not specifically trained in the working memory realm. EEG monitoring of these studies supports the proposed mechanism of enhancing cortical connectivity and efficiency and connectivity in task-associated networks [155].

Transcranial magnetic stimulation: High-frequency stimulation (3 Hz rTMS) of the affected hemisphere area with stroke, for example, may decrease inhibitory effects in the perilesional area. The premotor cortex may unmask circuitry that remains functional but inhibited and lead to cortical reorganization. Hyperactivity or excitability may be present in the unaffected hemisphere, which may respond to low-frequency stimulation (1 Hz rTMS). This has been shown to be effective for aphasia. Investigation into Broca's aphasia after stroke, applying low-frequency stimulation (1 Hz rTMS) to the right hemisphere in the equivalent region to Broca's area or Brodmann's area 45, has demonstrated improvement in dysnomia. This has been interpreted as modulation by rTMS of maladaptive consequences in the contralesional hemisphere (Figure 10.2) [156,157].

Cefaly device: The noninvasive transcutaneous supraorbital nerve stimulation (t-SNS) device Cefaly (Cefaly Technology, Herstal, Belgium) was shown by a double-blind randomized controlled trial to be effective in episodic migraine, and has gained FDA approval. The efficacy and safety ratio was especially favorable in comparison to prophylactic antimigraine medications. Apart from migraine treatment and prevention, of perhaps more significance was a PET scan study after three months of daily t-SNS treatment for migraine, which revealed an improvement in orbitofrontal hypometabolism

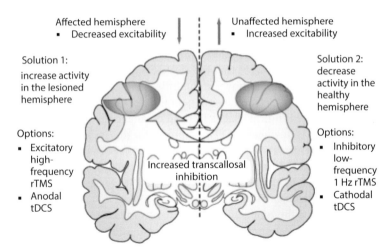

Figure 10.2 Brain stimulation with device-based therapies: tDCS and TMS.
Reproduced by permission from Springer Nature from Fregni F, Pascual-Leone A. Technology insight: noninvasive brain stimulation in neurology – perspectives on the therapeutic potential of rTMS and tDCS. *Nat Clin Pract Neurol* 2007;3:383–393.

and frontotemporal regions from baseline. The Cefaly device mechanism of action may be through a neuromodulation of pain control and limbic circuitry. Applications beyond migraine, such as TBI and frontotemporal lobe syndromes, for example, may develop, given these findings [158–160].

Mirror Neuron Therapy and Rehabilitation

Mirror visual feedback (MVF) therapy has been shown to be effective in treating a variety of neurological deficits, including stroke-related limb paresis, phantom limb pain, anxiety, and complex regional pain syndromes in controlled case series [161,162]. Postulated mechanisms of action include a rehabilitative effect of the visuomotor tract that promotes the "unlearning of the learned paralysis," whereby neurons and their fiber tracts are in an inhibited state and the "unlearning" is promoted by using a mirror [163]. This has been attributed to the mirror neuron system, which fosters interactions between the vision, proprioceptive, and motor modalities. Limb weakness after stroke may be related to both fiber tract damage and so-called learned paralysis [164]. Similarly, the technique termed "action observation treatment" activates circuits by observation that are similar to those that would perform the actual movement [165].

Neuropharmacological Manipulation of the Frontal Subcortical Circuitry

A number of well-conducted trials with positive outcomes, capitalizing on the ascending brainstem neurotransmitter systems, have been reported in several specific neurological syndromes.

Amantadine and Severe TBI

A randomized controlled multinational trial of minimally conscious or vegetative state patients administered amantadine 100–200 mg BID; by week four these patients showed faster recovery as measured by the disability rating scale. The mechanism of action was presumed presynaptic release facilitation, and postsynaptic reuptake blockade with an upregulation of dopaminergic transmission in nigrostriatal (arousal), mesolimbic (conation), and mesocortical (attention) circuitry [166].

Methylphenidate and Moderate to Severe TBI

Methylphenidate success in moderate to severe TBI has been reported in the context of a randomized controlled trial, with specific improvement noted for the core frontal component of attention and speed of information processing [167].

Trazodone and Frontotemporal Lobe Disorders

Trazodone, a selective serotonin reuptake inhibitor, has agonistic effects on 5HT1A, 5HT1C, and 5HT2 receptors, as well as being a blocking agent of the histamine (H1) and adrenergic alpha 1 and alpha 2 receptors. From meta-analyses, frontotemporal lobe syndrome patients are regarded as having primarily a serotonergic neurotransmitter deficit in addition to a dopaminergic deficit, and not involving acetylcholine and norepinephrine. A randomized controlled trial of trazodone (300 mg daily) showed significant improvement as measured by the neuropsychiatric inventory score, predominantly a behavioral improvement rather than in cognition [168,169].

Serotonergic Therapy and Stroke (Motor Deficit)

The early combination of fluoxetine and physiotherapy in stroke patients led to improved motor recovery by three months. The FLAME (fluoxetine for motor recovery after acute ischemic stroke) trial tested this combination in patients with moderate to severe motor deficit. The presumed mechanism of action is thought to include trophic factors and modulation of spontaneous brain plasticity by fluoxetine, but remains conjectural [170].

Neuropsychiatric Component Treatment

Most neurological syndromes have one or more neuropsychiatric illness components, such as anxiety, depression, and compulsion disorders. There is an increased emphasis on neurobiology of brain disorders, more attention to the newer neuroimaging modalities, and employing dimensional scales rather than categorical diagnoses such as provided by the DSM V [171]. The lack of biomarkers for neuropsychiatric syndromes, the integration of neuroradiology, basic neuroscience, neurogenetics, and epigenetics to help establish a diagnosis based on pathophysiology and etiology is emerging. Previously, psychiatric classifications led to the dichotomization of illnesses, when many might be more appropriately configured as dimensional traits with a range of presentations that may overlap with normality and be consistent with keeping a polygenic mode of inheritance. DSM V diagnoses often include a number of comorbidities that may be attributed to a diagnostic artifact with the underlying pathophysiology often due to a single entity. Contemporary psychiatric medication mechanisms of actions are usually beyond the boundaries of categorical DSM diagnoses [172].

New Treatment Insights from Understanding Brain Wiring

Multitasking refers to being engaged in two or more activities at the same time. Typically, one activity, whether cognitive or motor, is mundane and relatively automatic, and is performed by the basal ganglia circuitry. The other activity is more demanding, requiring executive and attentional input by the PFC. The automaticity of the basal ganglia circuitry sometimes fails, such as in Parkinson's disease. Instituting rhythms such as with music therapy or visual aids such as patterned lines on the floor may dramatically improve a Parkinsonian gait [173].

References

1. Pribram KH, King JS, Pierce TW, Warren A. Some methods for dynamic analysis of the scalp recorded EEG. *Brain Topogr* 1996;8:367–377.

2. Hattar S, Liao HW, Takao M, Berson DM, Yau KW. Melanopsin-containing retinal ganglion cells: architecture, projections, and intrinsic photosensitivity. *Science* 2002:295:1065–1070.

3. Tang GY, Ip AK, Siu AW. Pinoline and N-acetylserotonin reduce glutamate-induced lipid peroxidation in retinal homogenates. *Neurosci Lett* 2007;412:191–194.

4. LeGates TA, Fernandez DC, Hattar S. Light as a central modulator of circadian rhythms, sleep and affect. *Nat Rev Neurosci* 2014;14:443–545.

5. Masri S, Sassone-Corsi P. The circadian clock: a framework linking metabolism, epigenetics and neuronal function. *Nat Rev Neurosci* 2013;14:69–75.

6. Nielsen T, Levin R. Nightmares: a new neurocognitive model. *Sleep Med Rev* 2007;11:295–310.

7. Coolidge FL, Wynn T. The effects of the tree-to-ground sleep transition in the evolution of cognition in early *Homo*. *Before Farming* 2006;4:1–18.

8. Diekelmann S, Born J. The memory function of sleep. *Nat Rev Neurosci* 2010;11:114–126.

9. Benfey OT. August Kekulé and the birth of the structural theory of organic chemistry in 1858. *J Chem Educ* 1958;35:21–23.

10. Walker M. *Why We Sleep*. Scribner, New York, 2017.

11. Xie L, Kang H, Xu Q, et al. Sleep drives metabolic clearance from the adult brain. *Science* 2013;342:373–377.

12. Sterniczuk R, Theou O, Rusak B, Rockwood K. Sleep disturbance is associated with incident dementia and mortality. *Curr Alzheimer Res* 2013;10(7):767–775.

13. Yaffe K, Laffan AM, Harrison SL. Sleep-disordered breathing, hypoxia, and risk of mild cognitive impairment and dementia in older women. *JAMA* 2011;306:613–619.

14. Jagust WJ, Mormino EC. Lifespan brain activity, β-amyloid and Alzheimer's disease. *Trends Cogn Sci* 2011;15:520–526.

15. Ooms S, Overeem S, Besse K, et al. Effect of 1 night of total sleep deprivation on cerebrospinal fluid β-amyloid 42 in healthy middle-aged men: a randomized clinical trial. *JAMA Neurol* 2014;71:971–977.

16. Jike M, Itani O, Watanabe N, et al. Long sleep duration and health outcomes: a systematic review, meta-analysis and meta-regression. *Sleep Med Rev* 2017. doi: 10.1016/j.smrv.2017.06.011.

17. Beggs JM, Timme N. Being critical of criticality in the brain. *Front Physiol* 2012;3. doi: 10.3389/fphys.2012.00163.

18. Tagliazucchi E, Balenzuela P, Fraiman D, Chialvo DR. Criticality in large scale brain fMRI dynamics unveiled by a novel point process analysis. *Front Physiol* 2012;3. doi: 10.3389/fphys.2012.00015.

19. Bak P, Tang C, Wiesenfeld K. Self-organized criticality: an explanation of the 1/f noise. *Phys Rev Lett* 1987;59:381–384.

20. Pearlmutter BA, Houghton CJ. A new hypothesis for sleep: tuning for criticality. *Neural Comput* 2009;21(6):1622–1641.

21. Pearlmutter BA, Houghton CJ. Dreams, mnemonics and tuning for criticality. *Behav Brain Sci* 2013;36:625–626.

22. Lhal O, Wispel C, Willigens B, Pietrowsky R. An ultra short episode of sleep is sufficient to promote declarative memory performance. *Sleep Res* 2008;17:3–10.

23. Naska A, Oikonomou E, Trichopoulou A, Psaltopoulou T, Trichopoulos D. Siesta in healthy adults and coronary mortality in the general population. *Arch Intern Med* 2007;167:296–301.

24. Buysse DJ. Sleep health: can we define it? Does it matter? *Sleep* 2014;37(1):9–17.

25. Raz L, Knoefel J, Bhaskar K. The neuropathology and cerebrovascular mechanisms of dementia. *J Cereb Blood Flow Metab* 2016;36:172–186.

26. Elwood P, Galante J, Pickering J, et al. Healthy lifestyles reduce the incidence of chronic diseases and dementia: evidence from the Caerphilly cohort study. *PLoS One* 2013;8(12):e81877. doi: 10.1371/journal.pone.0081877.

27. Van Praag H. Neurogenesis and exercise: past and future directions. *Neuromolecular Med* 2008;10(2):128–140.

28. Buchman AS, Boyle PA, Yu L, et al. Total daily physical activity and the risk of AD and cognitive decline in older adults. *Neurology* 2012;78(17):1323–1329.

29. Sofi F, Valecchi D, Bacci D, et al. Physical activity and risk of cognitive decline: a meta-analysis of prospective studies. *J Intern Med* 2011;269:107–117.

30. Cotman CW, Berchtold NC, Christie LA. Exercise builds brain health: key roles of growth factor cascades and inflammation. *Trends Neurosci* 2007;30:464–472.

31. Rhodes JS, van Praag H, Jeffrey S, et al. Exercise increases hippocampal neurogenesis to high levels in mice. *Behav Neurosci* 2003;117:1006–1016.

32. Boecker H, Sprenger T, Spilker ME, et al. The runner's high: opioidergic mechanisms in the human brain. *Cereb Cortex* 2008;18:2523–2531.

33. Raichlen DA, Foster AD, Gerdeman G, Seillier A, Giuffrida A. Wired to run: exercise induced endocannabinoid signaling in humans and cursorial mammals with implications for the "runner's high." *J Exp Biol* 2013;215:1331–1336.

34. Kaminsky LA, Arena R, Myers J. Reference standards for cardiorespiratory fitness measured with cardiopulmonary exercise testing: data from the Fitness Registry and the Importance of Exercise National Database. *Mayo Clinic Proceedings* 2015;90:1515–1523.

35. Sedaghat S, Cremers LGM, de Groot M, et al. Lower microstructural integrity of brain white matter is related to higher mortality. *Neurology* 2016;87:927–934.

36. Au R, Massaro JM, Wolf PA, et al. Association of white matter hyperintensity volume with decreased cognitive functioning: the Framingham Heart Study. *Arch Neurol* 2006;63:246–250.

37. Pumprla J, Howorka K, Groves D, Chester M, Nolan J. Functional assessment of heart rate variability: physiological basis and practical applications. *Int J Cardiol* 2002;84:1–14.

38. Nauman J, Nes BM, Lavie CJ, et al. Prediction of cardiovascular mortality by estimated cardiorespiratory fitness independent of traditional risk factors: the HUNT study. *Mayo Clin Proc* 2017;92:218–227.

39. De Lorgeril M, Salen P, Martin JL, et al. Mediterranean diet, traditional risk factors and the rate of cardiovascular complications after myocardial infarction: final report of the Lyon Diet Heart Study. *Circulation.* 1999;99:779–785.

40. Estruch M, Ros E, Salas-Slavdo J, et al. Primary prevention of cardiovascular disease with a Mediterranean diet. *N Engl J Med* 2013;368:1279–1290.

41. Köbe T, Witte AV, Schelle A, et al. Combined omega-3 fatty acids, aerobic exercise and cognitive stimulation prevents decline in gray matter volume of the frontal, parietal and cingulate cortex in patients with mild cognitive impairment. *NeuroImage* 2016;131:226–238.

42. Sarris J. Nutritional medicine as mainstream in psychiatry. *Lancet Psychiatry* 2015;2:271–274.

43. Ngandu T, Lehtisalo J, Solomon A, et al. A 2 year multidomain intervention of diet, exercise, cognitive training, and vascular

risk monitoring versus control to prevent cognitive decline in at-risk elderly people (FINGER): a randomised controlled trial. *Lancet* 2015;385:2255–2263.

44. Bredesen DE, Amos EC, Canick J, et al. Reversal of cognitive decline in Alzheimer's disease. *Aging* 2016;8:1250–1258.

45. Bredensen DE. Reversal of cognitive decline: a novel therapeutic program. *Aging* 2014;6:707–717.

46. Iqbal R, Anand S, Ounpuu S, et al. Dietary patterns and the risk of acute myocardial infarction in 52 countries: results of the INTERHEART study. *Circulation* 2008;118;1929–1937.

47. O'Donnell MJ, Xavier D, Liu L, et al. Risk factors for ischemic and intracerebral hemorrhagic stroke in 22 countries (Interstroke study): a case control study. *Lancet* 2010;376:112–123.

48. Gardener H, Scarmeas N, Gu Y, et al. Mediterranean diet and white matter hyperintensity volume in the Northern Manhattan Stroke Study. *Arch Neurol* 2012;69:251–256.

49. Scarmeas N, Stern Y, Mayeaux R, et al. Mediterranean diet and mild cognitive impairment. *Arch Neurol* 2009;66:216–225.

50. Hansen CP, Overvad K, Olsen KC, et al. Adherence to a healthy Nordic diet and risk of stroke: a Danish cohort study. *Stroke*. 2017;48(2):259–264.

51. De Vany A. *The New Evolution Diet.* Rodale, New York, 2011.

52. Willcox BJ, Willcox DC, Todoriki H, et al. Caloric restriction, the traditional Okinawan diet, and healthy aging: the diet of the world's longest-lived people and its potential impact on morbidity and life span. *Ann NY Acad Sci.* 2007;1114:434–455.

53. Rosedale R, Westman EC, Konhilas JP. Clinical experience of a diet designed to reduce aging. *J Appl Res* 2009;9:159–165.

54. Kossoff EH, Cervenka MC, Henry BJ, Haney CA, Turner Z. A decade of the modified Atkins diet (2003–2013): results,

insights, and future directions. *Epilepsy Behav* 2013;29:437–442.

55. Banting W. *Letter on Corpulence, Addressed to the Public*, 3rd edn. Harrison, London, 1864.

56. Teicholz N. *The Big Fat Surprise: Why Butter, Meat and Cheese Belong in a Healthy Diet.* Simon & Schuster, New York, 2014.

57. Noakes, T. *Lore of Nutrition: Challenging Conventional Dietary Beliefs.* Penguin, Random House, Cape Town, 2018.

58. Lindbergh S. *Food and Western Disease: Health and Nutrition from an Evolutionary Perspective.* Wiley-Blackwell, Oxford, 2010.

59. Pallister T, Spector TD. Food: a new form of personalized (gut microbiome) medicine for chronic diseases? *JR Soc Med.* 2016;109(9):331–336.

60. Vaynman S, Ying Z, Wu A, Gomez-Pinilla F. Coupling energy metabolism with a mechanism to support brain derived neurotrophic factor mediated synaptic plasticity. *Neuroscience* 2006;139:1221–1234.

61. Nawa H, Carnahan J, Gall C. BDNF protein measured by a novel enzyme immunoassay in normal brain after seizure: partial disagreement with mRNA levels. *Eur J Neurosci* 1995;7:1527–1535.

62. Torres-Aleman I. Insulin-like growth factors as mediators of functional plasticity in the adult brain. *Horm Metab Res* 1999;31:114–119.

63. Johnson-Farley NN, Patel K, Kim D, Cowen DS. Interaction of FGF-2 with IGF-1 and BDNF in stimulating Akt, EFK and neuronal survival in hippocampal cultures. *Brain Res* 2007;1154:40–49.

64. Akbar M, Calderon F, Wen Z, Kim HY. Docosahexaenoic acid: a positive modulator of Akt signaling in neuronal survival. *PNAS* 2005;102:10858–10863.

65. Mattson, MP, Moehl K, Gena N, Schmaedick M, Cheng A. Intermittent metabolic switching, neuroplasticity and brain health. *Nat Rev Neurosci* 2018;19:81–94.

66. Fabrigoule C, Letenneur L, Dartigues JF, et al. Social and leisure activities and risk of dementia: a prospective longitudinal study. *J Am Geriatric Soc* 1995;43:485–490.

67. Wang HX, Karp A, Winblad B, Fratiglioni L. Late-life engagement in social and leisure activities is associated with a decreased risk of dementia: a longitudinal study from the Kungsholmen project. *Am J Epidemiol* 2002;155:1081–1087.

68. Scarmeas N, Levy G, Tang MX, Manly J, Stern Y. Influence of leisure activity on the incidence of Alzheimer's disease. *Neurology* 2001;57:2236–2242.

69. Kellert SR, Wilson EO. *The Biophilia Hypothesis*. Shearwater Book, Washington, DC, 1984.

70. Pergrams ORW, Zaradic PA. Evidence for a fundamental and pervasive shift away from nature-based recreation. *PNAS* 2008;105:2295–2300.

71. Finlayson C. The water optimization hypothesis and the human occupation of the Mid-Latitude Belt in the Pleistocene. *Quat Int* 2013;300:22–31.

72. Nichols WJ. *Blue Mind*. Little Brown & Co., New York, 2014.

73. Immordino-Yang MH, Christodoulou JA, Sing V. Rest is not idleness. *Perspect Psychol Sci* 2012;7:352–364.

74. Van Den Heuvel MP, Stam CJ, Kahn RS, Pol HEH. Efficiency of functional brain networks and intellectual performance. *J Neurosci* 2009;29:7619–7624.

75. Kaplan S. The restorative benefits of nature: toward an integrative framework. *J Environ Psychol* 1995;15:169–182.

76. Atchley RA, Strayer DL, Atchley P. Creativity in the wild: improving creative reasoning through immersion in natural settings. *PLoS One* 2012;7:1–3.

77. Li Q, Otsuka T, Kobayashi M, et al. Acute effects of walking in forest environments on cardiovascular and metabolic parameters. *Eur J Appl Physiol.* 2011;111:2845–2853.

78. Tsunetsugu Y, Miyazaki Y. Measurement of absolute hemoglobin concentrations of prefrontal region by near-infrared time resolved spectroscopy: examples of experiments and prospects. *J Physiol Anthropol Appl Human Sci* 2005;24:469–472.

79. Selhub EM, Long AC. *Your Brain on Nature*. Wiley, Mississauga, 2012.

80. MacKerron G, Mourato S. Happiness is greater in natural environments. *Global Environ Change* 2013;23:992–1000.

81. Li Q, Kobayashi M, Wakayama Y, et al. Effect of phytoncide from trees on human natural killer cell function. *Int J Immunopathol Pharmacol* 2009;22(4):951–959.

82. McConnell AR, Brown CM, Shoda TM, Stayton LE, Martin CE. Friends with benefits: on the positive consequences of pet ownership. *J Pers Soc Psychol* 2011;101:1239–1252.

83. Burton A. Dolphins, dogs, and robot seals for the treatment of neurological disease. *Lancet Neurol* 2013;12:851–852.

84. Bernabei V, De Ronchi D, La Ferla T, et al. Animal-assisted interventions for elderly patients affected by dementia or psychiatric disorders: a review. *J Psychiatr Res* 2013;47:762–773.

85. Shibata T, Wada K. Robot therapy: a new approach for mental healthcare of the elderly – a mini review. *Gerontology* 2013;57:378–386.

86. Rehn T, Handlin L, Uvnäs-Moberg K, Keeling LJ. Dogs' endocrine and behavioral responses at reunion are affected by how the human initiates contact. *Physiol Behav* 2014;124:45–53.

87. Killingsworth MA, Gilbert DT. A wandering mind is an unhappy mind. *Science* 2010;330:932.

88. Teasdale JD, Segal ZV, Williams JM, et al. Prevention of relapse/recurrence of major depression by mindfulness-based cognitive therapy. *J Consult Clin Psychol* 2000;68:615–623.

89. Kabat-Zinn J, Lipworth L, Burney R. The clinical use of mindfulness meditation for the self regulation of chronic pain. *J Behav Med* 1985;8:163–190.

90. Goldin P, Ramel W, Gross J. Mindfulness training and self-referential processing in social anxiety disorder: behavioral and neural effects. *J Cogn Psychother* 2009;23:242–257.

91. Bormann JE, Hurst S, Kelly A. Responses to Mantram Repetition Program from veterans with posttraumatic stress disorder: a qualitative analysis. *J Rehabil Res Dev* 2013;50(6):769–784.

92. Schutte NS, Malouff JM. A meta-analytic review of the effects of mindfulness meditation on telomerase activity. *Psychoneuroendocrinology* 2014;42:45–48.

93. Kang DH, Jo HJ, Jung WH. The effect of meditation on brain structure: cortical thickness mapping and diffusion tensor imaging. *Soc Cogn Affect Neurosci* 2013;8:27–33.

94. Hasenkamp W, Barsalou LW. Effects of meditation experience on functional connectivity of distributed brain networks. *Front Hum Neurosci* 2012;6:38.

95. Holzel BK, Carmody J, Vangel M, et al. Increases in regional brain gray matter density. *Psychiatry Res Neuroimaging* 2011;191:36–43.

96. Holzel BK, Ott U, Hempel H, et al. Differential engagement of anterior cingulate and adjacent medial frontal cortex in adept meditators and non meditators. *Neuroscience Lett* 2007;421:16–21.

97. Luders E, Toga AW, Leore N, Gaser C. The underlying anatomical correlates of long term meditation: larger hippocampal and frontal volume of gray matter. *Neuroimage* 2009;45:672–678.

98. Ryff CD, Singer BH, Dienberg Love, G. Positive health: connecting well being with biology. *Philos Trans R Soc London, Ser B* 2004;359:1383–1394.

99. Lewis GJ, Kanai R, Rees G, Bates TC. Neural correlates of the good life: eudaimonic well being is associated with insular cortex volume. *Scan* 2014;9:615–618.

100. Hwang JP, Lee TW, Tsai SJ, et al. Cortical and subcortical abnormalities in late onset depression with history of suicide attempts investigated with MRI and voxel based morphometry. *J Geriatr Psychiatry Neurol* 2010;23:171–184.

101. Mithen SJ. *The Prehistory of the Mind: A Search for the Origins of Art, Religion, and Science.* Thames and Hudson, London, 1996.

102. Bergman TJ. Speech-like vocalized lip smacking in geladas. *Curr Biol* 2013;23:R268–R269.

103. Freeman W. A neurobiological role for music in social bonding. In: Wallin NL, Merker B, Brown S (eds.), *The Origins of Music.* MIT Press, Cambridge, MA, 2000.

104. Mithen SJ. *The Singing Neanderthals: The Origins of Music, Language, Mind and Body.* Harvard University Press, Cambridge, MA, 2006.

105. Patel AD. Language, music, syntax and the brain. *Nat Neurosci* 2003;6:674–681.

106. Thaut MH, McIntosh GC, Rice RR. Rhythmic facilitation of gait training in hemiparetic stroke rehabilitation. *J Neurol Sci* 1997;151:207–212.

107. Thaut MH, McIntosh KW, McIntosh GC, Hoernberg V. Auditory rhythmicity enhances movement and speech motor control in patients with Parkinson's disease. *Functional Neurol* 2001;16:163–167.

108. Hurst CP, Rice RR, McIntosh GC, Thaut MH. Rhythmic auditory stimulation in gait training for patients with traumatic brain injury. *J Music Ther* 1998;35:228–241.

109. Tomlinson G. *A Million Years of Music: The Emergence of Human Modernity.* Zone Books, New York, 2015.

110. Zatorre RJ, Salimpoor VN. From perception to pleasure: music and its neural substrates. *PNAS* 2013;110:10430–10437.

111. Koelsch S. Brain correlates of music-evoked emotions. *Nat Rev Neurosci* 2014;15:170–180.

112. Barbas H, Bunce JG, Medalla M. Prefrontal pathways that control attention. In: Stuss DT, Knight RT (eds.), *Principles*

of Frontal Lobe Function, 2nd edn. Oxford University Press, Oxford, 2013.

113. Plutchik R. *The Psychology and Biology of Emotion.* Harper Collins, New York, 1994.

114. Juslin PN. What does music express? Basic emotions and beyond. *Front Psychol* 2013:4:596.

115. Koelsch S. Towards a neural basis of music related emotions. *Trends Cogn Sci* 2010;14(3):131–137.

116. George EM, Coch D. Music training and working memory: an ERP study. *Neuropsychologica* 2011;49:1083–1094.

117. Burunat I, Alluri V, Toiviainen P, Numminen J, Brattico E. Dynamics of brain activity underlying working memory for music in a naturalistic condition. *Cortex* 2014;57:254–269.

118. Clark CN, Downey LE, Warren JD. Brain disorders and the biological role of music. *Scan* 2014. doi: 10.1039/scan.

119. Patel AD. The evolutionary biology of musical rhythm: was Darwin wrong? *PLoS Biology* 2014;12:1–5.

120. Salimpoor VN, Benovoy M, Larcher K, Dagher A, Zatorre RJ. Anatomically distinct dopamine release during anticipation and experience of peak emotion to music. *Nat Rev Neurosci* 2011;14(2):257–262.

121. Schlaug G. Musicians and music making as a model for the study of brain plasticity. *Prog Brain Res* 2015;217:37–55. doi: 10.1016/bs.pbr.2014.11.020.

122. Sarkamo T, Tervaniemi M, Soinila S, et al. Amusia and cognitive deficits after stroke: is there a relationship? *Ann NY Acad Sci* 2009;1169:441–445.

123. Boden-Albala B, Litwak E, Elkind MS, Rundek T, Sacco RL. Social isolation and outcomes post stroke. *Neurology* 2005;64:1888–1892.

124. Ikeda A, Iso H, Kawachi I, et al. Social support and stroke and coronary artery disease: the JPHC study cohorts II. *Stroke* 2008;39:768.

125. Spiegel D, Sephton SE. Psychoneuroimmune and endocrine pathways in cancer: effects of stress and support. *Semin Clin Neuropsychiatry* 2001;6:252–265.

126. Strating MMH, Suurmeijer TPBM, Van Schuur WH. Disability, social support and distress in rheumatoid arthritis: results from a thirteen year prospective study. *Arthritis Care Res* 2006;55:736–744.

127. Cohen SD, Sharma T, Acquaviva K, et al. Social support and chronic kidney disease: an update. *Adv Chronic Kidney Dis* 2007;14:335–344.

128. Weil ZM, Normal GJ, Barker JM, et al. Social isolation potentiates cell death and inflammatory responses after global ischemia. *Mol Psychiatry* 2008;13:913–915.

129. Alexander GM, Farris S, Pirone JR, et al. Social and novel contexts modify hippocampal CA2 representations of space. *Nat Commun* 2016;7:10300.

130. Kandel ER. *The Age of Insight.* Random House, New York, 2012.

131. Hitti FL, Siegelman SA. The hippocampal CA2 region is essential for social memory. *Nature* 2014;508:88–92.

132. Karelina K, Stuller KA, Jarrett B, et al. Oxytocin mediates social neuroprotection after cerebral ischemia. *Stroke* 2011;42: 3606–3611.

133. Nowak M. *Super-Cooperators: Altruism, Evolution and Why We Need Each Other to Succeed.* Simon and Schuster, New York, 2011.

134. Hauser OP, Rand DG, Peysakhovich A, Nowak MA. Cooperating with the future. *Nature* 2014;511:220–223.

135. Wuchty S, Jones BF, Uzzi B. The increasing dominance of teams in production of knowledge. *Science* 2007;316(5827):1036–1039.

136. Uzzi B, Dunlap S. How to build your network. *Harv Bus Rev* 2005;83:53–60.

137. Uzzi B. A social network changing statistical properties and the quality of human innovation. *J Phys A: Math Theor* 2008;41:224023.

138. Koscik TR, Tranel D. Brain evolution and human neuropsychology: the inferential brain hypothesis. *J Int Neuropsychol Soc* 2012;18(3):394–401.

139. Grau C, Ginhoux R, Riera A, et al. Conscious brain-to-brain communication in humans using non invasive technologies. *PLoS One* 2014;9:1–6.

140. Pollet T, Robers SG, Dunbar RI. Use of social network sites and instant messaging does not lead to increased offline social network size, or to emotionally closer relationships with offline network members. *Cyberpsychol Behav Soc Netw* 2011;14:253–258.

141. Ekman P. *Emotions Revealed: Recognizing Faces and Feelings to Improve Communication and Emotional Life.* St Martin's Griffin, New York, 2003.

142. Dobson SD. Socioecological correlates of facial mobility in nonhuman anthropoids. *Am J Phys Anthropol* 2009;139:413–420.

143. Von Der Heide R, Skipper LM, Kobusicky E, Olsen IR. Dissecting the uncinate fasciculus: disorders, controversies and a hypothesis. *Brain* 2013;136:1692–1707.

144. Lebel C, Beaulieu C. Longitudinal development of human brain wiring continues from childhood into adulthood. *J Neurosci* 2011;31:10937–10947.

145. Köbe T, Witte AV, Schnelle A, et al. Combined omega-3 fatty acids, aerobic exercise and cognitive stimulation prevents decline in gray matter volume of the frontal, parietal and cingulate cortex in patients with mild cognitive impairment. *Neuroimage* 2016;131:226–238.

146. Podewils LJ, Guallar E, Kuller LH, et al. Physical activity, APOE genotype, and dementia risk: findings from the Cardiovascular Health Cognition Study. *Am J Epidemiol* 2005;161:639–651.

147. Akerlund E, Esbjörnsson E, Sunnerhagen KS, Björkdahl A. Can computerized working memory training improve impaired working memory, cognition and psychological health? *Brain Inj* 2013;27(13–14):1649–1657.

148. Taub E, Uswatte G, Mark VW. The functional significance of cortical reorganization and the parallel development of CI therapy. *Front Hum Neurosci* 2014;8:396.

149. Rojas JCF, Gonzalez-Lima F. Neurological and psychological applications of transcranial lasers and LEDs. *Biochemical Pharmacology* 2013;86:447–457.

150. Edwards CA, Kouzani A, Lee KH, Ross EK. Neurostimulation devices for the treatment of neurologic disorders. *Mayo Clin Proc* 2017;92:1427–1444.

151. Giocomo LM, Hasselmo ME. Neuromodulation by glutamate and acetylcholine can change circuit dynamics by regulating the relative influence of afferent input and excitatory feedback. *Mol Neurobiol* 2007;36(2):184–200.

152. Liu J, Fang J, Wang Z, et al. Transcutaneous vagus nerve stimulation modulates amygdala functional connectivity in patients with depression. *J Affect Disord* 2016;205:319–326.

153. Carreno FR, Frazer A. Vagal nerve stimulation for treatment-resistant depression. *Neurotherapeutics* 2017;14(3):716–727.

154. Sun L, Peräkylä J, Holm K, et al. Vagus nerve stimulation improves working memory performance. *Clin Exp Neuropsychol* 2017;39(10):954–964.

155. Jones KT, Peterson JD, Blacker KJ, Berryhill ME. Frontoparietal neurostimulation modulates working memory training benefits and oscillatory synchronization. *Brain Res* 2017;15;1667:28–40.

156. Fregni F, Pascual-Leone A. Technology insight: noninvasive brain stimulation in neurology – perspectives on the therapeutic potential of rTMS and tDCS. *Nat Clin Pract Neurol* 2007;3:383–393.

157. Bashir S, Mizrahi I, Weaver K, et al. Assessment and modulation of neuroplasticity in rehabilitation with transcranial magnetic stimulation. *PM R.* 2010;2(1202): S253–S268.

158. Fumal A, Laureys S, Di Clemente L, et al. Orbitofrontal cortex involvement in chronic analgesic-overuse headache evolving from episodic migraine. *Brain.* 2006;129:543–550.

159. D'Ostillo K, Thibaut A, Laureys S, et al. Cerebral FDG uptake changes after supraorbital transcutaneous electrical stimulation with the Cefaly® device in patients with migraine. Poster at international headache conference, Valencia, Spain, May 14–17, 2015.

160. Riederer F, Penning S, Schoenen J. Transcutaneous supraorbital nerve stimulation (t-SNS) with the Cefaly device for migraine prevention: a review of the available data. *Pain Ther* 2015;4:135–147.

161. Ramachandran VS, Altschuler EL. The use of visual feedback, in particular mirror visual feedback, in restoring brain function. *Brain* 2009;132;1693–1710.

162. McCabe CS, Haigh RC, Ring EF, et al. A controlled pilot study of the utility of mirror visual feedback in the treatment of complex regional pain syndrome (type 1). *Rheumatology* 2003;42:97–101.

163. Sütbeyaz S, Yavuzer G, Sezer N, Koseoglu BF. Mirror therapy enhances lower-extremity motor recovery and motor functioning after stroke: a randomized controlled trial. *Arch Phys Med Rehabil* 2007;88:555–559.

164. Franceschini M, Agosti M, Cantagallo A, et al. Mirror neurons: action observation treatment as a tool in stroke rehabilitation. *Eur J Phys Rehabil Med* 2010;46:517–523.

165. Sale P, Franceschini M. Action observation and mirror neuron network: a tool for motor stroke rehabilitation. *Eur J Phys Rehabil Med* 2012;48:313–318.

166. Giacino JT, Whyte J, Bagiella E, et al. Placebo-controlled trial of amantadine for severe traumatic brain injury. *N Engl J Med* 2012;366:819–826.

167. Willmott C, Ponsford J. Efficacy of methylphenidate in the rehabilitation of attention following traumatic brain injury: a randomised, crossover, double blind, placebo controlled inpatient trial. *J Neurol Neurosurg Psychiatry* 2009;80:552–557.

168. Huey E, Putnam K, Grafman J. A systematic review of neurotransmitter deficits and treatments in frontotemporal dementia. *Neurology* 2006;66:17–22.

169. Lebert F, Stekke W, Hasenbroek C, Paquir F. Frontotemporal dementia: a randomized controlled trial with trazodone. *Dement Geriatr Cogn Disord* 2004;17:355–359.

170. Chollet F, Tardy J, Albucher JF, et al. Fluoxetine for motor recovery after acute ischemic stroke (FLAME): a randomised placebo-controlled trial. *Lancet Neurol* 2011;10:123–130.

171. Hyman S. DSM IV and V and integration of neuroscience. *Nature Rev Neurosci* 2007;8:725–732.

172. Carlat DJ. *Unhinged: The Trouble with Psychiatry – A Doctor's Revelations about a Profession in Crisis*. Free Press, New York, 2010.

173. Salvucci DD, Taatgen NA. *Multitasking Mind*. Oxford University Press, New York, 2011.

Sense of Self Disorders

Sense of self disorders underlie many important features of human interactions within societies. Such a network is disrupted in many brain disorders, most notably frontotemporal lobe dementias. Many other pathological as well as physiological disorders may fall within the spectrum of altered sense of self, including delusional misidentification disorders, transcendental states, post-stroke anosognosia (denial of illness), and conversion disorders. Criminality in some of these syndromes may not be applicable in the normal sense. Criminal responsibility requires both performing a particular act and knowledge of the quality and nature of the act. The diagnosis and understanding of these syndromes is challenging but important to delineate because of the potential of uncoupling of "the sense of self."

The progressive escalation of our mirror neuron system enhanced our ability to read the minds of others, likened to a kind of "human Wi-Fi" system regarded by some as the "big bang of human evolution" [1,2]. The deficits relating to this expansive circuitry may provide us with critical insights and clues in diagnosis and management of frontal lobe pathologies we encounter today. Field-dependent behaviors (FDBs) are central and an underlying component of many frontal syndromes. FDBs are among the most common frontal lobe syndromes, most often seen in the first few days to weeks after stroke, but may occur with any lesion affecting the frontal and frontal subcortical circuitry [3–5]. A large clinical series reported by the author confirmed these to be among the most common behavioral sequelae after frontal injury and envisaged the underlying pathophysiology as an uncoupling of the mirror neuron system with loss of the inhibitory influence of the inferior orbitofrontal systems [6].

The loss of autonomy from the environment and consequently proneness to environmental stimuli or FDB is thought to be due to a mechanism of circuits being "released" that are normally inhibited by the inferior frontal lobes. A medial frontal, anterior cingulate, and parietal circuitry imbalance has been correlated with the more simple type of imitation behaviors. An orbitofrontal–limbic imbalance has been associated with disinhibitory behavior and dysociality, whereas stereotypical behavior is associated with disruption of the basal nuclei and the prefrontal cortex circuitry [7,8]. Different imitation complexities are subserved by different cerebral networks. From an evolutionary point of view, familiar imitation is mediated by an inferior frontal–posterior parietal–superior temporal circuit, whereas novel imitation is vested in a prefrontal and left posterior cerebellum which interacts with the familiar imitation circuit [9].

Table 11.1 Classification of field-dependent behavior syndromes; elementary and more complex forms

More elementary forms	Imitation behavior – actions spontaneously imitated by the person
	Utilization behavior – compulsive manipulation of objects in the immediate environment
	Echolalia – spontaneously repeating syllables, words, or sentences
More complex forms	Various environmental-dependency syndromes
	Forced hyperphasia – spontaneously calling out by the person of signs and verbiage such as road signs
	Zelig-like syndrome – attempts to appear or behave similar to people around them to foster acceptance
	Echoing approval – simply agreeing or disagreeing during conversation without regard to understanding the question
	Oral spelling behavior – a compulsion to spell out words used during discourse
	Exaggerated startle responses
	Command-automatism and echopraxia to television – the individual responds to commands by television actors or acts as if they are part of the cast
	Forced collectionism
	Echoplasia – an involuntary tracing or copying of the outlines or contours of objects or persons
	Excessive television watching
	Response to next-patient stimulation – speaking for a person, lying next to them in hospital, when questioned by medical personal, for example
	Hypermetamorphosis – marked tendency to attend and react to all visual stimuli
	Obsessive compulsive disorder and Tourette's syndrome

Source: adapted from [6] with permission of Taylor & Francis Ltd, www.tandfonline.com

The diagnosis of FDB is particularly important as the impaired personal autonomy in a person with otherwise relatively intact cognitive functioning and actively employed, as is often the case, may have dire consequences. The importance of Lhermitte's studies of the various FDBs was the realization that these various imitation behaviours constituted the earliest manifestations of signs associated with the various frontal pathologies [3]. As noted in Chapter 5, FDBs may involve several different frontal regions and the clinical manifestations may be of a more elementary or more complex nature (Table 11.1).

Closely tied to losing one's autonomy from the environment due to a disruption of the mirror neuron circuitry is the concept of free will. Such persons are no longer able to regulate the "automatic" responses to either external or internal stimuli. These may take the form of mimicking behaviors and speech of others, eating what others are eating, or imitating the accents of another's accent or culture. Various sociopathies may arise as the normal internal stimuli of anger may transform into rage attacks, violent outbursts, sexual drives, or lead to inappropriate remarks and actions toward others, and addictions, such as to pornography. The normal internal drive and need to urinate may precipitate this to occur in public places, with little or no concern for who may be in the immediate vicinity. Hunger pangs may trigger an immediate ingestion of food. The latter may be particularly disruptive when such persons eat off another person's plate of food, consume huge portion sizes, or have a stereotypy of food preferences – often sweet items such as ice creams which may be ingested in copious amounts.

Inappropriate behavior now becomes more understandable as the sight of something may elicit almost automatic, unchecked responses. A marked frontal dissonance of behaviors versus relatively intact cognition is common, with profound implications for diagnostic delays and perplexing to the patient's families. Disconcerting statements such as "driving through a red light is unlawful, but I may do so" may not be uncommon. Within the author's registry, another unusual admonition by a person as their primary presenting problem was "I live in squalor." This was described as allowing the dirty dishes to pile up in the kitchen for long periods of time, not picking up the dog's excrement in the house, and allowing many bags of refuse to accumulate in the house. In contradistinction to this behavioral "squalor syndrome," screening neuropsychological testing was normal in this person and a frontotemporal lobe syndrome secondary to traumatic brain injury (TBI) was etiologically relevant. The right orbitofrontal cortex in particular is associated with handling appropriate inhibitory responses. When affected by degenerative processes, including the loss of VEN cells, excessive drinking, not always of alcohol but also of water resulting in polydipsia, excessive eating, smoking, becoming a spendthrift, becoming sexually indiscriminate, and gambling tendencies may all manifest. The right anterior temporal lobe has a close association with the right inferior frontal lobe through the uncinate fasciculus. When affected by the behavioral variant of FTD, for example, loss of empathy may ensue with the disturbing behavioral consequences of the patient showing little or no concern for a spouse or loved one when in pain, suffering injury, or even terminally ill. Right amygdala involvement may present with even more startling behaviors, such as losing fear of threatening individuals, wild animals, and snakes. Interoceptive information from the body, including the central pain-processing circuitry – which includes the medial anterior PFC and predominantly the right anterior insula – may also be affected. This causes incongruent responses to their own pain as well as the pain others may portray. Such people may be oblivious to their own injuries and have a marked stifling of their pain, as portrayed in the movie *Concussion*, based on the true story of a football player who engaged in many years of self-mutilation, including pulling his own teeth, prior to committing suicide [10].

Criminalization in the context of frontotemporal syndromes has been reported in up to 25 percent of cases [11]. A notable case presentation to the author was that of a middle-aged man with a five-year college education presenting with a seizure that was subsequently attributed to a right frontal lobe arteriovenous malformation. Within four months post-removal by craniotomy, the family noted altered personality traits, behavioral changes, and many instances of social ineptitude, including public indecency for which he was incarcerated. Neuropsychological testing (NPT) was performed at the request of his attorney, concerned about the possibility of so-called organic brain disease. NPT was within the normal range save for mild executive impairment, with a number of domains in the superior range. Subsequent behavioral neurological testing delineated profound abnormalities with a diagnosis of frontotemporal lobe syndrome made according to the criteria of the Rascovsky et al., Frontal Behavioral Inventory (FBI), and Frontal Systems Behavior Examination (FRSBE). The markedly abnormal FBI and FRSBE scores were corroborated by neuroimaging evidence of a large, right inferior frontal encephalomalacea related to the arteriovenous malformation and its surgical removal (Figure 11.1). He was released from incarceration on the basis of loss of sense of

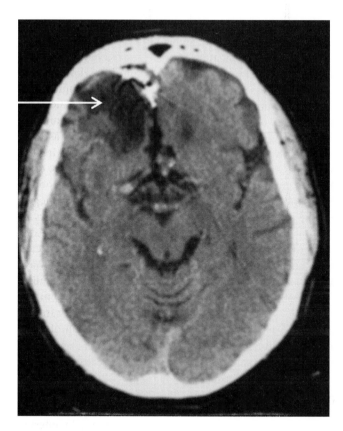

Figure 11.1 MRI brain scan of right frontal encephalomalacea (arrow) post arteriovenous malformation surgery with normal to above-average neuropsychological scores but with profound behavioral abnormalities including disinhibition and social and emotional dysregulation.

self relating to his frontotemporal lobe syndrome, buttressed by a comprehensive treatment plan, cognitive rehabilitation, and appropriate monitoring. There may be a marked cognitive and behavioral neurological dissonance with frontal lobe lesions that may lead to overlooking organic brain disease and may be associated with varying degrees of disorders of loss of sense of self. The emergence of criminal behavior in adults with an otherwise respectable past should prompt the consideration of frontotemporal lobe syndromes, as such behavior may be the initial or earliest sign of the disorder. People so affected may also require different legal processing rather than the standard US legal "insanity defense" [12].

Pertinent Evolutionary Aspects

One of the defining features of human evolution included a tripling of brain volume compared to extant apes. This was tempered only by the concomitant adoption of bipedalism, with the obligatory narrowing of the pelvis forcing a limitation on the passage of the larger head during birth. Several million years later, the surge in connectivity that enabled culture and language occurred, with the three most proximate precipitating factors including frugivory, socialization, and the aqua–arboreal phase of marine and lacustrine seafood/shellfish consumption. The latter occurred more than once in our evolution, with one of the phases about 8 mya, shortly after the "planet of the apes" phase and most recently during the Marine Isotope stage 6, about 180 kya in southern Africa. Socialization first became important with the ancestral primate lineage and evolved further, after which elaboration in episodic memory, autononetic memory, and prospective memory followed. That social brain processes, such as interpersonal skills, relations, and empathy can become disentangled and uncoupled is not surprising – hence the concept of loss of sense of self disorders or sense of agency (SOA) disorders.

Although the frontal lobes had acquired their present modern configuration and size by ~300 kya, the parietal lobes only acquired modern human dimensions during the last ~150 kya. The precuneal component of the parietal lobes, in particular, is of key importance in our super-connectivity. This has been associated with the understanding of the self in relation to others and the world around us, as well as being implicated in mental imagery and simulation. Together with the precuneus, the intraparietal sulcus and frontoparietal networks integrate visuospatial functions, memory, and self-awareness. The precuneus is a major hub of the default mode network, in addition to its key role in visuospatial and other more recent human cognitive specializations [13]. Neurophysiological correlates of the precuneus and its circuitry include processing of self-awareness, and episodic memory as well as consciousness [14]. From a neurobiological point of view, the key neural correlates of loss of sense of self lie in the connectivity between prefrontal regions that initiate action and the parietal regions that mediate the monitoring of perceived events [15]. The insula also has an important role in social emotions and empathy, as a role of the sentient self, as well as being the most common anatomical site of injury related to Takotsubo cardiomyopathy. Neurocardiological sequelae after stroke or TBI, usually to the right insula, may cause cardiac damage or milder reversible sequelae such as recoverable damage or stress cardiomyopathy [16]. A working clinical classification of loss of sense disorders is as follows:

1. Physiological and reversible altered sense of self manifestations:
   - migraine related out-of-body experiences (autoscopy)
   - transcendental meditation and paranormal experiences
   - sleep-related automatisms (sleepwalking, REM sleep behavior disorders).

2. Frontal hub lesions and decreased activity:
   - frontotemporal lobe syndromes and loss of sense of agency
   - frontotemporal lobe dementias (FTDs) and loss of sense of agency.

3. Decreased sense of self and precuneus hub lesions:
   - minimally conscious state
   - vegetative state.

4. Partial decreased sense of self disorders:
   - anosognosia and related syndromes
   - xenomelia (body integrity identity disorder)
   - phantom limb syndromes.

5. Altered (diaschisis)
   - delusional misidentification syndromes or content-specific delusions
   - out-of-body experiences (autoscopy), post-stroke, hypoxic, or cardiac arrest
   - alien hand syndrome
   - hysteria and so-called functional disorders.

6. Increased (diaschisis)

    • FTD, subtype of primary semantic aphasia variant and augmented right hemisphere function such as emergence of visual art aptitude and creativity

    • Geschwind-Gastaut syndrome (interpersonal viscosity, loquacity, hypergraphia, hyposexuality)

    • savant syndromes.

Self-control of personality and behavior may be mediated by the neural circuitry within the dorsal frontomedial cortex and anterior insula [17]. On the other hand, circuitry involved in the generation of intentional actions includes the cingulate motor area, supplementary motor area (SMA) and pre-SMA [18,19]. Electrophysiologically, the readiness potential (Bereitschaftspotential) in the SMA of the frontal lobe precedes movement by about one second [20]. Inhibition of endogenously generated intentional actions has been shown by fMRI studies to involve a network of dorsomedial frontal area (BA 9) and the anterior insula. This may be the neural substrate of inhibiting intentions or a veto process, but raises the possibility of initiation of inhibition having a non-conscious component, in the same way that the initiation of action has a non-conscious component. Identifying the neural processes of free will and those that veto such a function are of fundamental importance to society and ethical reflections, with profound legal ramifications [21,22].

Physiological states include a range of de-realization phenomena reported by migraineurs, including autoscopic experiences that are transient and reversible. We have already examined the capricious nature of neurotransmitter system impacts on the prefrontal cortex, which fluctuate with normal physiological stimuli. Rational choice may be heavily influenced by hormonal levels and fluctuations in these levels may have significant neuro-economical consequences. Coates and Herbert cite the responses of City of London male traders and their cognitive and behavioral influenced decisions related to cortisol and testosterone fluctuations, which may influence the rationality of stock market transactions. Elevated testosterone correlated with profitability, economic return, and a tendency to inflate the markets upward, and was associated with increased risk taking. Cortisol, on the other hand, was elevated with risk aversion and market plunges, and amplified when a market was down-trending [23].

Robert Lustig's impactful disquisition on our susceptibility to our biochemical endowment has perhaps the most profound lessons of all for us [24]. He cogently elucidates how the three areas of the brain that generate all emotions – the reward pathway or what feels good mediated by dopamine (in turn releasing endogenous opioids), the contentment pathway mediated by serotonin, and the stress, fear, and memory pathway – are prone to manipulation that may frequently be subliminal. For example, many different signals generate reward (dopamine), including gambling, excessive internet use, positions of power, shopping, erotic pursuits, alcohol, and processed foods, most notably sugar. An excess of dopamine leads to addiction.

Hedonic substances used to be rare and hard to come by. With respect to our current-day addiction to sugar, this represents an evolutionary relic from our frugivorous primate past with our major sustenance being fruit containing sugar and sometimes alcohol when overripe. Nowadays, processed food, the majority of it containing excess sugar, together with technology use, leads to addictions to these, with impaired sleep and metabolic syndromes and depression. The serotonergic pathway associated with contentment and happiness is dependent on dietary tryptophan intake (an essential amino acid) found in eggs, poultry, fish, spinach, and walnuts – and not in fast foods or processed foods. Hence, perhaps unwittingly we have succumbed to a form of dysevolution. "We spend money on hedonic pleasures, trying to make ourselves happy and in the process drive dopamine, reduce dopamine receptors, increase cortisol and reduce serotonin to ever further distance ourselves from our goal. The cognitive dissonance between our expectations and our reality is deafening." Lustig goes on to detail how the processed food industry – which is worth $1.46 trillion (compared with alcohol at $308 billion and the gaming industry at $92 billion) – exploits sugar in particular, the most easily obtained hedonic substance, leading to about 50 percent of the US population having some form of chronic metabolic disease (heart disease, diabetes, obesity, cancer). About half of our sugar intake is found in regular foods from which we unwittingly consume excess sugar. He goes on to state: "We are our biochemistry, whether we like it or not. And our biochemistry can be manipulated, sometimes naturally and sometimes artificially, sometimes by ourselves and sometimes by others, sometimes for good and sometimes for ill." The price tag is staggering, with the US health system having a budget of $3.2 trillion, and 75 percent of usage being related to chronic metabolic disease, 75 percent of which is preventable. This translates into the wasting of $1.8 trillion on preventable health problems [25]. Lustig's proposal for averting our chronic illness, depression, addiction, unhappiness, and potential national bankruptcy are summarized in his 4 Cs of contentment: connect, contribute, cope, cook [24]. Not surprisingly, there is extensive overlap with the five brain fitness rules elaborated in Chapter 10 and summarized in the online resource available at www.cambridge.org/execmind.

Perhaps the most dramatic examples of loss of sense of self are those conditions in which only wakefulness is evident, but the response from the person is either absent or marginal. Persistent vegetative state (PVS) refers to a syndrome of disconnection of different cortical networks. Clinical recovery into a minimally conscious state (MCS) or full consciousness has been seen with functional restoration of the corticothalamocortical connections. Both PVS and MCS are characterized by wakefulness with either no response to environmental stimuli (PVS) or a partial response (MCS). Precuneal hypoactivity has also been correlated with recovery. In Adrian Owen's famous demonstration of a woman in an MCS being requested to imagine playing tennis or walking about her house, the same circuit activation was present as in normal people. Moreover, with recovery from MCS, precuneal metabolism normalized [26]. Anecdotal, albeit transient, recovery has been reported with pharmacological agents, including amantadine, zolpidem, and baclofen, which include both central nervous stimulants and depressants [27].

Many different partial examples of loss of sense of self disorders are known. The anosognosia (Greek, *nosos* meaning disease and *gnosis* meaning knowledge) group of disorders present quite commonly after right hemisphere damage, usually stroke-related, during which a denial of illness or deficit of hemiplegia may be expressed. This may be either partial, with underestimation of deficit, or an emphatic denial of any weakness at all. Many variations may accompany anosognosia and include allied conditions such as somatoparaphrenia in which, aside from denial of weakness, some attribute the affected limb or limbs to another person [28–30]. Another variation is anosodiaphoria, in which an indifference or strange lack of concern for the paretic arm or leg is noted, sometimes also called insouciance, of French origin. Yet another variant, asomatognosia, refers to a denial of ownership of the, usually left, arm; less often this affects the left leg [31,32].

Perhaps the most dramatic is xenomelia, whereby an expressed desire is made for amputation of the healthy left arm or leg by a person with right superior parietal impairment or lesion. The right superior parietal lobe is responsible for integrating the multimodal sensory inputs for the creation of body image. Hypothetically it is presumed that the tactile information of the arm remains but fails to be incorporated into the composite body image, leading to the desire for amputation [33]. Other terms or similar syndromes include apotemnophilia and body integration disorder.

Conversion Disorders and Hysteria

The neurobiology of conversion paresis or disorder is emerging and understanding is growing. Hypoactivity of the right temporoparietal junction (TPJ) has also been reported in conversion disorder. Other functional imaging findings have included hypoactivity of the precuneus in the medial parietal lobe and increased activity of the lateral parietal supramarginal gyrus and SMA for the organization of motor control [34]. Both a ventrolateral PFC activity increase – that may be related to input from the amygdala – and a right frontal activation with inhibition of the sensorimotor circuitry have been recorded [35]. This has led to a hypothesis that motor conversion disorder may be viewed as abnormal activation of amygdala activity (stress, threats, adverse experience-related) with downstream influences on the SMA region where motor movement plans and their initiation take place, and a non-conscious response inhibition [36,37].

Delusional Misidentification Syndromes (DMIS)

These syndromes are also referred to as content-specific delusion syndromes and relate to situations in which the person may incorrectly identify a person either as familiar or as a stranger, or incorrectly state their location (such as saying they are at home when in fact they are in hospital). More than a dozen different DMIS have been identified. These include the following:

- Capgras syndrome: the belief that a familiar individual, or even the individual themselves, has been replaced by an imposter (hypoidentification).
- Fregoli's syndrome: a person, familiar to the person in question, is regarded as impersonating and in so doing is presenting themselves as a stranger (hyperidentification).
- Intermetamorphosis: two people, both of whom are known to the person in question, have interchanged their identities
- Reduplicative paramnesias: chimeric type – the claim of being in one's private home while actually lying in hospital.
- Extravagant spatial localization: the individual claims to be in a place other than the location at time of interview.
- Place reduplication: the belief that there are two identical places of the same name but in geographically different regions.
- De Clerambault's syndrome: a belief by the person of being loved by an individual of higher socioeconomic status.
- Doppelgänger syndrome: the person believes they have a twin or duplicate.
- Othello syndrome: the mistaken belief that their spouse is engaging in unfaithful pursuits.

- Ekbom syndrome (parasitosis): the belief of being infested by insects.
- Cotard's syndrome: the belief that one is demised.
- Dorian Gray syndrome: the belief of being immune to aging.
- Lycanthropy: a belief of being periodically transformed into an animal, usually a wolf.

Most of these syndromes occur in association with stroke, TBI, schizophrenia, and dementia, and the responsible lesion is usually a right frontal lesion, although subcortical lesions such as right caudate nucleus have been implicated [38–41].

Recent advances in understanding the pathophysiology were reported by Darby et al. using lesion network mapping techniques. Their group showed that a single lesion can lead to complex symptoms, signs, and syndromes based on the lesion location within the connectome. Both right frontal and the retrosplenial cortex were functionally connected in all the cases studied, causing the various delusional misidentifications [42].

Alien Hand Syndromes

Disinhibitory control syndromes may take the form of some unusual presentations, such as the alien hand or anarchic hand syndromes. With such syndromes, either the hand or arm behaves autonomously. This may take the form of inadvertently hitting the bed partner while recumbent or inadvertently grabbing objects. With the latter example, one hand can be seen to interfere with the function of the other hand while performing a task, by making opposing movements. A fork laden with food on its way to the person's mouth may suddenly be interrupted and grabbed by the other hand, for example. These are not voluntary actions and are non-conscious. Several alien hand subtypes have been identified, including frontal, parietal, corpus callosal, and ictal.

The frontal variant alien hand syndromes involve grasping or reaching actions, and difficulty with releasing a grasp. The posterior parietal syndromes present with an incoordinate withdrawal from contact (parietal avoidance syndrome) that may be the opposite to the grasping action typical of the frontal variant. With the corpus callosal type, an inter-manual conflict between the two hands of the person may be observed, with the two hands performing approximately opposite actions (also termed diagnostic ideomotor apraxia). The ictal alien hand presentation occurs only during seizural activity. From the pathophysiological point of view, a primary motor cortex isolation from the premotor area has been inferred from fMRI studies [43–46].

Hodological Syndromes of Hyperfunction with Improved Behaviors, Skills, and Aptitudes

Brain lesions may present with syndromes related to hypo- or hyperfunction of the area involved or the brain circuitry affected, as well as hypo- or hyperfunction of remotely connected (diaschisis) regions. This is the nature of brain connectomics. Proposed explanatory hypotheses include Kapur's paradoxical functional facilitation in which one brain region reverses inhibition in another region or regions, with compensatory amplification of function with augmentation in specific brain functions [47]. A number of well-published examples are discussed below.

Visual artistic aptitude ability may emerge in association with neurodegenerative processes often affecting the left temporal lobe. Examples include frontotemporal lobe disorders presenting with semantic or logopenic aphasia syndromes, the primary progressive aphasia syndromes with Alzheimer's disease, as well as other conditions such as post-stroke lesions, Parkinson's, migraine, and epileptic syndromes [48]. Emergent literary artistic prowess has been described after impairment involving the right temporal lobe [49]. Visuospatial creativity syndromes have also been described, such as an acquired architectural brilliance also described with FTD syndromes [50].

At times both improved emotional interaction, increased empathy, and an increase in humor may occur, particularly after right frontal lesion, often stroke-related [51]. Although loss of empathy is relatively common, occurring particularly with FTD, the opposite syndrome, one of hyperempathy, was reported in a patient after elective right amygdalohippocampectomy for treatment-resistant epilepsy [52]. Dreaming has already been noted to be a critical brain function for emotional regulation and enhancing interpersonal skills and societal understanding. The widespread network involved includes profound visual imagery in most dreams, the latter of which can be lost as a result of brain lesions [53].

The delusional misidentification syndromes as already mentioned are encountered primarily with right frontal lesions, but are best explained by the connectomal diaschisis [54]. Savant syndromes may emerge or become apparent after brain lesions, often involving the left hemisphere. A number of more common prodigious abilities are consistently encountered in such instances, including proficiency in visuospatial skills, mathematics, calendar counting, music, and art. In addition, less common abilities may be encountered, including synesthesia, hyperlexia, language (polyglots), adeptness in navigation and statistical skills, as well as proficiency with respect to vision, smell, and time appreciation. Hence the syndrome presentations of savant people may take the form of acquired, prodigious, sudden, splinter, or talented subtypes [55].

Both the Geschwind-Gastaut syndrome (GGS) and Klüver–Bücy syndrome are manifestations of FTDs. GGS features include a viscous personality, metaphysical preoccupations, hypergraphia, hyperlexia, loquacity, hyperreligiosity (increased intensity and increased alternative religious exploration), and altered physiological parameters. The viscous personality in particular is regarded as the principal component of GGS and includes circumstantiality of their communication and an over-inclusive verbosity during interpersonal discussions. An unusual excess of detailed information is characteristic as well as "interpersonal adhesiveness" leading to a prolongation of interpersonal encounters [56–59].

The hypergraphia can present with excessive writing, painting, or drawing. The metaphysical preoccupations present with relatively sudden intense intellectual, philosophical, moral, and religious interests. The latter can take the form of increased intensity and increased alternative religious exploration. Physiological alterations include mostly hyposexuality, as well as changes related to aggression and fear. Although regarded as uncommon, it may be more frequent but the components and synthesis into the syndrome may present difficulties. To date the best semi-quantitative assessment tool is the Bear Fedio Inventory [60].

With regard to the legal implications of loss of sense of self disorders, these have largely followed the English M'Naghten's Case of 1843 that relates to a presumed mentally disordered defendant. The accused may accordingly be judged "not guilty by reason of insanity" or at times "guilty but insane." The sentence may consequently be confinement and treatment within a secure hospital facility or some other punitive measures. This insanity defense system is followed in most English-speaking countries, including the USA, although not all states do so [61]. As far as treatment is concerned, there is increasing evidence for neurostimulation and hypnosis-related therapy methods, as discussed in Chapter 10.

References

1. Arbib M. From mirror neurons to complex imitation in the evolution of language and tool use. *Ann Rev Anthropol* 2011;40:257–273.

2. Ramachandran VS. *The Tell-Tale Brain*. W.W. Norton, New York, 2011.

3. Lhermitte F, Pillon B, Seradura M. Human autonomy and the frontal lobes. Part 1: imitation and utilization behavior – a neuropsychological study of 75 patients. *Ann Neurol* 1986;19:326–334.

4. De Renzi E, Cavalleri F, Facchini S. Imitation and utilization behavior. *J Neurol Neurosurg Psychiatry* 1996;61:396–400.

5. Besnard J, Allain P, Aubin G, et al. A contribution to the study of environmental dependency phenomena: the social hypothesis. *Neuropsychologia* 2011;49:3279–3294.

6. Hoffmann M. The panoply of field dependent behavior in 1436 stroke patients: the mirror neuron system uncoupled and the consequences of loss of personal autonomy. *Neurocase* 2014;20(5):556–568.

7. Bien N, Roebuck A, Goebel R, Sack AT. The brain's intention to imitate: the neurobiology of intentional versus automatic imitation. *Cerebral Cortex* 2009;19:2338–2351.

8. Rizzolatti G, Fabbri Destro M, Cattaneo L. Mirror neurons and their clinical relevance. *Nat Clin Pract Neurol* 2009;5:24–34.

9. Subiaul F. Mosaic cognitive evolution: the case of imitation learning. In: Broadfield D, Yuan M, Schick K, Toth N (eds.) *The Human Brain Evolving*. Stone Age Institute Press, Gosport, IN, 2010.

10. *Concussion,* 2015, Columbia Pictures, Director Peter Landesman.

11. Liljegren M, Naasan G, Temlett J, et al. Criminal behavior in frontotemporal lobe dementia and Alzheimer disease. *JAMA Neurol* 2015;72(3):295–300.

12. Diehl-Schmid J, Perneczky R, Koch J, Nedopil N, Kurz A. Guilty by suspicion? Criminal behavior in frontotemporal lobar degeneration. *Cogn Behav Neurol* 2013;26(2):73–77.

13. Bruner E, Preuss TM, Chen X, Rilling JK. Evidence for expansion of the precuneus in human evolution. *Brain Struct Funct* 2017;222(2):1053–1060.

14. Cavanna AE, Trimble MR. The precuneus: a review of its functional anatomy and behavioral correlates. *Brain* 2006;129:S64–S83.

15. Haggard P. Sense of agency in the human brain. *Nat Rev Neurosci* 2017;18:197–208.

16. Chen Z, Venkar P, Seyfried D, et al. Brain–heart interaction: cardiac complications after stroke. *Circ Res* 2017;121(4):451–468.

17. Northoff G, Bermpohl F. Cortical midline structures and the self. *Trends Cogn Sci* 2004;8:102–107.

18. Ball T, Schreiber A, Feige B, et al. The role of higher-order motor areas in voluntary movement as revealed by high-resolution EEG and fMRI. *NeuroImage* 1999;10:682–694.

19. Nachev P, Rees G, Parton A, et al. Volition and conflict in human medial frontal cortex. *Curr Biol* 2005;15:122–128.

20. Shibasaki H, Hallett M. What is the Bereitschaftspotential? *Clin Neurophysiol* 2006;117:2341–2356.

21. Brass M, Haggard P. To do or not to do: the neural signature of self-control. *J Neurosci* 2007;27(34):9141–9145.

22. Libet B, Gleason CA, Wright EW, Pearl DK. Time of conscious intention to act in relation to onset of cerebral activity

(readiness-potential): the unconscious initiation of a freely voluntary act. *Brain* 1983;106:623–642.

23. Coates JM, Herbert J. Endogenous steroids and financial risk taking on a London trading floor. *PNAS* 2008;105:6167–6172.

24. Lusting RH. *The Hacking of the American Mind: The Science behind the Corporate Takeover of our Bodies and Brains.* Avery, New York, 2017.

25. Centers for Medicare and Medicaid Services 2015–2025 Projections of National Health Care Expenditures Data, July 13, 2016 www.coms.gov/newsroom/mediareleasedatabase/press-releases/2016.

26. Owen AM, Coleman MR, Boly M, et al. Detecting awareness in the vegetative state. *Science* 2006;313:1402.

27. Pistoia F, Mura E, Govoni S, Fini M, Sarà M. Awakenings and awareness recovery in disorders of consciousness: is there a role for drugs? *CNS Drugs* 2010;24(8):625–638.

28. Paulig M, Weber M, Garbelotto S. Somatoparaphrenia: a positive variant of anosognosia for hemiplegia. *Nervenarzt* 2000;71(2):123–129.

29. Appelros P, Karlsson GM, Seiger A, Nydevik I. Neglect and anosognosia after first-ever stroke: incidence and relationship to disability. *J Rehabil Med* 2002;34:215–222.

30. Critchley M. *The Parietal Lobes.* Hafner Press, London, 1953.

31. Critchley M. Personification of paralyzed limbs in hemiplegics. *BMJ* 1955;2(4934):284–286.

32. Critchley M. Misoplegia, or hatred of hemiplegia. *Mt Sinai J Med* 1974;41:82–87.

33. McGeoch PD, Brang, D, Song T, et al. Xenomelia: a new right parietal lobe syndrome. *J Neurol Neurosurg Psychiatry* 2011;82:1314–1319.

34. Van Beilen M, de Jong BM, Gieteling EW, Renken R, Leenders KL. Abnormal parietal function in conversion paresis. *PLoS One* 2011;6(10):e25918.

35. Voon V, Gallea C, Hattori N, et al. The involuntary nature of conversion disorder. *Neurology* 2010;74:223–228.

36. Cojan Y, Waber L, Carruzzo A, Vuilleumier P. Motor inhibition in hysterical conversion paralysis. *Neuroimage* 2009;47(3):1026–1037.

37. Voon V, Brezing C, Gallea C, et al. Emotional stimuli and motor conversion disorder. *Brain* 2010:133;1526–1536.

38. Devinsky O. Delusional misidentifications and duplications: right brain lesions, left brain delusions. *Neurology* 2009;72:80–87.

39. Larner AJ. Delusion of pregnancy in frontotemporal lobar degeneration with motor neurone diseases. *Behav Neurol* 2008;19:199–200.

40. Forstl H, Almeida OP, Owen AM, Burns A, Howard R. Psychiatric, neurological and medical aspects of misidentification syndromes: a review of 260 cases. *Psychol Med* 1991;21(4):905–910.

41. Feinberg TE, Roane DM. Misidentification syndromes. In: Feinberg TE, Farah MJH (eds.), *Behavioral Neurology and Neuropsychology.* McGraw Hill, New York, 1997.

42. Darby RR, Laganiere S, Pascual-Leone A, Prasad S, Fox MD. Finding the imposter: brain connectivity of lesions causing delusional misidentifications. *Brain* 2017;140:497–507.

43. Denny-Brown D. The nature of apraxia. *J Nerv Ment Dis* 1958;126:9–32.

44. Graff-Radford J, Rubin MN, Jones DT, et al. The alien limb phenomenon. *J Neurol* 2013;260(7):1880–1888.

45. Scepkowski LA, Cronin-Golomb A. The alien hand: cases, categorizations, and anatomical correlates. *Behav Cogn Neurosci Rev* 2003;2(4):261–277.

46. Carrazana E, Rey G, Rivas-Vazquez R, Tatum W. "Ictal" alien hand syndrome. *Epilepsy Behav* 2001;2(1):61–64.

47. Kapur N. Paradoxical functional facilitation in brain behavior research: a critical review. *Brain* 1996;119:1775–1790.

48. Schott GD. Pictures as a neurological tool: lessons from enhanced and

emergent artistry in brain disease. *Brain* 2012;135:1947–1963.

49. Miller B. *The Frontotemporal Lobe Dementias.* Oxford University Press, New York, 2013.

50. Förstl H, Immler G, Seitz M, Hacker R. Ludwig II, King of Bavaria: a royal medical history. *Acta Psychiatr Scand* 2008;118(6):499–502.

51. Pell MD. Judging emotion and attitudes from prosody following brain damage. *Prog Brain Res* 2006;156:303–317.

52. Richard-Mornas A, Mazzietti A, Koenig O, et al. Emergence of hyper empathy after right amygdalohippocampectomy. *Neurocase* 2013. doi: 10.1080/13554794.2013.826695.

53. Peña-Casanova J, Roig-Rovira T, Bermudez A, Tolosa-Sarro E. Optic aphasia, optic apraxia and loss of dreaming. *Brain Lang* 1985;26:63–71.

54. Christodoulou GN, Magariti M, Kontaxakis VP, Christodoulou NG. The delusion misidentification syndromes: strange, fascinating and instructive. *Curr Psychiatry Rep* 2009;11:185–189.

55. Treffert DA. *Islands of Genius.* Jessica Kingsley Publishers, London, 2010.

56. Gastaut H. Etude electroclinique des episodes psychotiques survenanten dehors des crises cliniques chez les epileptiques. *Rev Neurol* 1956;94:587–594.

57. Waxman SG, Geschwind N. Hypergraphia in temporal lobe epilepsy. *Neurology* 1974;24:629–636.

58. Trimble M, Mendez MF, Cummings JL. Neuropsychiatric symptoms from the temporolimbic lobes. *J Neuropsychiatry Clin Neurosci* 1997;9:429–438.

59. Trimble M, Freeman A. An investigation of religiosity and the Geschwind Gastaut syndrome in patients with temporal lobe epilepsy. *Epilepsy Behav* 2006;9:407–414.

60. Bear DM, Fedio P. Quantitative analysis of interictal behavior in temporal lobe epilepsy. *Arch Neurol* 1977;34:454.

61. United Kingdom House of Lords Decisions. "Daniel M'Nagthen's case. May 26, June 19, 1843." British and Irish Legal Information Institute.

Chapter 12

Implications for You and Society

As humans we have a fervent desire to acquire knowledge that is hedonically linked, underscoring the importance from an evolutionary point of view. However, knowledge acquisition and its assimilation to our current erudition is a time-consuming process. Our brains "light-up" when we seek knowledge. The acquisition of information has been a major focus in human evolution, a process that in various disciplines may span many decades. The mean age of Nobel prize winners in chemistry, physiology, and physics is 71. What may be the implications of how and when to retire?

Where Have our Brains Come from and Where Are We Going?

The geophysical, climatological, and astrophysical events explored in the introductory chapters forged our bodies and brains, which consequently became attuned to the basic rhythms of life. In response to light, the suprachiasmatic nucleus (SCN) in the hypothalamus, the central pacemaker, keeps 24-hour time and tracks seasonal time. Linked to the SCN are multiple peripheral body clocks, expressing a network of clock genes that influence sleep, metabolism, and the immune system. With about 10 percent of the cellular genome concerned with circadian oscillation rhythms, the SCN and peripheral tissue body clocks influence molecular networks through transcriptional factors that act as epigenetic modifiers, which can influence memory and cognition. Light exposure variances are risk factors for cardiovascular disease, metabolic diseases, and depression [1,2]. The legacy we have inherited and that we have to abide by is to keep our 1.5 kg brain, comprising 100 billion neurons, one trillion glial cells, 700 km of blood vessels, and 150 000 km of fibers, functioning in peak condition. Brain fitness and maintenance rules, discussed in detail in Chapter 10, represent the best and most effective methods we have. What of our further cognitive development, given that we are living longer and increasingly emphasizing protracted intellectual pursuits? Some clues may come from our brain development thus far.

Our perceptual processing was primarily chemosensory during early mammalian evolution, then visually predominant during the primate era, and now the socially challenging polyadic ambiguities place a premium on our cognitive computations. This has led to a more deductive type of processing and extrapolations from environmental and conspecific (other members of a species) information, as conceptualized in Koscik and Tranel's Inferential Brain Hypothesis [3] and Subiaul's Reinterpretation Hypothesis [4]. The frontotemporal connections from the ventromedial and orbitofrontal PFC to the amygdala, anterior and lateral temporal lobes expanded as evidenced by comparative neuroanatomy of the uncinate fasciculus [5]. Beyond the brain's intra-connectivity, our brain's circuitry has extended beyond our skulls, as encapsulated in Malafouris's Blind Man's Stick Hypothesis and material engagement theory. He envisaged a two-way brain–environment interaction of materials and objects, with both the brain and the environment exerting plasticity effects on each other, likened to a type of cognitive scaffold, cognitive prostheses, or metaplasticity [6,7]. The understanding of such mechanisms is helpful for gaining insights for potential treatment. Overall cognitive performance correlates with the efficiency of our cerebral networks, in particular the default mode network [8]. The integrity of our networks can be maintained and even improved by abiding by the brain health edicts depicted in Chapter 10. Monitoring and measurement of these networks can be performed by resting-state network evaluations by fMRI and mathematical network analysis and with "precision medicine," based on n-of-1 trials discussed below. The trend in human evolution has been a remarkable spiraling networking, beginning with intracortical connectivity, progressing to networking and interaction with the minds of others or intercortical connectivity, to present-day brain–machine interfaces. Preliminary studies have even documented brain-to-brain communication in the absence of our customary sensory and motor circuitry [9]. At a more simplistic, clinical level, testing the principal network functions, all of which are dependent on central hub processing and which are susceptible to failure, involves the measurement of attention, inhibition, executive function, and working memory. These can all be responsive to the interventions mentioned in Chapter 10.

An evolutionary perspective of information processing posits that the amount of information that can be processed about environmental factors or conspecifics per unit time correlates with survival or success in an activity. At the brain level, this requires new information being matched with as many memory repositories as possible, in the least amount of time allowed, by the physical constraints of neurotransmission. Predictably, the zeal we have within us for knowledge acquisition is linked to our hedonic reward circuitry. However, not only is the extent of information acquisition crucial, but so is the method of its acquisition. The mere seeking of novelty information, termed diversive curiosity, as occurs with electronic media "web surfing," for example, is less "neurobiologically resilient" than that acquired through epistemic curiosity. Epistemic knowledge (Greek; epistemology, knowledge discourse) acquisition is postulated to be associated with more integrated knowledge storage mechanisms combined with knowledge already laid in long-term storage within brain. This involves more expansive brain circuitry being activated in the process, and at the same time more accessible transmodally. The premise is that the more informed one is in today's world, the better one's decisions will be [10–12]. Because of the demands on our brain's processing, with limited working memory capacity, we have outsourced to external storage devices ever since the creation of the Blombos Cave and Pinnacle Point artifacts from ~75 kya in South Africa. The incised lines and engravings on bone and stone found in these sites are thought to be records of natural cycles, perhaps tides or lunar cycles [13]. These and other cognitive advances have enabled a marked escalation in our capacity for learning, and human societies evolved by cultural evolution since that time, with no other obvious biological brain changes during that time. Nowadays we have become "hyperpersonalized," with access to different social media platforms on a 24/7 basis, and globally we are gathering data at the rate of 5 exabytes (an exabyte is 10^{18} bytes) every two days. By 2020 we will have amassed over 35 zettabytes (10^{21} bytes), in what Eric Topol calls a data deluge, storing data on cloud computing server farms [14].

Since the dawn of civilization and more so with Western cultures, intellectual inquiry has been pursued in two major directions, the sciences and the humanities [15]. These two divides, in turn, have fractured further into dozens of different disciplines. From the foregoing chapters it was readily apparent how multiple unrelated scientific, as well as humanities, disciplines each contributed unique insights into human brain development (Figure 0.1). However, interdisciplinary interaction tends to be sporadic rather than commonplace, as depicted by Van Noorden in a recent *Nature* review article. Although interdisciplinary pursuits are considered decisive by scientists, policy-makers and funding agents still commit limited funding. Although an increase has been documented since the 1980s, an analysis of over 35 million papers in the Web of Science ascribed to 14 principal disciplines, with 143 subspecialties, a disparity remains with some enterprising and others not. For example, when characterized in four quadrants, the most interdisciplinary included social medicine studies, general biology, geriatrics, and physiology; the least interdisciplinary included statistics, international relationships, virology, economics, nuclear and particle physics, astronomy and astrophysics, and inorganic chemistry. Particularly notable in the latter, least interdisciplinary group, was clinical medicine [16]. The merging of the sciences and humanities may not only inform each other, but catapult disciplines ahead.

Eric Kandel, winner of the Nobel prize in physiology or medicine in 2000, at the age of 71, represents a lustrous example of how a life's dedication to neuroscience as well as the arts provides increasing opportunities for one discipline to inform the other. Amassing the knowledge base, he has to make sense of two such vast disciplines and their close relationships, took many decades of intellectual pursuit. Both of his landmark books about fostering the neuroscience and art interaction, *The Age of Insight* and *Reductionism in Art and Brain Science*, are erudite and resplendent examples of bridging this divide and nurturing their mutual beneficence [17,18]. He proposed that both science and art have used a reductionist approach as a way of simplifying a process and breaking it down into more elementary components. Close collaboration and sometimes the merging of disciplines can lead to quantum leaps in the understanding of the natural world and the human mind. For example, our response to abstract art differs markedly to our response to figurative art, with the former influencing a top-down process that involves our emotions, creativity, and imagination by a reductionizing processing of images in terms of color, lines, and form. Because our brains process color, movement, depth, and form in different circuits within the cortex, our emotional reaction to color, for example, may vary depending on the context and mood. Both color and facial interpretation are important to the brain, as face patches and color patches lie adjacent to each other. Isbell's snake-detection hypothesis and the evolution of trichromatic color vision in primates may be relevant to the profound effect that color has on our emotional repertoire. The circuitry processing these functions includes the inferior temporal cortical and color-processing regions and face patches with direct connectivity to the hippocampal memory functions and amygdala emotion-processing areas. The inferior temporal cortex also connects to the nucleus accumbens, the ventrolateral PFC, the orbitofrontal PFC, and the medial temporal lobe. These regions and their accompanying circuitry contribute to the crucial role of facial processing and recognition. Color processing also influences behavior, as well as positive and negative emotions, and recognition and categorization of different objects [19]. Abstract paintings captivate our imagination and engage our brain's top-down processing mechanism, including the default mode network of the brain. In general, the DMN is activated when we are in repose, recalling events, memories, listening to music, and when engaged in introspection. The DMN is considered to be a preconscious activity lodged between the conscious and non-conscious processing states of our minds. Functional MRI imaging has revealed that the DMN is activated especially during aesthetic experiences of art. Abstract art can also impart a profound sense of spirituality for some who contemplate such works of art [20].

With the average age of Nobel prize winners being 71, the obvious inference is that the longer we keep our minds functioning in optimum condition, the more we can contribute to society, whether these be our intellectual institutions or any other societal domain. Connecting the disparate scientific and humanities disciplines with our brains often requires half a dozen decades or more. The scourges of our most common diseases (cardiovascular disease, stroke, cancer, metabolic disease) counter such achievements at the very time when we are able to benefit most from our acquired knowledge base. Notwithstanding the overall decrease in brain size in the last 10 000–20 000 years, we are currently experiencing a global pandemic of neurological diseases. Globally, the burden of neurological diseases has increased dramatically within the last 25 years, and in 2015 they were the leading disease group in terms of disability-adjusted life years (DALYs). The major entities include stroke, dementias (Alzheimer's, vascular dementias, frontotemporal, Lewy body disease), migraine, meningitis, encephalitis, Parkinson's disease, multiple sclerosis, motor neuron disease, epilepsy, drug rebound headache syndromes, and a miscellaneous group [21].

Accurate diagnosis preempts effective treatment and management. However, in general medicine, diagnostic errors are the leading category of paid medical malpractice claims, accounting for 6–17 percent of adverse events and are more than twice as likely to result in the death of a patient compared to other claims [22]. Several factors contribute to diagnostic error. Electronic health records have had the unfortunate side-effect of "note bloat" in the quest for maximum "documentation" to substantiate claims and remuneration. This profoundly impedes assimilation of vast quantities of data, cognitive overload, and hence clinical reasoning, as well as effective communication among multiple providers. It is an undeniable fact that absolute diagnostic certainty in medicine is not achievable, no matter how much information is at hand. Hypothesis-driven diagnoses and pathophysiological insights are the mainstay cognitive assertions that drive treatment programs. Even more alarming is the deluge of diagnostic tools that provide ever more information points to assimilate with a patient's symptoms and signs – at the same time that the clinical interview and examination are being compromised and downscaled. Yet, the face-to-face interview, establishing empathy and rapport with a patient, remains the most important and reliable tool for a clinician in avoiding medical errors and adverse events [23].

How we measure our results and how we value performance indicators is sometimes to blame. The quantification of performance and obsession with the numbers may at times obscure the real problem at hand. In his book *The Tyranny of Metrics*, Muller gives examples from various disciplines and organizations about how surgical scorecards relate to increased morbidity and mortality, and how some police homicide records reflect a downtrend when there was really an increase [24].

Nowhere are these concerns more relevant than with brain disorders. Neurological and more specifically frontal lobe disorders are replete with examples of diagnostic imprecision and errors. The very source of the information – the patient – has to be questioned at times. Some with higher cortical function impairment may even deny the presence of major deficits, such as occurs with anosognosia, or diminish the importance of a deficit (anisodiaphoria). Someone with Alzheimer's disease may have no complaints whatsoever. In addition to the patient, the doctor and the brain may also get it wrong. Cognition normally fluctuates during the day, even in normal as well as in impaired people from hour to hour, and problems may only manifest when fatigue, medication, or metabolic upset occurs. Neurological lesions may also be "silent" to both the doctor and the patient, as exemplified by silent strokes depicted by MRI imaging or PET brain imaging. The latter may even reveal an extensive Alzheimer's pattern in otherwise cognitively intact people in the setting of high cognitive reserve. A clinician's technical examination skills may be error-prone and lead to a diagnostic error and subsequent ill-placed treatment. Groopman mustered more than a dozen types of errors that doctors may make in patient evaluation [25].

Leading cognitive and behavioral neurologists have consistently intimated that single-case reports satiated with hundreds of data points relating to histories, clinical features, cognitive findings, and laboratory and neuroimaging data have made the most breakthroughs in neurology. Classic examples include the case of motor aphasia (Broca's aphasia) described by Paul Broca [26], Harlow's case of Phineas Gage and frontal lobe syndromes [27], patient HM and memory syndromes [28], and Ramachandran's cases of synesthesias and phantom limb pain syndromes [29,30]. Population-based medicine has generally had dismal results in neurological and psychiatric disorders. Many examples can be cited, but perhaps one of the most telling is the European Agency decision against the use of cholinesterase inhibitors: "Donepezil is not cost effective, with benefits below minimally relevant thresholds. More effective treatments than cholinesterase inhibitors are needed for Alzheimer's disease" [31]. The new personalized medicine approach, precision medicine, and n-of-1 trials may be opening up a new era of neurotherapeutics.

An unappealing statistic for those prescribed a statin for stroke or cardiovascular disease prevention, for example, is that very few are likely to benefit. Population-based medicine and large randomized controlled trials do not translate very well into therapies for an individual patient. Taking an example from some of the most commonly prescribed drugs today, such as Lipitor, with sales of over $13 billion per year, 3 percent of people on placebo versus 2 percent taking Lipitor had a cardiac infarct. In simple terms this translates into, for every 100 patients that are taking Lipitor, one patient benefits and 99 do not. A similar scenario played out with another lipid-lowering drug, Crestor, with a 4 percent versus 2 percent placebo drug effect – benefiting 2 out of 100 patients. Plavix and aspirin both reduce stroke similarly, but the former costs about $4 per day, while enteric-coated aspirin costs about $7 for 120 tablets. However, Plavix became the second largest drug for this purpose, with global sales over $9 billion dollars by 2010 [32,33]. Another factor is the uncertainty, even with the most revered clinical trial design, the double-blind randomized controlled clinical trial. In a review of high-impact clinical journals, John Ioannidis of Tufts University concluded that most published findings to date are false and cannot be replicated, in what has been termed a replication crisis [34]. Many reasons have been offered, with one criticism being an overreliance on p-values, with a value of 0.05 being insufficient with inadequate attention to confidence intervals and effects sizes. In addition, Nuzzo has recommended that probability should refer to a tenable outcome, rather than the frequency of an outcome [35]. The concern about the validity of clinical research relating to chronic diseases, especially, was also voiced by Marcia Angell, former editor in chief of the *New England Journal of Medicine*, in her book, *The Truth about the*

Drug Companies: How They Deceive Us and What to Do about It [36]. Munafo and Smith have opined that even when experiments are repeated by independent researchers, only ~40 percent of published findings can be replicated. They propose a triangulation method be employed whereby different approaches address the same experimental question; the approaches have their biases pointing in opposite directions and the results from more than two procedures with their differing key sources of bias are compared [37].

Topol envisages a new era of theranostics in which there is integrated use of diagnostic biomarkers, a therapy and a sensor, with digitized evaluation of effect or titration accomplished by digital and wireless sensors. Medical interventions or therapies that are effective for the majority of people with a particular chronic condition have not been successful, with number-to-treat type of data generally uninspiring. A focus on an individual's unique biology, metabolism, and response to pharmaceutical agents has prompted the emergence of precision and personalized medicine [38–40]. An increasingly popular method for determining optimal therapy for a particular person are *n*-of-1 trials. Several *n*-of-1 trials may be pooled and combined, as well as performing meta-analyses of these trials as reported by Yelland et al. [41]. Current electronic monitoring devices can be configured to be indiscernible to the user and are already widely used in monitoring cardiac issues such as arrhythmias, glucose and diabetes control, and physical activity. From the *n*-of-1 to the *n*-of-billions is conceived as being a distinct possibility if we can combine series of *n*-of-1 trials by digitizing the information on people into datasets with baseline and post-intervention data [42].

Increasingly, innovative precision medicine research is contributing to advances in clinical medicine by garnering hundreds of data points about one individual, rather than a few data points from thousands of individuals. In a classic demonstration of a double-blind, randomized, placebo-controlled, single patient (*n*-of-1) trial, Brefel-Courbon et al. demonstrated the paradoxical efficacy of the hypnotic zolpidem in awakening a young woman from a two-year coma, corroborated by PET brain scan improvement [43]. Inflammatory bowel disease, which is frequently characterized by alteration in gut microbes, termed a dysbiotic expansion of one or more bacterial species (Enterobacteriaceae for example), was inhibited by tungstate treatment through the inhibition of molybdenum (tungsten replacing molybdenum) cofactor dependent microbial mechanisms, which are active during the inflammation phase [44].

Another obstacle nowadays is the fragmented nature of our disciplines and at times the lack of interdisciplinary effort. Clinical medicine has been shown to be one of the lowest-ranking disciplines in this regard [16]. On the contrary, interdisciplinary collaboration has been correlated with the most success [45]. At the same time, prescription drug costs represent the fastest growing fraction of rising healthcare costs, having risen sixfold in the period 1990–2008 to reach the current estimated value of at $234.1 billion. An increase in the number of adverse events, emergency visits, and hospital re-admissions has been correlated to these cost factors and related nonadherence to medications [46].

Neurodegenerative disease or cerebrovascular disease are not reversed by "pill therapy," but by making brain health a priority, such as performing a reconciliation of brain health performance measures. This constitutes what is termed "disease modifying therapies." In a recent study by Micha et al., physical exercise and ten dietary factors were related to approximately 45 percent of deaths due to cardiometabolic disease [47] and physical exercise can attenuate neuroinflammation, a key process in many neurological diseases [48–50]. To help buttress against the effects of aging and the increased incidence of neurological disease while getting older, "brain padding" or cognitive reserve measures remain by far the most effective approach.

Executive Health and Executive Communication

The human penta-sensory (vision, hearing, touch, smell, taste) systems process approximately 11 million bits of information per second. The conscious mind, however, is capable of processing only 16–50 bits per second [51]. Hence the vast majority of sensory information is processed non-consciously or subconsciously, estimated to comprise of ~95 percent of cognitive activity, with conscious activity the remaining 5 percent [52,53]. Many critical survival-related reflexes and decisions are made by the much more rapid, evolutionarily more ancient, non-conscious processing that proceeds out of our awareness. These neuronal reflexes, nevertheless, constitute our inherent neural heritage. As a considerable portion of communication occurs at a non-conscious level, to benefit from our non-conscious processing capabilities optimum communication between us necessarily has to take place in each other's company, or face-to-face. We have a multimodal communication system with at least ten output channels including gaze signaling eyes, pupillary alterations, facial expressions and micro-expressions, body posturing and gesturing, language, and prosody in language expression. Other less often used modalities include musicality, visual arts, and olfaction. For example, visual processing in terms of eye gaze interpretation is a socially important sign and assists in the analysis of another's mind. This circuitry is linked to the mirror neuron system which gives us a "theory of mind" to help assess the intentional states of others [54]. Humans have evolved much larger and wider eyes, with a greater proportion of visible sclera or the "whites of the eyes," the latter of which is unique among primates and enhances direction of gaze appraisal. Identification of eyeball trajectories, such as sideways glimpses, may signify either interest or be cause for suspicion; excessive blinking may reflect a stressed individual, or one that is lying [55]. Pupillary signals are less easily appreciated and are registered non-consciously, as pupillary control is independent of conscious control. Pupillary dilation is associated with pleasant images and constriction with unpleasant images. Together, both eye signaling and pupillary size allow insights into the states of mind of our conspecifics or colleagues [56–58]. The estimates of thousands of different facial expressions we are supposedly capable of may be debatable, but that we are capable of many is certain as is that our expressions to some extent mirror what we are thinking [59]. Perhaps more important are the very fleeting facial micro-gestures (duration ~1/5 of a second), also subconscious, that are indicative of certain behaviors such as lying. Other subconscious, automatic-type expressions include a genuine smile, for example, which differs to a forced smile [60]. From facial electromyographic muscle analysis we know that we tend to mimic facial expressions of people we face in conversation or interact with, and positive and negative emotional reactions may also be reflected non-consciously [61]. Gesturing is a normal accompaniment of social discourse and augments spoken language and assists by freeing up working memory during narration [62,63]. Several different hand to face gestures may be encountered, such as covering the mouth, rubbing one's nose, eyes, or neck, or scratching an ear – all correlated with potential lying [64]. Similarly, body language and posturing may reflect reservation, potential aggression, or impatience [65]. Another output modality, the melodic intonation of speech, or prosody, may intimate the opposite meaning to the literary one, depending on the accentuation, and is a vital component to comprehend during social discourse. Olfaction (smell) may seemingly play a minor role, or no role at all, in social interaction and communication. It remains important, though, as similar to sound, the information is spatially unconstrained and, unlike vision, does not require focusing on a particular object. Without the need for attention, concentration, or focus, these two senses are permanently "online" and remain critical alerting responses for both environmental and social proceedings, with information generally processed non-consciously. For example, aromas influence our minds and may modulate our other four senses, even while sleeping. Emotional responses can be directly affected by pleasant or unpleasant odors. Human chemosensory signaling therefore remains a factor in modulating or regulating emotions and emotional communication [66–69].

Causes of communication failure are multifactorial. Although a young adult's word lexicon numbers 50 000–70 000 words, we are also capable of thousands of different facial expressions and thousands of different body postures [69,70]. Our senses and signaling modes evolved with these competencies because of the very dynamic social interaction we were part of [71]. Lack of sociality, or a dysociality, has many detrimental consequences, such as depression, anxiety, and overall increased cardiovascular morbidity and mortality, and is most dramatically portrayed when afflicted with frontotemporal lobe dementia [72]. Although attention is critical to language, it is limited as we can only attend to a small fraction of the incoming sensory data and hence multitasking is a misnomer, as tasks can really only be performed sequentially. It is difficult to engage in more than one "control demanding activity" at a time – driving a vehicle while talking on a cell phone may be common, but may lead to inattention blindness equated to drunk driving [73,74]. Attention is impaired in those with lack of sleep, brain vascular disease, and attention deficit disorder.

From an evolutionary point of view, reliance on dependable universal senses such as sound or smell serve to signal opportunity or danger. Brain networks may fail due to intra-connectivity failure due to hub malfunction. The major brain hubs, also termed rich hubs, have long-range connections as opposed to more locally situated provincial hubs. These major hubs mediate the core components of our higher cognitive functions, namely attention, executive function, and working memory. Consequently, they are the most energy-consuming brain components. They are therefore also the most vulnerable and affected by energy supply failure due to metabolic, vascular, or traumatic brain injury. They may also fail transiently in physiological states such as sleep deprivation, fatigue, stress, and migraine. They are also termed "hot spots" in the "hub vulnerability hypothesis" of Crossley et al. [75]. Maintaining one's hubs at optimal functional capacity is among the most important rudiments of communication. In addition to maintaining one's intra-connectivity and avoidance of hub failure, we can maintain peak attention, executive function, and working memory by adhering to the brain fitness principles of physical exercise, sleep hygiene, brain foods, socialization, and cognitive exercise, detailed in Chapter 10. Maintaining interconnectivity for optimal social communication using your various sensory inputs and multimodal outputs enhances and augments interpersonal communication and helps avert social alienation and compromised work performance.

We are wired to chatter using the combination of the human communication output and as part of our socialization. The circuitry involved is linked to hedonic reward systems, dopamine neurotransmitter predominant, but also involves opioid and cannabinoid (marijuana stimulates these too) circuitry. The most proximate cause is that these have become entrained to seek out activities and nurture such that they are crucial for survival. When deprived of these, we may suffer mental illness or physical illnesses such as withdrawal states. The rich, holistic, face-to-face interpersonal communication systems and methods we evolved with, over tens of millions of years of evolutionary sculpting of our brain circuitry, are largely absent when using only the literary or written narrative communication. The "fragmented" message sent by texting, typing, or tweeting does not launch the "feel good" hormones and euphoric neurotransmitter effects and may lead to a dysociality, with loss of health-protective effects as well as occasionally an important business deal. Communication modes, however, are complementary, with each having their advantages and disadvantages, with narrative written or electronic instructions best for stepwise technical instructions or directions, for example. Deliberating on a major business deal or with interpersonal or intimate issues, deployment of our multisensory and multichannel communication competencies would be most advantageous. A more protracted face-to-face meeting, often in serene environments away from the workplace, over dinner in what may be termed a "fireside chat," are common practices that facilitate optimum communication.

Preparing for the Stewardship of our Planet

Because the frontal circuitry (specifically the uncinate fasciculus) responsible for societal and emotional health only matures well into the fourth decade, students in their formative years are especially susceptible to the ravages of lost sleep, suboptimal diet, and addiction [76] (Figure 12.1). Interneurons, with their inhibitory functions, are incorporated

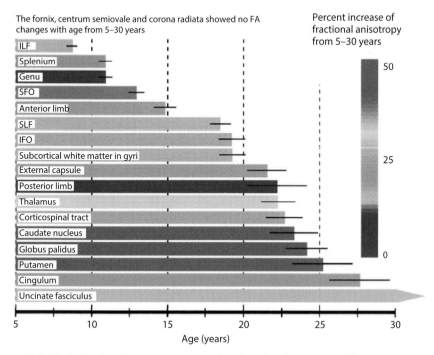

Figure 12.1 Principal brain white matter tract maturation determined by magnetic diffusion tensor imaging. *Source:* Lebel C, Walker L, Leemans A, Phillips L, Beaulieu C. Microstructural maturation of the human brain from childhood to adulthood. *Neuroimage* 2008;40:1044–1055. Reproduced with permission from Elsevier.

into the complex circuitry of the human brain much later and also mature later than the excitatory neurons in the developing human brain, as measured by Zhong et al. in more than 2300 single-cell recordings of the human prefrontal cortex. These provide critical inhibition relevant to conditions characterized by excitatory–inhibition imbalances, such as social cognitive syndromes, autism, and schizophrenia [77].

Aside from sleep-related memory formation, which is important for passing examinations in school and college students, perhaps even more important is the role of sleep in emotional regulation. Sleep deprivation has been linked to an approximate 60 percent increase in amygdala emotional reactivity, with the PFC inhibitory braking effect relatively diminished and in turn linked to many psychiatric disturbances. Impaired sleep or dyssomnia is a known trigger for a number of psychiatric disorders, including bipolar disease, neurological diseases such as Alzheimer's, and increased infections due to immunological compromise [78,79]. Sleep disrupts the critical emotion-building and -repairing processes. This is normally accomplished by REM dreaming activity, which archives important and salient daytime experiences into long-term memory circuits and attempts reconciliation and contemplation of emotionally charged daytime experiences. The words of Matthew are particularly apt: "REM sleep stands between rationality and sanity," quoted from in his landmark book, *Why We Sleep* [80]. During REM, our emotional circuitry is modulated and calibrated and in so doing maintains our ability to identify important social cues, such as eye signaling, facial expressions, and bodily gestures, that are such an important part of the socioemotional interaction among people and for fostering the healthy emotional intelligence that is key to success in life. Added to this is pervasive smartphone use and social media, used by scholars and students today, that have the net effect of what Sherry Turkle has termed a "flight from conversation that is also a flight from self-reflection, empathy and mentorship." In an example cited by her, of a student summer camp experiment in which the use of electronic devices was banned, children showed increased empathy toward their fellows after only five days bereft of their gadgets. Similar to the processed food industry and its deleterious effects on our brain health, this is now compounded by a "digital diet" that is also addictive, with empathy and compassion compromised by up to 40 percent in a college student study [81].

Aircraft pilots and medical residents are among some of the professionals that frequently transgress nature's day–night rhythms. The former industry has strict hours to compensate for this disruption, but medical residents are perhaps the most sleep-deprived professionals, with a notorious sleep deficit. With regard to medical residents, this emanated from ill-conceived legacies dating to the time of William Stewart Halsted, Chief of Surgery, 1889, a cocaine addict whose sleep-deprived work ethic has been associated with current-day residency program work schedule organization. Mounting research relating to such schedules is startling. For example, residents are 36 percent more likely to commit serious errors if working shifts totaling 30 hours or more, and 1 in 20 will be responsible for the demise of a patient due to their sleep deprivation. As noted in earlier in this chapter, medical errors are a national health priority and the third leading cause of death in the USA, following cardiovascular disease and cancer [82–84]. The profound cognitive–behavioral dissonance that can be part of a normal-appearing person, such as the CEO of a large corporation or perhaps even a national figurehead – has far-reaching ramifications. The solutions are self-evident. Make sleep hygiene a priority, base work schedules on individual chronotypes, and use electronic tracking devices to monitor sleep and the lack thereof, with automobile sleep detectors for driving.

The maintenance rules for a healthy brain should begin in childhood and never lapse. However, it is never too late, with studies showing benefit even when first initiated in middle and older ages. From the seventh and eighth decades of one's lifetime is the juncture at which the complement of accumulated knowledge can be assimilated with that already known and a contribution to the human arts and sciences can be made, or rather, the consilience of knowledge.

References

1. Masri S, Sassone-Corsi P. The circadian clock: a framework linking metabolism, epigenetics and neuronal function. *Nat Rev Neurosci* 2013;14:69–75.

2. LeGates TA, Fernandez DC, Hattar S. Light as a central modulator of circadian rhythms, sleep and affect. *Nat Rev Neurosci* 2014;14:443–545.

3. Koscik TR, Tranel D. Brain evolution and human neuropsychology: the inferential brain hypothesis. *J Int Neuropsychol Soc* 2012;18:394–401.

4. Subiaul F, Barth J, Okamoto-Barth S, Povinelli DJ. Human cognitive specialization. In: Kaas J (ed.), *Evolution of Nervous Systems: A Comprehensive Review*, Elsevier, New York, 2007.

5. Gottfried JA, Zald DH. On the scent of human olfactory orbitofrontal cortex: metanalysis and comparison to non-human primates. *Brain Res Rev* 2005;50:287–304.

6. Malafouris L. Beads for a plastic mind: the "blind man's stick" (BMS) hypothesis and the active nature of material culture. *Cambridge Archaeol J* 2008;18:401–414.

7. Malafouris L. Between brains, bodies and things: tectonoetic awareness and the extended self. *Phil Trans R Soc B* 2008;363:1993–2002.

8. Van den Heuvel MP, Stam CJ, Kahn RS, Hulshoff Pol HE. Efficiency of functional brain networks and intellectual performance. *J Neurosci* 2009;29:7619–7624.

9. Grau C, Ginhoux R, Riera A, et al. Conscious brain-to-brain communication in humans using non-invasive technologies. *PLoS One* 2014;9:1–6.

10. Berlyne DE. Uncertainty and epistemic curiosity. *Br J Psychol* 1962;53:27–34.

11. Leslie I. *Curious: The Desire to Know and Why your Future Depends on It.* Basic Books, New York, 2014.

12. Kringelbach MI, Vuust P, Geake J. The pleasure of reading. *Interdiscip Sci Rev* 2008;33:321–333.

13. Soriano S, Villa P, Delagnes A, et al. The Still Bay and Howiesons Poort at Sibudu and Blombos: understanding Middle Stone Age technologies. *PLoS One* 2015;10(7):e0131127.

14. Topol E. *The Creative Destruction of Medicine.* Basic Books, New York, 2012.

15. Snow CP. *Two Cultures and the Scientific Revolution: Rede Lecture*, Cambridge University Press, Cambridge, 1961.

16. Van Noorden R. Interdisciplinary research by the numbers. *Nature* 2017;525:306–307.

17. Kandel ER. *The Age of Insight.* Random House, New York, 2012.

18. Kandel ER. *Reductionism in Art and Brain Science: Bridging the Two Cultures.* Columbia University Press, New York, 2016.

19. Lafer-Sousa R, Conway BR, Kanwisher NG. Color-biased regions of the ventral visual pathway lie between face and place selective regions in humans, as in macaques. *J Neurosci* 2016;36(5):1682–1697.

20. Vessel EA, Starr GG, Rubin N. The brain on art: intense aesthetic experience activates the default mode network. *Front Hum Neurosci* 2012;6:66.

21. GBD 2015. Neurological Disorders Collaborator Group. Global, regional, and national burden of neurological disorders during 1990–2015: a systematic analysis for the Global Burden of Disease Study 2015. *Lancet Neurol* 2017;16:877–897.

22. National Academies of Science, Engineering and Medicine. *Improving Diagnosis in Healthcare.* The National Academies Press, Washington, DC, 2015.

23. Verghese A, Charlton B, Kassirer JP, Ramsey M, Ioannidis JP. Inadequacies of physical examination as a cause of medical errors and adverse events: a collection of vignettes. *Am J Med* 2015;128:1322–1324.

24. Muller JZ. *The Tyranny of Metrics.* Princeton University Press, Princeton, NJ, 2018.

25. Groopman J. *How Doctors Think.* Houghton Mifflin Co., New York, 2008.

26. Broca P. Nouvelle observation d'aphémie produite par une lésion de la moitié postérieure des deuxième et troisième circonvolution frontales gauches. *Bulletin de la Société Anatomique* 1861;36:398–407.

27. Harlow JM. Passage of an iron rod through the head. *Boston Med Surg J* 1848;39:389–393.

28. Preilowski B. Remembering an amnesic patient (and half a century of memory research). *Fortschr Neurol Psychiatr* 2009;77:568–576.

29. Ramachandran VS, Brang D, McGeoch PD. Dynamic reorganization of referred sensations by movements of phantom limbs. *Neuroreport* 2010;21(10):727–730.

30. Brang D, Ramachandran VS. Survival of the synesthesia gene: why do people hear colors and taste words? *PLoS Biol.* 2011;9(11):e1001205.

31. Courtney C, Farrell D, Gray R, et al. Long term donepezil treatment in 565 patients with Alzheimer's disease (AD2000): randomised double-blind trial. *Lancet* 2004;363(9427):2105–2115.

32. Topol EJ, Shork NJ. Catapulting clopidogrel pharmacogenomics forward. *Nat Med* 201;17:40–41.

33. Mukherjee D, Topol EJ. Pharmacogenomics in cardiovascular diseases. *Prog Cardiovasc Dis* 2002;44:479–498.

34. Ioannidis JPA. Why most published research findings are false. *PLoS Med* 2005;2(8):e124.

35. Nuzzo R. Statistical errors. *Nature* 2014;506:150–152.

36. Angell M. *The Truth about the Drug Companies.* Random House, New York, 2005.

37. Munafo MR, Smith GD. Repeating experiments is not enough. *Nature* 2018;553;399–401.

38. Jorgensen JT. New era of personalized medicine: a 10-year anniversary. *Oncologist* 2009;14(5):557–558.

39. Jorgensen JT. Are we approaching the post-blockbuster era? Pharmacodiagnostics and rational drug development. *Expert Rev Mol Diagn* 2008;8(6):689–695.

40. Hu SX, Foster T, Kieffaber A. Pharmacogenomics and personalized medicine: mapping of future value creation. *Biotechniques* 2005;39(10 Suppl.):S1–S6.

41. Yelland MJ, Nikles CJ, McNairn N, et al. Celecoxib compared with sustained-release paracetamol for osteoarthritis: a series of n-of-1 trials. *Rheumatology* 2007;46(1):135–140.

42. Lillie EO, Patay B, Diamant J, et al. The n-of-1 clinical trial: the ultimate strategy for individualizing medicine? *Per Med* 2011;8(2):161–173.

43. Brefel-Courbon C, Payoux P, Ory F, et al. Clinical and imaging evidence of zolpidem effect in hypoxic encephalopathy. *Ann Neurol* 2007;62:102–105.

44. Zhu WM, Winter MG, Byndloss MX, et al. Precision editing of the gut microbiota ameliorate colitis. *Nature* 2018;553:208–211.

45. Wuchty S, Jones BF, Uzzi B. The increasing dominance of teams in production of knowledge. *Science* 2007;316(5827):1036–1039.

46. Castellon YM, Bazargan-Hejazi S, Masatsugu M, Contreras R. The impact of patient assistance programs and the 340B pricing program on medication cost. *Am J Manag Care* 2014;20(2):146–150.

47. Micha R, Penalvo JL, Cudhea F, et al. Association between dietary factors and

mortality from heart disease, stroke and type 2 diabetes in the United States. *JAMA Neurology* 2017;317:912–924.

48. Spielman LJ, Little JP, Klegeris A. Physical activity and exercise attenuate neuroinflammation in neurological diseases. *Brain Res Bull* 2016;125:19–29.

49. Motl RW, Pilutti LA. Is physical exercise a multiple sclerosis disease modifying treatment? *Expert Rev Neurother* 2016;16:951–960.

50. Maliszewska-Cyna E, Lynch M, Oore JJ, Nagy PM, Aubert I. The benefits of exercise and metabolic interventions for the prevention and early treatment of Alzheimer's disease. *Curr Alzheimer Res* 2017;14:47–60.

51. Laughlin SB, Sejnowksi TJ. Communication in neuronal networks. *Science* 2003;301:1870–1874.

52. Attwell D, Laughlin SB. An energy budget for signaling in the grey matter of the brain. *J Cereb Blood Flow Metab* 2001;21:1133–1145.

53. Hassin RR, Uleman JS, Bargh JA, *The New Unconscious*. Oxford University Press, Oxford, 2005.

54. Wicker B, Perrett DI, Baron-Cohen S, et al. Being the target of another's emotion: a PET study. *Neuropsychologia* 2003;41(2):139–146.

55. Ten Brinke L, Porter S. Cry me a river: identifying the behavioral consequences of extremely high-stakes interpersonal deception. *Law Hum Behav* 2012;36(6):469–477.

56. Kobayashi H, Kohshima S. Unique morphology of the human eye and its adaptive meaning: comparative studies on external morphology of the primate eye. *J Hum Evol* 2001;40:419–435.

57. Hess EH. Pupil size as related to interest value of visual stimuli. *Science* 1960;132(3423):349–350.

58. Kret ME, Tomonaga M, Matsuzawa T. Chimpanzees and humans mimic pupil-size of conspecifics. *PLoS One* 2014;9:e104886.

59. Ekman P. Facial expression and emotion. *Am Psychol* 1993;48:384–392.

60. Ekman P, Sorenson ER, Friesen WV. Pan-cultural elements in facial displays of emotion. *Science* 1969;164(3875):86–88.

61. Dimberg U, Thunberg M. Empathy, emotional contagion, and rapid facial reactions to angry and happy facial expressions. *Psych J* 2012;1(2):118–127.

62. Johannesson A. The gestural origin of language; evidence from six "unrelated" languages. *Nature* 1950;166(4210):60–61.

63. Aboitiz F, García R. Merging of phonological and gestural circuits in early language evolution. *Rev Neurosci* 2009;20(1):71–84.

64. Pease A, Pease B. *The Definitive Book of Body Language.* Bantam Books, New York, 2006.

65. Ekman P. Biological and cultural contributions to body and facial movements. In: Blacking J (ed.), *Anthropology of the Body.* Academic Press, London, 1977.

66. Frasnelli J, Collignon O, Voss P, Lepore F. Crossmodal plasticity in sensory loss. *Prog Brain Res* 2011;191:233–249.

67. Schredl M, Atanasova D, Hörmann K, et al. Information processing during sleep: the effect of olfactory stimuli on dream content and dream emotions. *J Sleep Res* 2009;18:285–290.

68. Barnes DC, Chapuis J, Chaudhury D, Wilson DA. Odor fear conditioning modifies piriform cortex local field potentials both during conditioning and during post-conditioning sleep. *PLoS One* 2011;6 e18130.

69. Ekman P. *Emotions Revealed: Recognizing Faces and Feelings to Improve Communication and Emotional Life,* 2nd edn. Owl Books, Henry Holt & Co., New York, 2003.

70. Mehrabian A, Deese, J. Significance of posture and position in the communication of attitude and status relationships. *Psychological Bull* 1969;71:359–372.

71. Seyfarth RM, Cheney DL. The evolution of language from social cognition. *Curr Opin Neurobiol* 2014;28:5–9.

72. Brüne M. *Textbook of Evolutionary Psychiatry: The Origins of Psychopathology.* Oxford University Press, Oxford, 2008.

73. Strayer DL, Turrill J, Cooper JM, et al. Assessing cognitive distraction in the automobile. *Hum Factors* 2015;57(8):1300–1324.

74. Strayer DL, Johnston WA. Driven to distraction: dual-task studies of simulated driving and conversing on a cellular phone. *Psychological Science* 2001;12:462–466.

75. Crossley NA, Mechelli A, Scott J, et al. The hubs of the human connectome are generally implicated in the anatomy of brain disorders. *Brain* 2014;137:2382–2395.

76. Lebel C, Walker L, Leemans A, Phillips L, Beaulieu C. Microstructural maturation of the human brain from childhood to adulthood. *Neuroimage* 2008;40:1044–1055.

77. Zhong S, Zhang S, Fan X, et al. A single cell RNA-seq survey of the developmental landscape of the human prefrontal cortex. *Nature* 2018;555:524–528.

78. Sterniczuk R, Theou O, Rusak B, Rockwood K. Sleep disturbance is associated with incident dementia and mortality. *Curr Alzheimer Res* 2013;10(7):767–775.

79. Gildner TE, Liebert MA, Kowal P, Chatterji S, Snodgrass J. Sleep duration, sleep quality, and obesity risk among older adults from six middle-income countries: findings from the study on global ageing and adult health (SAGE). *Am J Hum Biol* 2014. doi: 10.1002/ajhb.22603.

80. Walker M. *Why We Sleep.* Scribner, New York, 2017.

81. Turkle S. *Reclaiming Conversation: The Power of Talk in a Digital Age.* Penguin Books, New York, 2015.

82. Lockley SW, Barger LK, Avas NT, et al. Effects of health care provider work hours and sleep deprivation on safety and performance. *Jt Comm J Qual Patient Saf* 2007;33(11 Suppl.):7–18.

83. Gupta A, Synder A, Kachalia A, et al. Malpractice claims related to diagnostic errors in the hospital. *BMJ Qual Saf* 2017. doi: 10.1136/bmjqs-2017-006774.

84. Mansukhani MP, Kolla BO, Surani S, et al. Sleep deprivation in resident physicians, work hour limitations, and related outcomes: a systematic review of the literature. *Postgrad Med* 2012;124:241–249.

Index